Hospice Palliative Home Care and Bereavement Support

Lorraine Holtslander
Shelley Peacock • Jill Bally
Editors

Hospice Palliative Home Care and Bereavement Support

Nursing Interventions and Supportive Care

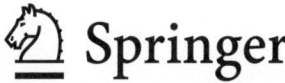

Editors
Lorraine Holtslander
College of Nursing
University of Saskatchewan
Saskatoon
SK
Canada

Shelley Peacock
College of Nursing
University of Saskatchewan
Saskatoon
SK
Canada

Jill Bally
College of Nursing
University of Saskatchewan
Saskatoon
SK
Canada

ISBN 978-3-030-19534-2   ISBN 978-3-030-19535-9 (eBook)
https://doi.org/10.1007/978-3-030-19535-9

© Springer Nature Switzerland AG 2019
This work is subject to copyright. All rights are reserved by the Publisher, whether the whole or part of the material is concerned, specifically the rights of translation, reprinting, reuse of illustrations, recitation, broadcasting, reproduction on microfilms or in any other physical way, and transmission or information storage and retrieval, electronic adaptation, computer software, or by similar or dissimilar methodology now known or hereafter developed.
The use of general descriptive names, registered names, trademarks, service marks, etc. in this publication does not imply, even in the absence of a specific statement, that such names are exempt from the relevant protective laws and regulations and therefore free for general use.
The publisher, the authors, and the editors are safe to assume that the advice and information in this book are believed to be true and accurate at the date of publication. Neither the publisher nor the authors or the editors give a warranty, expressed or implied, with respect to the material contained herein or for any errors or omissions that may have been made. The publisher remains neutral with regard to jurisdictional claims in published maps and institutional affiliations.

This Springer imprint is published by the registered company Springer Nature Switzerland AG
The registered company address is: Gewerbestrasse 11, 6330 Cham, Switzerland

~ I dedicate this work to my parents and grandparents for their unconditional love and care ~

LFH

~ I dedicate this work to my mother, Sheila, for all her love and support ~

SCP

~ I dedicate this work to my parents who showed me the endless possibilities of love, joy, and commitment ~

JMGB

Preface

This unique book places emphasis on providing a resource for registered nurses working in hospice palliative care in peoples' homes and the community and also incorporates literature related to palliative care in acute healthcare settings, as part of the overall services and supports required. Very few resources exist which specifically address hospice palliative care in the home setting, despite the fact that most palliative care occur outside the hospital setting and are primarily supported by unpaid family caregivers. An overview of the unique concerns for individuals and families, as well as specific nursing interventions, from all ages and many contexts, is an excellent support for nursing students and practicing registered nurses alike. The overall learning objectives for this resource book include:

1. Understand current trends, theories, and models and their relevance to provide excellent hospice palliative care in the community.
2. Describe the concept of hope and its relevance in providing care to persons and families living with life-threatening or life-limiting conditions.
3. Explore the role of the family caregiver across the spectrum of ages and conditions and the best evidence for supporting them in their important role.
4. Analyze the "palliative approach to care" that meets the needs of many noncancer populations, such as people living with dementia and those with heart failure.
5. Evaluate current trends and needs for supporting families with children with life-threatening and life-limiting conditions and the spectrum of pediatric palliative care.
6. Compare evidence-informed approaches and current global trends in palliative care specific to home-based care in the community, exploring differences and similarities across countries and healthcare systems.
7. Describe bereavement support for family caregivers, including inequities, consequences, coping, and costs of caring.

Overview of the Book

This resource book is laid out with four specific sections to situate the work of registered nurses in hospice palliative home care. The first section, Section A, Introduction and Overview, begins with a chapter by Dr. Kelly Penz and Lisa Tipper to reveal the consequences for nurses and other formal caregivers working in hospice palliative home care. Providing care at the end of life has the potential to impact quality of life, especially when registered nurses are contending with perceived gaps in care and inadequate pain and symptom management. This chapter offers evidence-informed personal and organizational strategies to improve self-care and supportive work environments that foster wellness for these care providers. Sherrill Miller, a bereaved family caregiver, has provided a beautiful chapter, complete with four images, that explores her journey in providing palliative home care for her husband. Sherrill provides examples of emails she sent and received that supported both her family and friends and her own journey, particularly the way this writing contributed to how she reinvented her life after caregiving.

The section then moves onto setting the context of hospice palliative care from an international perspective. The chapters include works from Canada, New Zealand, Nigeria, the United Kingdom, and the United States. Dr. Agatha Ogunkorode outlines the unique challenges facing Nigeria and other under-resourced countries when considering their approach to hospice palliative care services and supports. More palliative care centers are urgently needed especially considering the incidence and mortality rates of cancer in low-resourced countries. Drs. Elaine Stevens and Stuart Milligan have examined home palliative care in the United Kingdom and Europe, the birthplace of the modern hospice movement. Even in the United Kingdom, challenges remain in access to, and coordinating of, services for the ever-increasing demand for quality palliative care. Dr. Chad Hammond and Sharon Baxter, from the Canadian Hospice Palliative Care Association, outline their findings from wide consultations across Canada to identify models, priorities, and current actions to implement a *palliative approach to care*. Transformation is needed to meet the demand, and the goal is an integrated palliative approach to care across all settings and available to all people with life-limiting conditions in their homes and communities. A New Zealand perspective of pediatric palliative care is provided by Karyn Bycroft and Rachel Teulon, who have included the cultural heritage of the indigenous Māori people and the importance of collaborative partnerships as a basis to provide care for all. The aim of pediatric palliative care is to support children and their families as close to home as possible. Dr. Cindy Tofthagen, Ann Guastella, and Jessica Latchman have provided a chapter focused on the development of hospice and palliative care in the United States, including current issues and potential solutions for the ever-increasing need for these services. The definitions of hospice and palliative care unique to the United States are provided as well as the emerging trends, such as telehospice and telemedicine, which have the potential to revolutionize healthcare, especially for those at home with limited access to services. To close the section, Mary Ellen Walker examines palliative care from a global perspective and provides a high-level overview of palliative care needs and services throughout the world. She has identified key issues, such as a lack of access, especially for those living in low- and middle-income countries, and a lack of education, medication, funding, and policies for implementation. Practical solutions, models, and essentials for providing adequate palliative care are contained in this chapter and throughout the section.

Section B, Evidence-Informed Nursing Interventions, is comprised of five chapters and represents a compilation of successful, evidence-informed interventions used with, and for, persons requiring hospice palliative home care. These interventions include family caregivers who support those who are living with life-threatening and life-limiting illnesses, those who are dying persons, and those who have transitioned into bereavement. In the first chapter in this section, Dr. Lorraine Holtslander describes the experiences of older adults during bereavement and presents the Finding Balance Intervention which was developed and tested through research. He uses a case study to illustrate the use of the tool in clinical practice and introduces select resources to inform care with older adults, bereaved after losing a spouse to cancer. In the following chapter, Drs. Jill Bally and Meridith Burles present research leading to the Keeping Hope Possible Toolkit and provide a description of the toolkit. A case vignette is presented to demonstrate the use of the Keeping Hope Possible Toolkit in supporting parents of children with life-threatening or life-limiting illnesses during uncertain and often traumatic informal caregiving experiences. Furthermore, Drs. Shelley Peacock and Melanie Bayly describe the limited support provided for bereaved spousal carers of persons with dementia, particularly when a family member dies in long-term care, and provide insight into the development of the Reclaiming Yourself tool, aimed at older adult spouses of persons with dementia. The goal of supporting spouses to positively navigate their bereavement is realized through the presentation of a powerful case study in which the authors illustrate how bereaved spousal carers of persons with dementia can use the Reclaiming Yourself tool.

In the subsequent chapter, Dr. Wendy Duggleby describes the development of the Living with Hope Program from research exploring the experience of hope of older persons receiving palliative home care. The Living with Hope Program is an evidence-informed, easy-to-use, self-administered intervention that can potentially increase hope and improved quality of life of persons receiving palliative home care. The final chapter in this section by Drs. Cindy Tofthagen and Sherry S. Chesak focuses on COPE (creativity, optimism, planning, and expert information), a psycho-educational intervention that teaches problem-solving skills to help manage symptoms and other problems that persons with cancer may encounter at home. Clinical trials have demonstrated that COPE improves quality of life and alleviates cancer caregiver burden and distress for family caregivers of persons with cancer at the end of life.

Section C, Innovative Approaches Specific to Disease and Community Setting, presents six different contexts where hospice palliative home care is used. Drs. Rhoda MacRae and Margaret Brown, with Professor Debbie Tolson, provide an in-depth consideration of dementia and its causes, in particular the challenges with defining advanced dementia where hospice palliative care is vitally needed to support and guide quality person-centered care. Their chapter considers the complexity of the dementia context and provides a meaningful discussion of the need for a hospice palliative care approach to support persons with dementia to live well until their death by preventing and minimizing stress and distress. The next chapter by Alexandra Hodson presents the significance of a hospice palliative care approach for persons with advanced stages of heart failure and their family caregivers. Persons with heart failure experience debilitating symptoms and, as such, benefit from the support of their family caregivers over what is usually an unpredictable disease course. Hodson examines the hospice palliative care needs of the person with heart failure as well as their family caregiver and extends the discussion into the bereavement period.

Following this, Dr. Kristen Haase describes the ALERT (ask, listen, engage, reflect/reorient, and time) model, a research-derived model that is intended to guide registered nurses as they work with and support people diagnosed with cancer, and focuses the chapter on the experiences of older adults; many older adults are beginning to use smart phones and Internet-based information across their illness (including the need for hospice palliative care and end of life), and the ALERT model optimizes support of persons with cancer to better engage with Internet information. The next chapter focuses on the context of residential long-term care settings. Drs. Genevieve Thompson and Shelley Peacock present the notion that all persons are deserving of a good death and that persons should live well until they die. This notion is supported by utilizing a palliative care philosophy to guide the care practices within residential long-term care homes considering the significant needs presented by the residents. A palliative care philosophy in residential long-term care homes is of benefit to all residents, whether they are actively dying or not. The next chapter, as presented by Dr. Meridith Burles and Professor Cindy Peternelj-Taylor, provides an overview of a human rights approach that aims to guide correctional healthcare practice. The authors consider various relational and contextual factors that influence palliative care and identify strategies using a model of care that registered nurses might adopt to enhance the effectiveness of palliative care provision for this vulnerable population. In the same vein as persons living and dying in residential long-term care homes, incarcerated persons are deserving of a good death and should be supported to live well until they die.

The final chapter in Section C considers the specific context of children with life-threatening or life-limiting illnesses. Dr. Jill Bally, Nicole Smith, and Dr. Meridith Burles present the importance of addressing the various needs (physical, emotional, cultural, spiritual, and psychosocial) of a family when faced with the possibility of a child's death. Dr. Bally and colleagues' intention is to explore family experiences when a child is diagnosed and in treatment for a life-threatening or life-limiting illness, an experience that significantly disrupts the normal order of life. Moreover, Dr. Bally and colleagues include a unique commentary on the considerations of Canadian Indigenous families within this context. Registered nurses are in key positions to be part of the impetus to improve pediatric hospice palliative care for families.

Section D, Looking Ahead, is the last section in this resource book and provides a reflection of the included chapters. Given the expertise and recommendations of

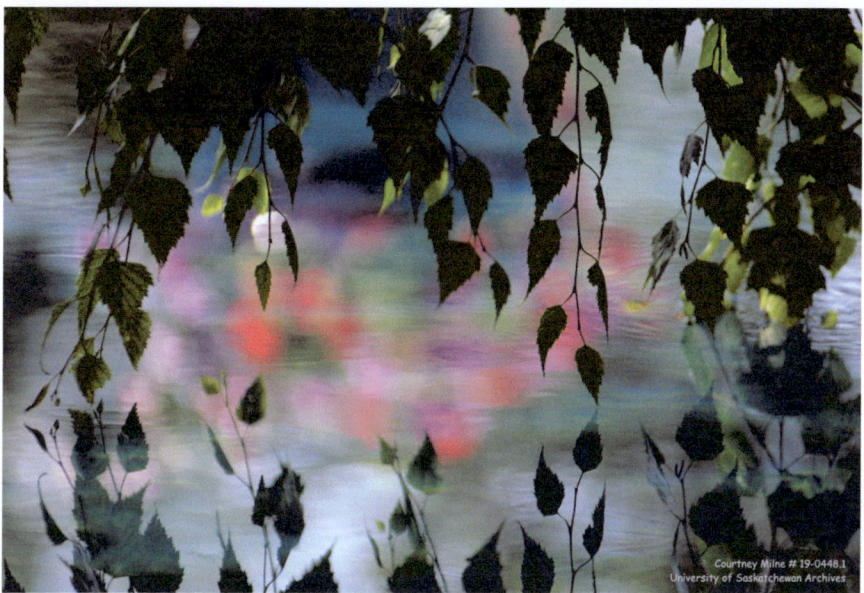

Fig. 1 Self-confidence, from the Pool of Possibilities # 19-0448.1 Image source: Courtney Milne Fonds, University of Saskatchewan Library, University archives and special collections

the chapter authors, the most important next steps for nursing students, registered nurses in practice, and nurse educators and researchers are presented for consideration. That is, the implications for nursing practice, education, and research are explored, and the readers are invited to move their nursing practice forward to the benefit of those in receipt of hospice palliative home care.

Terminology

The term or concept of hospice palliative home care is presented from each unique perspective of the authors throughout this book. While the authors may use slightly different terms, in essence, they are all referring to care that, at its core, strives to improve the quality of life for persons and their family living with life-threatening and life-limiting illness by providing timely diagnosis, adequate assessment of pain and treatment for the same, support for the various needs that arise over the course of the illness and with decision-making, and person- and family-centered care. Hospice palliative home care is not limited to care provided at the end of life but rather is an overarching philosophy to guide the provision of person- and family-centered care (Fig. 1).

Saskatoon, SK, Canada
Lorraine Holtslander
Shelley Peacock
Jill Bally

Acknowledgements

We gratefully acknowledge the work of Ms. Mary Ellen Walker for all her support in drawing the chapters of this book together. This work would not have been possible without all of the contributing authors, thank you to each of you for your insightful chapters. As well, to all the patients, families, and study participants who teach us every day what hospice and palliative home care means to them and how we can continue to improve this important care. Lastly, each of us personally acknowledges the unconditional support of Dr. Wendy Duggleby over the course of our careers who enabled us to propose and edit this book.

Contents

1 **"Who Cares for the Caregiver?": Professional Quality of Life in Palliative Care**.. 1
Kelly Penz and Lisa Tipper
  1.1 Who Cares for the Caregiver? 2
  1.2 What Are Some of the Mental and Emotional Outcomes of Concern? 3
  1.3 Occupational Demands and Resources in Hospice, Palliative, and End-of-Life Care.. 5
  1.4 The Importance of Knowing Oneself: Recognizing Warning Signs 7
  1.5 The Good News: Compassion Satisfaction and Professional Quality of Life 8
  1.6 Personal and Organizational Strategies: Collaborating to Promote Provider Wellness 9
  1.7 Conclusions 13
  References... 14

2 **Family Caregiver Perspective: Navigating the Palliative Care Pathway—How an Email Chronicle Eased the Journey** 17
Sherrill Miller
  2.1 A Personal Odyssey...................................... 17
  2.2 A Phenomenological Process.............................. 19
  References... 33

3 **Global Perspectives on Palliative Care: Nigerian Context** 35
Agatha Ogunkorode
  3.1 Introduction 35
  3.2 Palliative Care 36
  3.3 Palliative Care in Nigeria................................. 37
  3.4 Challenges to Palliative Care Provision in Nigeria 37
  3.5 Prospects and the Way Forward............................ 38
  3.6 Integration of Palliative Care into the Mainstream Healthcare Delivery System in Nigeria...................... 39
  3.7 Education and Training of Healthcare Professionals............ 39

	3.8 Home-Based Care	39
	3.9 Psychosocial Care	41
	3.10 Making Available and Improving Access to Opioid Medication	41
	3.11 The Role of the Nurse	41
	3.12 Palliative Care for Women with Advanced Breast Cancer	42
	3.13 Conclusions	42
	References	43
4	**Home Palliative Care in the United Kingdom and Europe**	**45**
	Elaine Stevens and Stuart Milligan	
	4.1 Hospice Palliative Home Care in the United Kingdom	46
	4.2 Hospice Palliative Home Care in Europe	53
	4.3 Implications for Home Palliative Care	59
	4.4 Conclusion	59
	References	60
5	**Mapping a New Philosophy of Care: The State and Future of Implementing a Palliative Approach Across Canada**	**63**
	Chad Hammond and Sharon Baxter	
	5.1 What Is a Palliative Approach to Care?	63
	5.2 The Way Forward: A National Initiative to Promote a Palliative Approach	66
	5.3 CHPCA Stakeholder Surveys on Implementing a Palliative Approach	73
	5.4 The Way Forward, Phase II: We Know the Way, Now Let's Walk It Together	82
	5.5 Conclusions	83
	References	83
6	**Global Perspectives of Paediatric Palliative Care in the Home in Aotearoa, New Zealand**	**85**
	Karyn Bycroft and Rachel Teulon	
	6.1 Introduction to New Zealand (Aotearoa)	86
	6.2 Children's Palliative Care in New Zealand	87
	6.3 Provision of Care for Children	92
	6.4 Implications for Nursing Practice	95
	6.5 Implications for Nursing Education	101
	6.6 Implications for Nursing Research	101
	6.7 Conclusion	102
	References	102
7	**Perspectives on Hospice and Palliative Care in the United States**	**105**
	Cindy Tofthagen, Ann Guastella, and Jessica Latchman	
	7.1 Introduction and Background	105
	7.2 Costs of Hospice Services: Policy and Payment	108
	7.3 Ethical Issues in Hospice and Palliative Care	109
	7.4 Current Trends in Hospice Care in the United States	110

	7.5	Current Trends in Palliative Care	114
	7.6	Conclusions	117
		References	118
8	**Global Perspectives: Palliative Care Around the World**		**121**
	Mary Ellen Walker		
	8.1	Palliative Care Defined	122
	8.2	Global Palliative Care Needs and Access	123
	8.3	Barriers to Palliative Care Implementation	125
	8.4	Palliative Care as an Ethical Responsibility	127
	8.5	The Palliative Care Model	128
	8.6	Palliative Care Success Stories	132
	8.7	Nursing Considerations	132
	8.8	Conclusion	135
		References	135
9	**Finding Balance Through a Writing Intervention**		**137**
	Lorraine Holtslander		
	9.1	The Finding Balance Intervention Description	138
	9.2	Case Example	139
	9.3	Conclusions	140
		References	141
10	**Keeping Hope Possible**		**143**
	Jill M. G. Bally and Meridith Burles		
	10.1	Life-Limiting and Life-Threatening Illnesses: Family and Hope	143
	10.2	The Keeping Hope Possible Toolkit: An Intervention for Parents	144
	10.3	Case Vignette	149
	10.4	Conclusions	151
		References	151
11	**Reclaiming Yourself**		**153**
	Shelley Peacock and Melanie Bayly		
	11.1	For Whom the Intervention is Appropriate	153
	11.2	The Intervention	154
	11.3	Case Example	156
	11.4	Conclusions	158
		References	159
12	**Living with Hope Program**		**161**
	Wendy Duggleby		
	12.1	Older Persons Receiving Palliative Homecare	161
	12.2	Living with Hope Program	162
	12.3	Case Example	165
	12.4	Conclusions	166
		References	166

13 Creativity, Optimism, Planning, and Expert Advise (COPE): A Problem-Solving Intervention for Supporting Cancer Patients and Their Family Caregivers 169
Cindy Tofthagen and Sherry S. Chesak
13.1 Introduction 170
13.2 Summarizing COPE Research........................... 174
13.3 COPE and the Educate, Nurture, Advise, Before Life Ends (ENABLE) Intervention 176
13.4 Discussion 177
13.5 Conclusions 178
References... 178

14 Dementia 181
Rhoda MacRae, Margaret Brown, and Debbie Tolson
14.1 Global Prevalence 182
14.2 Risk Factors and Causes 182
14.3 Alzheimer's Disease..................................... 183
14.4 Vascular Dementia...................................... 183
14.5 Dementia with Lewy Bodies 184
14.6 Early/Young Onset Dementia 184
14.7 Frontotemporal Degeneration/Dementia (FTD) 185
14.8 Comorbidities and Dementia............................ 185
14.9 Dementia as a Dynamic Concept......................... 186
14.10 As Dementia Progresses 187
14.11 Terminology and Definitions 187
14.12 Defining Advanced Dementia 188
14.13 Features of Advanced Dementia 188
14.14 Palliative Care 189
14.15 Palliare... 190
14.16 Care Empathia 192
14.17 Fundamentals of Advanced Dementia Care............... 194
14.18 Preventing and Minimising Stress and Distress............ 195
14.19 Discussion 196
14.20 Conclusions 196
References... 197

15 Persons with Advanced Heart Failure: A Caregiver-Focused Approach 201
Alexandra Hodson
15.1 Background 201
15.2 Heart Failure in the Community 205
15.3 Practice Implications 207
15.4 Research Implications 210
15.5 Conclusion... 210
References... 211

16	**Development of a Model to Guide Conversations About Internet Use in Cancer Experiences: Applications for Hospice and Palliative Care**	213
	Kristen R. Haase	
	16.1 Method	214
	16.2 Findings	215
	16.3 The Model	216
	16.4 Discussion	219
	16.5 Conclusions	221
	References	221
17	**Long-Term Care**	223
	Genevieve Thompson and Shelley Peacock	
	17.1 Long-Term Care	224
	17.2 The Role of Palliative Care in Long-Term Care	226
	17.3 Implications for Practice, Policy, and Education	232
	17.4 Conclusions	233
	References	233
18	**When Home Is a Prison: Exploring the Complexities of Palliative Care for Incarcerated Persons**	237
	Meridith Burles and Cindy Peternelj-Taylor	
	18.1 Introduction	237
	18.2 Background	238
	18.3 Theoretical and Conceptual Considerations	239
	18.4 Nursing in Correctional Environments: A Model for Care	240
	18.5 The Correctional Client and Palliative Care	241
	18.6 The Nurse–Client Relationship	242
	18.7 Professional Role Development	244
	18.8 Treatment Setting	245
	18.9 Societal Norms	247
	18.10 The Need for Nursing Research	249
	18.11 Closing Thoughts	249
	References	250
19	**Pediatric Palliative and Hospice Care in Canada**	253
	Jill M. G. Bally, Nicole R. Smith, and Meridith Burles	
	19.1 Introduction	253
	19.2 Family Experiences and Need for Specialized Care	254
	19.3 Pediatric Hospice Palliative Care in Canada	256
	19.4 What Does Pediatric Hospice Palliative Care Look Like in Practice?	258
	19.5 Indigenous Perspectives in Canada	262
	19.6 Implications for Nursing Practice, Education, and Research ...	263
	19.7 Conclusion	266
	References	267
Looking Ahead		271

"Who Cares for the Caregiver?": Professional Quality of Life in Palliative Care

Kelly Penz and Lisa Tipper

Contents

1.1	Who Cares for the Caregiver?...	2
1.2	What Are Some of the Mental and Emotional Outcomes of Concern?......................	3
	1.2.1 Burnout...	3
	1.2.2 Compassion Fatigue...	4
1.3	Occupational Demands and Resources in Hospice, Palliative, and End-of-Life Care...	5
	1.3.1 What Are the Potential Job-Related Demands in HP/EOL Care?.....................	5
	1.3.2 What Are the Potential Job-Related Resources in HP/EOL Care?....................	6
1.4	The Importance of Knowing Oneself: Recognizing Warning Signs........................	7
1.5	The Good News: Compassion Satisfaction and Professional Quality of Life..............	8
1.6	Personal and Organizational Strategies: Collaborating to Promote Provider Wellness...	9
	1.6.1 Personal Strategies: Keeping Your Compassion Bank Account Filled..............	9
	1.6.2 Organizational Strategies: Creating Supportive Work Environments in Palliative Care...	11
1.7	Conclusions...	13
References...		14

K. Penz (✉)
College of Nursing, University of Saskatchewan, Regina, SK, Canada
e-mail: kelly.penz@usask.ca

L. Tipper
Saskatchewan Health Authority, Moose Jaw, SK, Canada

© Springer Nature Switzerland AG 2019
L. Holtslander et al. (eds.), *Hospice Palliative Home Care and Bereavement Support*, https://doi.org/10.1007/978-3-030-19535-9_1

The *Way Forward National Framework* is the result of a collaborative initiative lead by the Quality End-of-Life Care Coalition of Canada and calls for a system-wide shift of ensuring that Canadians have access to an integrated approach to palliative care within all practice settings, this philosophy of care is called "a palliative approach" [1]. According to the World Health Organization [2], "Palliative care is an approach that improves the quality of life of patients and their families facing the problems associated with life-threatening illness, through the prevention and relief of suffering by means of early identification and impeccable assessment and treatment of pain and other problems, physical, psychosocial and spiritual" (para. 1). Although often solely associated with care for the dying, models of palliative care recommend a duality approach that includes the gradual transition from a curative intent to end-of-life care, which also extends into the bereavement period [3].

Nurses and other formal caregivers are expected and ethically mandated to advocate for high-quality patient and family-centered HP/EOL care. However, formal caregivers (e.g., nurses, physicians, social workers, therapists) are increasingly having to deal with the considerable disparity between the growing demand for a palliative approach to care, and the capacity of the Canadian healthcare system and its' various care settings (e.g., home care, hospitals, long-term care) to fully implement this approach. There are concerns regarding the cumulative emotional/mental toll experienced by nurses and other formal caregivers who are more commonly witness to the pain and suffering of others, who are facing challenging workloads, and who may not have adequate personal and/or organizational resources to feel supported in their complex roles [4, 5]. Although it is important to acknowledge the numerous evidence-based community resources (e.g., handbooks, websites, support groups, volunteer services) designed to support palliative patients and family members, it is also crucial that the psychosocial needs of nurses and other formal caregivers are not overlooked, and that their professional quality of life is fully recognized as an ongoing priority.

1.1 Who Cares for the Caregiver?

We know that many who provide palliative nursing care view their work as a privilege as they strive to assist patients and families to journey throughout the illness trajectory and to help shape a more positive understanding of the process of dying [6]. Nurses are commonly driven by their own sense of "compassion empathy," which is a deeper form of empathy where they not only try to understand a person's predicament and feel *with* them, but they are spontaneously moved to help [7]. Even so, the expectations placed on these nurses are high, especially when they routinely deal with the physical, mental, and/or existential suffering of their patients. There is a Latin phrase written in the early second century AD by the Roman poet Juvenal (Satire VI, lines 347–348) which states "Quis custodiet ipsos custodes?" Though literally translated as "who will guard the guards themselves?," a variant translation that seems to shed light on the realities of nursing practice is, "who cares for the caregiver?" Nationally, we are seeing an increasing focus on the professional well-being and recognition of the occupational burdens placed on nurses and other formal caregivers. Reports of formal caregivers' experiencing depression rates double those of the general population, up to a third of nurses experiencing symptoms of Post-traumatic Stress Disorder (PTSD), and widespread burnout [8] are highly distressing. For nurses in palliative care, a particular quote comes to mind which states "the expectation that we can be immersed in suffering and loss daily and not be touched by it is as unrealistic as expecting to be able to walk through water without getting wet" ([9], p. 52). This philosophy suggests that caregivers "burn out" not because they don't care, but because they don't have time to grieve; with their own experiences of loss leaving them less reserves over time [9]. It is important that nurses and other formal palliative caregivers reflect on their own experiences of loss and some of the mental and emotional outcomes for which they may be at risk.

1.2 What Are Some of the Mental and Emotional Outcomes of Concern?

Although HP/EOL care is an area that many formal caregivers are drawn toward, experiencing the distress of others in the midst of organizational constraints may have a negative impact on nurses' mental and emotional well-being. In a study involving hospice nurses, 79% of them had moderate to high rates of compassion fatigue, with 83% indicating that they did not receive any type of debriefing/support after a patient's death [10]. Even in the midst of viewing one's work in hospice and palliative care as a privilege, nurses may still be experiencing the symptoms of compassion fatigue, especially when they feel solely responsible for the recipients of their care, such as in home healthcare [11]. For palliative care professionals, the experience of burnout is not a certainty, but should not be overlooked in relation to their overall well-being. Nurses and other formal caregivers who work in oncology care may also be at a higher risk for burnout than those who work in other settings [12]. There are many similar concepts that have been used to measure and describe the mental, emotional, and physical effects of occupational stress and working in the presence of suffering (e.g., burnout, compassion fatigue, vicarious trauma, post-traumatic stress disorder [PTSD]). The purpose of this chapter is not to debate which of these concepts are most relevant in the context of HP/EOL care, but to explore a few that may help nurses and other formal caregivers self-reflect on what they may be at risk for over time, or are actually experiencing in their current practice. Two of the concepts that will be described in more detail are burnout and compassion fatigue.

1.2.1 Burnout

Burnout is a term commonly used to describe the physical and emotional exhaustion that formal caregivers experience when they are overwhelmed in relation to their work. Most well recognized in this area are Christina Maslach and Susan Jackson, whose early work lead to the development of the Maslach Burnout Inventory (MBI). Burnout is defined as a prolonged psychological response to chronic organizational and interpersonal stressors on the job, made up of three key dimensions: (1) overwhelming exhaustion, (2) feelings of cynicism or detachment from the job, and (3) a sense of ineffectiveness and lack of accomplishment [13]. Burnout among nurses is a concern as they face increased workloads and pressure to provide quality HP/EOL care in settings that may not fully embrace or understand this philosophy of care. When nurses perceive that they are working to their full capacity and beyond on a regular basis (e.g., high demands), with limited resources, and/or inadequate training or support; this is when they are most at risk. Nurses' and other formal caregivers' experiences of burnout may also be amplified when they are experiencing higher personal stressors [14], and have less opportunity to rest, recover, and restore their sense of balance amidst the competing expectations often placed on them.

1.2.2 Compassion Fatigue

Compassion fatigue is a complimentary experience to burnout; however, it relates specifically to our interpersonal interactions with patients and their family members, especially in the presence of distress and suffering. Commonly referred to as "the cost of caring" or "the cost of caring too much," compassion fatigue describes the emotional and physical burden created by the impact of helping others in distress, which leads to a decreased capacity for empathy toward suffering in the future [15]. Another way of understanding the experience of compassion fatigue is to imagine the fuel gauge of a car sitting on the "E" line, where nurses are continuously striving to provide empathic care, but not having the time or support to be able to fully refuel. In a sense, they may struggle with feeling like they are "running on empty" [16].

Anyone who cares for others may develop a certain amount of compassion fatigue over time; however, there are some formal caregivers who may be at a higher level of risk. For example, those who work in more challenging areas of practice such as pediatric HP/EOL care, are dealing with the emotional toll of helping families cope with unexpected terminal illnesses or the deaths of young children or adolescents. Rural and remote nurses may also be at a higher risk for compassion fatigue as they typically live and work in their home communities and may have personal connections to the potential recipients of their care. In addition, rural and remote nurses are more likely to provide nursing care to patients across the illness trajectory, including from diagnosis through undergoing interventions, to care in their last days or hours. The challenge of these blurred personal/professional boundaries means that many rural and remote nurses may feel the ongoing expectation to maintain their formal caregiver roles but may also be contending with their own grief at the same time. Compassion fatigue tends to follow healthcare professionals from work setting to work setting, even if they make a change. One of the most challenging aspects of compassion fatigue is that it depletes caregivers' reserves for what brought them to their work in the first place; their empathy for others.

1.3 Occupational Demands and Resources in Hospice, Palliative, and End-of-Life Care

Although there is a commitment and shift toward better access and higher quality HP/EOL care, this is occurring within a healthcare context of formal caregivers "doing more with less." For example, the perception of having a finite amount of nursing personnel and resources leads to increased workloads, especially when there are few allowances for the increased time and commitment required when utilizing a palliative approach to care. Part of caring for our formal caregivers in HP/EOL care is developing a better sense of the specific demands and resources that they may be experiencing in their work. Nurses who provide this care may recognize that although most people want to die at home, in reality 70% of Canadian deaths still occur in hospital settings [17]. Canadian nurses are also contending with caring for an aging population and the medicalization of death/dying, where an overestimation of medicine's ability to prolong life is a common view among patients and their family members. Occupational stress, burnout, and compassion fatigue among formal caregivers may occur when the resources available to them are insufficient or inadequate, reducing their capacity to offset their often complex and competing demands. See Table 1.1 for a list of potential demands and resources that nurses are experiencing in HP/EOL care.

1.3.1 What Are the Potential Job-Related Demands in HP/EOL Care?

The *Job Demands-Resources Model* of occupational stress emphasizes the interplay of both the stressors and motivational characteristics of our work that have a potential impact on employee well-being [18]. Job demands are defined as the physical, psychological, social and/or organizational aspects of the job that require sustained cognitive and/or emotional effort and are associated with job-related stress [19]. Although occupational burdens are a reality for most formal caregivers, research suggests that those providing HP/EOL care experience unique demands [5]. Some examples include experiencing multiple and concurrent losses [5], dealing with difficult family dynamics and moral dilemmas (e.g., medical futility) [20], feeling

Table 1.1 Common job-related demands and resources in HP/EOL care [5, 20–29, 31, 32]

Job-related demands	Job-related resources
• Multiple/concurrent losses	• Supportive leadership
• Challenging family dynamics	• Collaborative team approach to care
• Complex pain/symptom management	• Peer/collegial support
• Moral dilemmas/medical futility	• Patient- and family-centered care
• Lack of competence/death anxiety	• Philosophy of palliative approach understood/embraced in care setting
• Conflicting goals of care (e.g., bias regarding opioid addiction)	• Caregiver autonomy
• Uncertainty surrounding MAiD	

unprepared to effectively manage pain and other symptoms [21], and personal discomfort regarding death and provision of bereavement care [22–24]. Even when nurses seek out professional development and education in HP/EOL care, they may contend with a misunderstanding of the goals surrounding palliation within their work setting, and lack of knowledge surrounding pain and symptom management among other formal caregivers and non-licensed personnel with whom they work [25, 26]. For example, dealing with personal biases regarding fears of opioid addiction in the context of palliative pain management is not uncommon. In some cases, pain assessment may be driven by outdated fallacies (i.e., if the patient is not exhibiting signs of pain there is the erroneous belief that they are not experiencing pain), despite overwhelming evidence to the contrary.

A more recent demand placed on nurses in this area is the increased media attention and often, the sole focus on Medical Assistance in Dying (MAiD). As of June 2016, changes occurred to the Criminal Code of Canada outlining that a person who is facing foreseeable death and meets certain eligibility criteria, can pursue an assisted death (Bill C-14) [27]. Although the legal provision of this service is an important discussion toward the end of life, many formal caregivers also see this as overshadowing the opportunity to improve public understanding of the principles of palliative care. There are also concerns that patients may be offered this service, even without their request, leading to a slippery slope of MAiD being the "proposed" option with neglect and lack of recognition of the true effectiveness of a palliative approach to care. The growing evidence suggests that some nurses who are involved in the provision of this service may view this as an aspect of holistic nursing care; however, others struggle with taking an active role in hastening death, with experiences of uncertainty and moral distress being an ongoing concern [28, 29]. For nurses and other formal caregivers who practice in HP/EOL care, the long-term impacts of being witness to patients' experiences of MAiD and providing bereavement care to the remaining family members are not yet fully understood.

1.3.2 What Are the Potential Job-Related Resources in HP/EOL Care?

Although the majority of nurses who provide HP/EOL care experience numerous demands related to their work, most remain highly engaged in their work, have high levels of job satisfaction, and stay in their chosen career path [11, 30]. Job resources are defined as the physical, psychological, social, and/or organizational aspects of the job that help to reduce the impact of complex job demands and stimulate professional growth [19]. In general, both personal and organizational resources play a role in protecting nurses from burnout and other negative work- and health-related outcomes. Some important resources for nurses in HP/EOL care include having trust in their work organizations and perceptions of supportive leadership [31], working in collaborative teams [4, 32], feeling emotionally supported by their peers/ colleagues [31], and having the autonomy to fully engage in patient/family-centered care [5]. In order for organizations and leaders to provide this support, they must have a genuine knowledge of the philosophy and principles surrounding HP/EOL care and recognize the ongoing challenges that nurses and other formal caregivers are currently facing in their roles.

1.4 The Importance of Knowing Oneself: Recognizing Warning Signs

For nurses and other formal caregivers in HP/EOL care, the risk for burnout and compassion fatigue increases when they perceive that they are lacking the physical or emotional energy to meet the cumulative demands placed upon them, often in the context of a lack of readily available resources. Every professional who chooses a career in HP/EOL care will likely develop an individual understanding of the work-related demands and resources that influence their practice, with their own personal stressors contributing to their level of risk over time. When exploring concepts such as compassion fatigue and burnout, a helpful method of self-reflection for formal caregivers is to imagine their own level of risk as warning signs on a continuum (Fig. 1.1) (based on [16, 33]).

Within a particular work setting, there will be, at any one point in time, many caregivers who are generally feeling well and fulfilled in their work (e.g., in the green zone), some may be experiencing symptoms of increasing severity (i.e., in the yellow zone), and a few may be entering the "red zone" with feelings of helplessness, and leading to a sense of being disconnected or depersonalization [33]. Some of the warning signs that formal caregivers are at risk for compassion fatigue and burnout may be physical (e.g., weakened immune system, exhaustion, insomnia) [33–35], behavioral (e.g., expressed anger or irritability, increased use of alcohol or drugs, difficulty separating work and personal lives) [33, 34, 36, 37], and/or psychological/emotional (e.g., depression, heightened anxiety, reduced empathy) [33, 34, 38, 39] in nature. A summary of potential warning signs within these three domains is displayed in Table 1.2.

It is vital that nurses and other formal caregivers in HP/EOL care are able to develop their own skills in self-reflection to sense what their own warning signs are, and where they might find themselves on this type of continuum at any given time. One of the most practical ways to self-reflect on ones' own risk for outcomes (i.e., compassion fatigue) is to visualize the continuum on a scale of 1 to 10, with 10 (height of the red zone) being the worst they have ever felt about their ability to

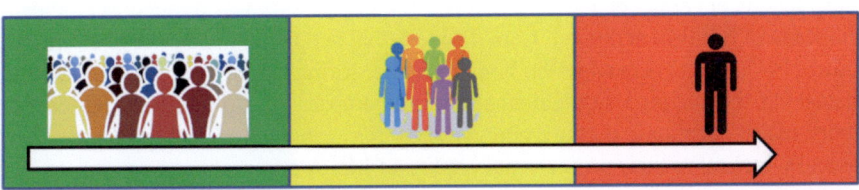

Fig. 1.1 Compassion fatigue continuum

Table 1.2 Warning signs on the compassion fatigue continuum [16, 33–39]

Physical	Behavioral	Psychological/emotional
• Weakened immune system • Headaches (i.e., stress induced) • Insomnia • Exhaustion • Somatization (i.e., physical symptoms of stress such as upset stomach)	• Expressed anger/irritability • Increased use of alcohol/drugs • Absenteeism/missing work • Struggle to separate work and personal life • Avoidance of certain patients/clients • Difficulty making decisions	• Heightened anxiety • Reduced empathy • Negative self-image (i.e., feeling unskilled) • Hypersensitivity to emotional material (e.g., news reports) • Depression

convey empathy/compassion and 1 (lowest level of the green zone) being the best they have ever felt [33]. This involves imagining what a 1 or 2 may look and feel like compared to somewhere in the middle, such as 4 or 5, up to imagining what a higher level of risk such as an 8 or 9 may look like for each individual. For example, someone who is approaching a 4 or 5 may find themselves being more distant from their colleagues or friends or may turn to alcohol more frequently [33] to escape feelings of grief or loss associated with their work. Those who are approaching a more concerning level of risk, for example toward an 8 or a 9, may find themselves calling in sick more often, ignoring text messages or phone calls, or feeling that they themselves are in crisis [33], making it difficult to respond professionally to the pain or suffering of their patients/clients. Being able to recognize that one's level of compassion fatigue or burnout is creeping up to the red zone is the most effective way to implement strategies immediately [16].

1.5 The Good News: Compassion Satisfaction and Professional Quality of Life

The good news is that more organizations and work settings are recognizing the importance of creating healthy healthcare workforces, and the positive impact this may have on the quality of life of patients and their family members. Some of the concepts recognized in the literature regarding HP/EOL care include work engagement and existential fulfillment [40], "joy in work" [41], workplace resilience [42], and "professional quality of life" [43]. A key aspect of a formal caregivers' professional quality of life is conceptualized as "compassion satisfaction" and may be particularly relevant for nurses who work in hospice, palliative, and end-of-life care [43]. In a recent concept analysis, compassion satisfaction was defined as an intrinsic sense of fulfillment derived from the work that people do in helping or caring for others [44]. When viewed in the bigger picture, formal caregivers are supported in balancing their compassion satisfaction and compassion fatigue, with reasonable work-related demands that are countered by the resources available to them, this actually makes up their professional quality of life. A comprehensive group of elements that precede or are viewed as necessary antecedents for formal caregivers to possess or aspire toward achieving an ongoing sense of compassion satisfaction in their work include the following [44]:

- Perception of caregiving as a calling.
- Empathetic caregiving relationship with care recipients and their family members.
- Importance of collegial support.
- Development of resilience.
- Healthy coping mechanisms.
- Practicing Self-Care.
- Aiming for work–life balance with adequate social supports.

When examining the above elements, it is important to recognize that there are both personal and organizational actions that are necessary to both support and build such traits within our nurses and other formal caregivers who are providing HP/EOL care.

1.6 Personal and Organizational Strategies: Collaborating to Promote Provider Wellness

The key to the success of creating healthy environments in HP/EOL care is to have leaders, practitioners, and organizations work together to support and promote provider wellness, and to reduce the tendency to solely focus on individual resiliency and personal coping abilities. If outcomes such as compassion fatigue and burnout are viewed as the "cost of caring," it is important that formal caregivers develop and rely on their own personal strategies of keeping their own "compassion bank accounts" filled so that they have the reserves to keep providing empathetic care over the course of their careers. Caring for the formal caregiver also involves collaboration and advocacy for the introduction of specific supports within organizations, and ongoing evaluation of their impact, relevance, and value. This chapter will conclude with an overview of potential personal and organization strategies designed to best support nurses in HP/EOL care.

1.6.1 Personal Strategies: Keeping Your Compassion Bank Account Filled

As often happens in many caring professions, nurses and other formal caregivers in HP/EOL care prioritize their patients, then their own family members/friends, with their own emotional and mental well-being viewed as less of a priority. Nurses in this field of practice may even feel guilty if they take personal time to experience their own grief/loss, with the cumulative effect having potential negative impacts over time [5]. Research regarding compassion fatigue supports the notion that the actions taken by formal caregivers to improve their own self-care are the cornerstone of prevention [16, 45]. Figure 1.2 summarizes some of the main personal strategies that nurses, and other formal caregivers may benefit from in terms of keeping their own "compassion bank accounts filled," and maintaining their reserves to provide quality HP/EOL care over time. A key aspect of working toward better

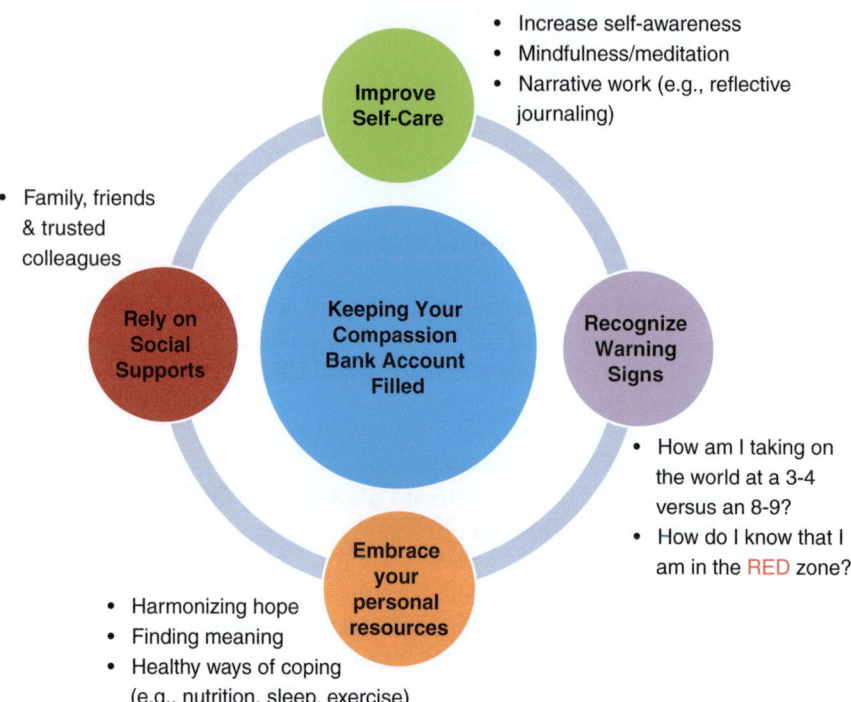

Fig. 1.2 Personal strategies: keeping your compassion bank account filled [4, 5, 16, 23, 33, 42, 46–49]

self-care is to develop ones' own skills in self-reflection personally and professionally [46] and finding a sense of meaning in ones' work [4, 5, 23].

Personal strategies identified as most helpful with the caring professions include increased self-awareness through mindfulness, meditation, and/or narrative work [47] such as reflective journaling [48]. Reflective journaling in particular may contribute to nurses' health and well-being in relation to their work in HP/EOL care [48]. Palliative care nurses who practice in community setting and had the opportunity to participate in reflective journaling indicated that it allowed them to reflect on what kept them hopeful when dealing with concurrent death/dying and loss and were able to disclose aspects of their experiences that they found most difficult [5, 48]. Reflective journaling also offered a focused strategy to reflect on the meaning they found in their work, which enhanced their ability to identify their own level of expertise and celebrating the differences they make in patients' or clients' lives [4, 5, 48].

Self-care also involves nurses developing a sense of what their own warning signs are [33], especially in the context of the competing demands experienced in community HP/EOL care, where resources are often perceived as limited. Nurses in these settings may be working alone or at a distance from their colleagues, and they may not wish to burden their own family members or friends with their own challenges in dealing with gaps in care, or organizational constraints [4]. As outlined in the section on warning signs [33], nurses and other formal caregivers need to take the time to reflect on where they are on the warning signs continuum. For example, what are their perceptions of their effectiveness in assisting during MAiD when they are at a 3 or 4 on the warning signs continuum? Or, when dealing with a series of losses in close succession of people who they knew personally, such as may occur in rural practice settings? What do these nurses experience when they are entering the red zone at an 8 or a 9?

Self-reflection may also assist nurses in identifying their own personal resources, which are unique to each individual. This may include reflecting on the meaning they find in their work [4, 5, 23], relying on healthy coping mechanisms (e.g., nutrition, sleep, exercise) [49] and reflecting on their own sense of hope or sense of resilience [4, 42] in the face of daily challenges. A particularly relevant personal resource for nurses in HP/EOL care is their own perceptions of hope as both sustaining them and motivating them to provide high-quality care [4]. A grounded theory study exploring nurses sense of hope in the context of palliative care delivery found that nurses were most concerned about "keeping hopeful in their work" when they were facing ongoing organizational constraints and competing goals/viewpoints from colleagues, patients, and/or family members when moving from a curative mindset to compassionate care toward the end of life [4]. They dealt with keeping hopeful through a process of "harmonizing their hope," with a focused effort on accepting that different perspectives and goals existed, and that it was possible to achieve a sense of harmony within themselves while acknowledging differences [4]. Finally, informal support networks are also vital in providing psychosocial support [46], with the importance of relying on family, friends, and trusted colleagues during times of increased emotional fatigue and/or distress. This is particularly important for nurses who work in rural and remote settings where strong bonds are commonly developed between colleagues and where caregivers rely on one another for encouragement and strength during particularly difficult times.

1.6.2 Organizational Strategies: Creating Supportive Work Environments in Palliative Care

Focusing on personal strategies and resources, while important, only goes so far in addressing nurses' overall professional well-being. From an organizational point of view, there must be recognition that nurses' maintenance of their own resilience in HP/EOL care delivery is not fully possible unless leadership also takes an active role in providing formal supports. There is a need to openly discuss and recognize the cumulative influence of complex job-demands in this area of practice, and that the risk for compassion fatigue and/or burnout in the workplace is a reality [34, 49]. Given that the organizational strategies designed to support formal caregivers are numerous and diverse within the literature, we have chosen to highlight those most relevant in the prevention of compassion fatigue [11, 16, 33, 46, 49, 50] (see Fig. 1.3).

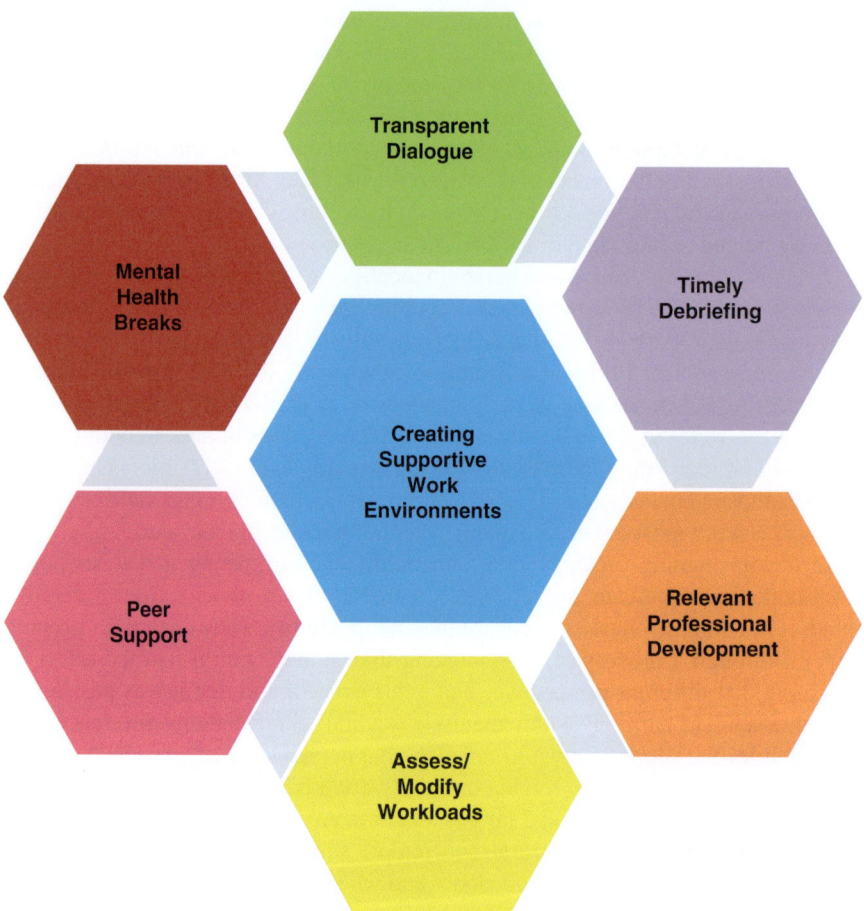

Fig. 1.3 Organizational strategies: creating supportive work environments in palliative care [11, 16, 33, 46, 49, 50]

Formal caregivers who are more likely to witness the pain and suffering of others need to be given opportunities to discuss their experiences through formal debriefing sessions at the time of, and in the immediate aftermath of difficult events [16, 33]. In a sense, they need to have safe spaces in which they can express their uncertainty of whether they made the "right" choices in their nursing care, and question subsequent patient outcomes, which allow them to normalize their experiences [46]. If this is offered on a regular basis, and becomes the norm, it also becomes the basis for an organizational culture of transparent dialogue [16]. Other organizational strategies might include mental breaks in the day [16], or even mental health days that can be utilized at particularly difficult times.

Although many nurses and formal caregivers rely on their colleagues for social support, formal "peer support" is a newer type of psychosocial counseling that is being adopted within healthcare settings. Peer support is defined as a formal relationship between two people who have a shared experience in common and focuses on the provision of emotional and social support [50]. Peer support programs utilize "peer" volunteers who are trained in various counseling techniques to provide support to others (e.g., colleagues) when needed. Similar to formal debriefing, those who seek peer support are counseled in the normalcy of what they might be feeling, with a focus on reframing their experiences and looking at them through a different lens. Additional organizational strategies include assessing nursing workloads on a regular basis and seeking ways to modify workloads within the limits of the practice setting [16].

Finally, professional development and continuing education opportunities that are relevant to HP/EOL nursing practice need to be offered using flexible modes of delivery and made accessible to all who would benefit and who desire to participate. There is a need for consultation with formal caregivers about the educational topics that are covered and are viewed as beneficial to assist them in their practice. For example, the educational needs for under-resourced rural nurses who provide HP/EOL care may be unique when compared to their urban counterparts who have regular access to formal HP/EOL care programs and/or teams. Particular topics of focus that may be more relevant in the context of HP/EOL care may include: interpersonal communication strategies regarding death and dying, advanced care planning, complex pain management, existential suffering and other overlooked symptoms (e.g., existential suffering), and trauma-informed care. A collaborative approach is necessary that involves individual practitioners, leadership, and work environments to improve organizational supports and promote formal caregivers' wellness.

1.7   Conclusions

The fact that many healthcare environments are prioritizing a palliative approach to care is highly encouraging, with nurses being at the forefront in the provision of this care. The rewarding aspects of this career pathway are undeniable as formal caregivers experience the privilege of being with their patients at a very unique period in their lives. In the midst of these rewarding experiences, we must also emphasize the need to "care for our caregivers" and to support them in their efforts to continue to provide high-quality HP/EOL care. Given that limited resources, competing demands, and experiences of compassion fatigue are viewed as the "cost of caring" in many areas of nursing practice, it is necessary to take a collaborative approach to assist nurses in maintaining their reserves to provide high-quality HP/EOL care over time. Nurses can take individual action to reflect on where they are at personally/professionally, participate in self-care activities, and rely on their peer and social support networks. Finally, actions taken by organizations and leadership toward developing more supportive work environments are crucial, which include positive efforts to fully foster an integrated approach to palliative care in all settings.

References

1. Canadian Hospice Palliative Care Association (CHPCA). The Way Forward National Framework: a roadmap for an integrated palliative approach to care, The Way Forward Initiative. 2015.
2. World Health Organization (WHO). *Palliative Care.* 2019. https://www.who.int/cancer/palliative/definition/en/.
3. Canadian Hospice Palliative Care Association (CHPCA). A model to guide hospice palliative care. Ottawa, ON: Canadian Hospice Palliative Care Association; 2013.
4. Penz K, Duggleby W. Harmonizing hope: a grounded theory study of the experience of hope of registered nurses who provide palliative care in community settings. Palliat Support Care. 2011;9(3):281–94. https://doi.org/10.1017/S147895151100023X.
5. Penz K, Duggleby W. It's different in the home... the contextual challenges and rewards of providing palliative nursing care in community settings. J Hosp Palliat Nurs. 2012;14(5):365–73.
6. Cottrell L, Duggleby W. The good death: an integrative literature review. Palliat Support Care. 2016;14:686–712. https://doi.org/10.1017/S1478951515001285.
7. Goleman D. Emotional intelligence: why it can matter more than IQ. London: Bloomsbury Publishing Plc; 1996.
8. Dragan V, Smith CM, Tepper J. Burnout in healthcare: what are we doing about it? [cited 2019 Feb 14]. https://healthydebate.ca/2018/09/topic/burnout-in-health-care.
9. Remen RN. Kitchen table wisdom stories that heal. New York, NY: Riverhead Books; 2006.
10. Abendroth M, Flannery J. Predicting the risk of compassion fatigue: a study of hospice nurses. J Hosp Palliat Nurs. 2006;8(6):346–56. https://doi.org/10.1097/00129191-200611000-00007.
11. Melvin CS. Historical review in understanding burnout, professional compassion fatigue, and secondary traumatic stress disorder from a hospice and palliative nursing perspective. J Hosp Palliat Nurs. 2015;17:66–72.
12. Martins Pereira S, Fonseca AM, Sofia Carvalho A. Burnout in palliative care: a systematic review. Nurs Ethics. 2011;18:317–26.
13. Maslach C, Leiter MP. Understanding the burnout experience: recent research and its implications for psychiatry. World Psychiatry. 2016;15(2):103–11. https://doi.org/10.1002/wps.20311.
14. Rizo-Baeza M, Mendiola-Infante SV, Sepehri A, Palazon-Bru A, Gil-Guillen VF, Cortes-Castell E. Burnout syndrome in nurses working in palliative care units: an analysis of associated factors. J Nurs Manag. 2018;2018:19–25. https://doi.org/10.1111/jonm.1250.
15. Figley CR. Compassion fatigue: toward a new understanding of the costs of caring. In: Stamm BH, editor. Secondary traumatic stress: self-care issues for clinicians, researchers, and educators. Baltimore, MD: The Sidran Press; 1995. p. 3–28.
16. Mathieu F. Running on empty: compassion fatigue in health professionals. Rehab & Community Care Medicine. 2007. http://www.compassionfatigue.org/pages/RunningOnEmpty.pdf
17. Canadian Institute for Health Information (CIHI). Health care use at the end-of-life in Western Canada. Ottawa: CIHI; 2007.
18. Demerouti E, Bakker AB, Nachreiner F, Schaufeli WB. The job demands-resources model of burnout. J Appl Psychol. 2001;86:499–512. https://doi.org/10.1037/0021-9010.86.3.499.
19. Schaufeli WB, Bakker AB. Job demands, job resources and their relationship with burnout and engagement: a multi-sample study. J Organ Behav. 2004;25(3):293–315. https://doi.org/10.1002/job.248.
20. Brazil K, Kassalainen S, Ploeg J, et al. Moral distress experienced by health care professionals who provide home-based palliative care. Soc Sci Med. 2011;71:1687–91.
21. Thacker KS. Nurses' advocacy behaviors in end-of-life nursing care. Nurs Ethics. 2008;15:174–85.
22. Melo CG, Oliver D. Can addressing death anxiety reduce health care workers' burnout and improve patient care? J Palliat Care. 2011;27:287–95.
23. Fillion L, Dupuis R, Tremblay I, et al. Enhancing meaning in palliative care practice: a meaning-centered intervention to promote job satisfaction. Palliat Support Care. 2006;4:333–44.

24. Vachon MLS, Sherwood C. Staff stress and burnout. In: Berger AM, Shuster JL, JHV R, editors. Principles and practice of palliative care and supportive oncology. Philadelphia, PA: Lippincott Williams & Wilkins; 2007. p. 667–83.
25. Estabrooks CA, Hoben M, Poss JW, Chamberlain SA, Thompson GN, Silvius JL, et al. Dying in a nursing home: treatable symptom burden and its link to modifiable features of work context. J Am Med Dir Assoc. 2015;16(6):515–20. https://doi.org/10.1016/j.jamda.2015.02.007.
26. Huskamp HA, Kaufmann C, Stevenson DG. The intersection of long-term care and end-of-life care. Med Care Res Rev. 2012;69(1):3–44.
27. Government of Canada. An act to amend the criminal code and make related amendments to other acts (medical assistance in dying). 2016. https://laws-lois.justice.gc.ca/PDF/2016_3.pdf.
28. Beuthin R, Bruce A, Scaia M. Medical assistance in dying (MAiD): Canadian nurses' experiences. Nurs Forum. 2018;2018(53):511–20. https://doi.org/10.1111/nuf.12280.
29. Lamb C, Evans M, Babenko-Mould Y, Wong A, Kirkwood K. Nurses' use of conscientious objection and the implications for conscience. J Adv Nurs. 2018;2018:1–9. https://doi.org/10.1111/jan.13869.
30. Pierce B, Dougherty E, Panzarella T, et al. Staff stress, work satisfaction, and death attitudes on an oncology palliative care unit, and on a medical and radiation oncology inpatient unit. J Palliat Care. 2007;23:32–9.
31. Slater PJ, Edwards S. Needs analysis and development of a staff well-being program in pediatric oncology, hematology, and palliative care services group. J Healthc Leaders. 2018;10:55–65.
32. Penz K. What are the potential factors that sustain registered nurses who provide home-based palliative and end-of-life care? J Hosp Palliat Nurs. 2008;10(5):295–303.
33. Mathieu F. The compassion fatigue workbook: creative tools for transforming compassion fatigue and vicarious traumatization. New York: Taylor and Francis Group; 2012.
34. Peters E. Compassion fatigue in nursing: a concept analysis. Nurs Forum. 2018;53(4):466–80. https://doi.org/10.1111/nuf.12274.
35. Coetzee S, Klopper H. Compassion fatigue within nursing practice: a concept analysis. Nurs Health Sci. 2010;12:235–43. https://doi.org/10.1111/j.1442-2018.2010.00526.x.
36. Sheppard K. Compassion fatigue: are you at risk? Am Nurs Today. 2016;11:53–5. https://www.americannursetoday.com. Accessed 23 Sept 2016
37. Harris C, Griffin TQ. Nursing on empty: compassion fatigue signs, symptoms, and system interventions. J Christ Nurs. 2015;32:80–7. https://doi.org/10.1097/CNJ.0000000000000155.
38. Nolte AG, Downing C, Temane A, Hastings-Tolsma M. Compassion fatigue in nurses: a metasynthesis. J Clin Nurs. 2017;26:4364–78. https://doi.org/10.1111/jocn.13766.
39. Perry B, Toffner G, Merrick T, Dalton J. An exploration of the experience of compassion fatigue in clinical oncology nurses. Can Oncol Nurs J. 2011;21:91–105. https://doi.org/10.5737/1181912x2129197.
40. Tomic M, Tomic E. Existential fulfilment, workload and work engagement among nurses. J Res Nurs. 2010;16(5):468–79. https://doi.org/10.1177/1744987110383353.
41. Perlo J, Balik B, Swensen S, Kabcenell A, Landsman J, Feeley D. IHI framework for improving joy in work, IHI white paper. Cambridge, MA: Institute for Healthcare Improvement; 2017.
42. Ablett JR, Jones RSP. Resilience and well-being in palliative care staff: a qualitative study of hospice nurses' experience of work. Psycho-Oncology. 2007;16:733–40.
43. Yilmaz G, Ustun B. Professional quality of life in nurses: compassion satisfaction and compassion fatigue. J Psychiatr Nurs. 2018;9(3):205–11. https://doi.org/10.14744/phd.2018.86648.
44. Sacco TL, Copel LC. Compassion satisfaction: a concept analysis in nursing. Nurs Forum. 2018;53(1):76–83.
45. Sanso N, Galiana L, Oliver G, Pascual A, Sinclair S, Benito E. Palliative care professionals' inner life: exploring the relationships among awareness, self-care, and compassion satisfaction and fatigue, burnout, and coping with death. J Pain Symptom Manag. 2015;50(2):200–7. https://doi.org/10.1016/j.jpainsymman.2015.02.013.

46. Brighton LJ, Selman LE, Bristowe K, Edwards B, Koffman J, Evans CJ. Emotional labour in palliative and end-of-life communication: a qualitative study with generalist palliative care workers. Patient Educ Couns. 2018:1–9. https://doi.org/10.1016/j.pec.2018.10.013.
47. Tend Academy. What is compassion fatigue? 2019 [cited 2019 Feb 14]. https://www.tendacademy.ca/wp-content/uploads/2018/05/what-is-compassion-fatigue-2018-05-20.pdf.
48. Penz K. Sidebar 2.1. Use of Canadian palliative care nurses' reflective journaling as contributing to nurses' health and wellbeing. In: Lindquist R, Snyder M, Tracy MF, editors. Complementary & alternative therapies in nursing. 7th ed. New York, NY: Springer Publishing Company; 2014. p. 21–2.
49. Rourke MT. Compassion fatigue in pediatric palliative care providers. Pediatr Clin N Am. 2007;54(2007):631–44. https://doi.org/10.1016/j.pcl.2007.01.004.
50. Kim S, Wendy M, Peer Leadership Group, Mental Health Commission of Canada. Guidelines for the practice and training of peer support. Calgary, AB: Mental Health Commission of Canada; 2013. http://www.mentalhealthcommission.ca

Family Caregiver Perspective: Navigating the Palliative Care Pathway—How an Email Chronicle Eased the Journey

Sherrill Miller

Contents

2.1	A Personal Odyssey..	17
2.2	A Phenomenological Process...	19
	2.2.1 Allegro to Caesura: A Break in the Music, to Pause, to Catch One's Breath......	20
	2.2.2 Entering Rubato: Stealing Time..	22
	2.2.3 Largo and Staccato: The Slow Bumpy Journey.................................	23
	2.2.4 Nocturne: The Night Journey..	24
	2.2.5 Recapitulation: A Retrospective Synthesis.....................................	27
	2.2.6 Reprise: An Elegy for the Ongoing Journey....................................	29
References...		33

2.1 A Personal Odyssey

My early education included an RN and BScN with a working background in various counselling settings including developing the role of Sexual Health Care Clinician at the Spinal Cord Injury Unit and GF Strong Rehabilitation Centre in Vancouver British Columbia, Canada, in the late 1970s. I think that early work with the devastating losses around paraplegia and quadriplegia primed me to begin to understand bereavement. I also pursued pre-medical studies and then work in psychiatric nursing. I eventually left health care to enter the business world, and later became the researcher, writer, and marketing manager of the photography company established by my husband, renowned Canadian photographer, Courtney Milne; we are pictured in Fig. 2.1. Together we travelled the world and created books, exhibitions and multimedia shows with sacred landscapes from all seven continents. When

---

S. Miller (✉)
Victoria, BC, Canada
e-mail: sherrill@landscapesofconsciousness.com

© Springer Nature Switzerland AG 2019
L. Holtslander et al. (eds.), *Hospice Palliative Home Care and Bereavement Support*, https://doi.org/10.1007/978-3-030-19535-9_2

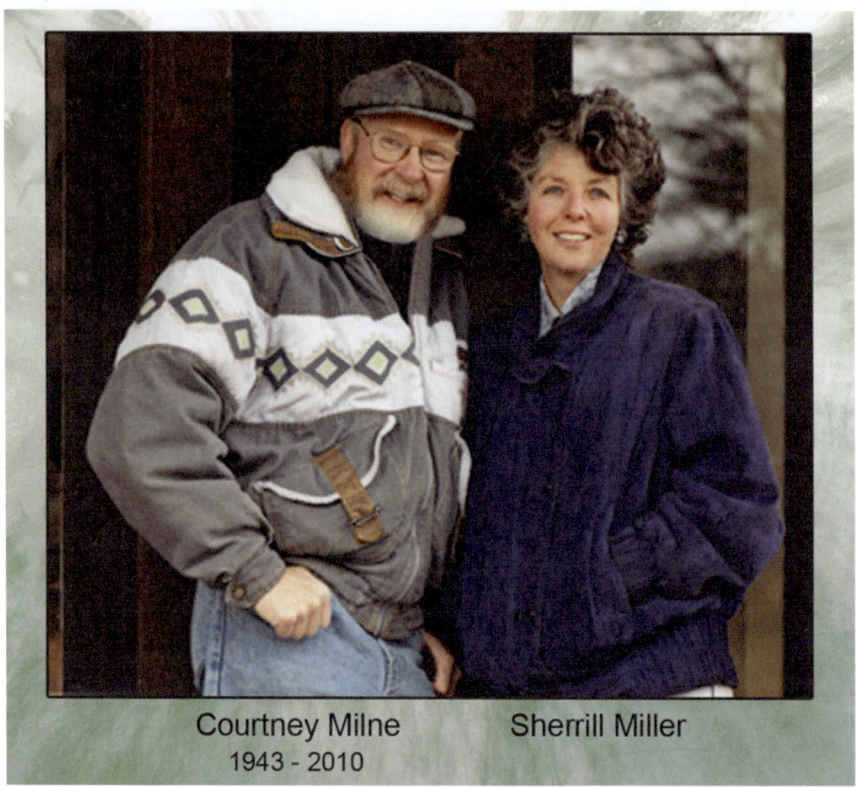

Fig. 2.1 Photo credit Gene Hattori. Image source: Courtney Milne Fonds. University of Saskatchewan Library, University Archives and Special Collections

Courtney was diagnosed with multiple myeloma in 2009, I became his primary caregiver, a situation I called 'coming full circle', in my being able to use my early specialty nursing training to assist him. During Courtney's illness, we both experienced significant losses and the grief associated with them. Our work together and our exotic lifestyle of travel and spiritual exploration was done. We turned to each other, to the land, and to a few close friends and family, but my heart also ached for our extended families and many friends and colleagues who were shocked and dismayed at how our incredibly creative life had taken a turn into darkness. I then discovered writing.

Writing as a therapeutic intervention during bereavement is often prescribed by counselling professionals [1]. Some people may write about a trauma or appeal to a higher power at their darkest moment. Writing during grief may encounter obstacles such as lack of time and diminished energy, difficulty focusing, and feelings of overwhelm. It may leave the grieving person feeling more stressed, especially when struggling to acknowledge an imminent death. In retrospect, my writing became a tool for both catharsis and desensitization to the pain of the journey. It kept me 'in the present', rather than mired in the losses of our past life. That said, at the time I was more aware of the need to share, rather than the unexpected outcomes that ultimately allowed me to gain perspective, deepen my own journey, and receive support through this connection with friends.

Now, looking back 9 years since the death of my husband, I think the desensitization was a bonus, as was the feeling that we were not alone through this mysterious and rocky journey. Courtney transitioned from a passionate, vibrant, physically active 64-year-old professional landscape photographer, to an invalid in the acute phase, and later to a paraplegic with limited ability to care for himself due to the pain and systemic weakness resulting from the myeloma lesions in his spine. It was a journey of acceptance and grace, nurtured by Courtney's ever-present sense of humour and our shared sense of hope and possibility. It was a dramatic invitation to employ our long established, but not fully tested beliefs and mantras, including 'correct, and continue', and 'this too shall pass'.

2.2 A Phenomenological Process

I think the value of this writing is best seen through a phenomenological approach, a sharing of my 'lived experience'. It seems to me that phenomenology seeks to portray the unique sense of self and highly personal experiences that perhaps can only be described as the *art* of living. Stories create a rich visual landscape of a lived life, allowing us to share at a deeper level. Telling a story has a bigger mythic impact—a more direct revelation of truth, which can never be fully understood through the words of the typical scientific research model. Perhaps there is no way we can truly and fully understand each other's journeys. The hidden essence must be felt, and the conversation kept open and evolving through personal narrative. Many cultures rely on ancient myths to understand life's deepest mysteries. The Irish call mythic storytelling "preparation by anecdote" [2]. John O'Donohue, the Celtic philosopher/priest said that our task on this earth is to find our "relentless originality". He suggests that no one else *sees* your life, *feels* your life, or *stands* on the same ground as you. No one else but you can really understand what that is like … and our uniqueness is both a privilege, and a burden [3]. So our stories are a way of sharing our essence.

I have also come to see our life on the palliative care journey as a musical metaphor. It is a symphony of many movements, with a variety of lyrical instrumental voices echoing back and forth, portraying the emotional ups and downs, weaving the texture of the life that is evolving. Courtney and I quickly relinquished the demands of our busy Allegro tempo work life—cheerful, brisk and lively—and transitioned to Rubato time, living in response to life, setting our own pace. Periods of Largo, Staccato, Nocturne, and Appassionato were revealed along the way… and finally, for me, an opportunity for Recapitulation and Reprise: to review, recognize, reinvent, and to make meaning in a new way.

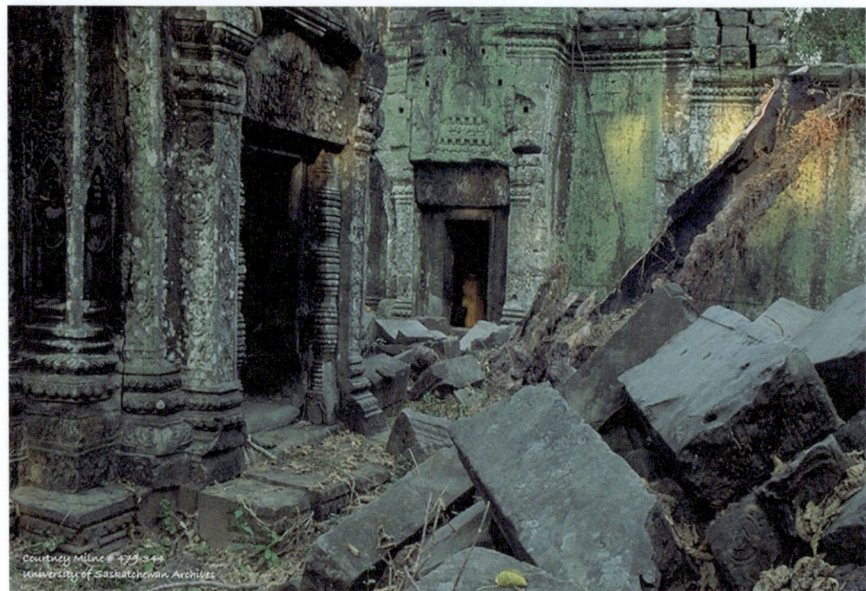

Fig. 2.2 # 479-344 Image source: Courtney Milne Fonds, University of Saskatchewan Library, University Archives and Special Collections

In a lecture to nursing students several years after Courtney died, I opened with:

What we are really talking about is brokenness—something like this temple portrays (Fig. 2.2) … broken bodies, broken lives, broken dreams. But I wonder—is there still a spiritual impulse here, despite the damage? Is there still a vestige of the sacred power it once had, despite the brokenness? Does it still carry the mystery and fullness of its individuality? Can we learn to love this mystery, and just be with it?

Perhaps this echoes the quote: "some things in life cannot be fixed—they can only be carried" [4]. I think that is very good advice for many times of life, but particularly for the Palliative Care Journey.

2.2.1 Allegro to Caesura: A Break in the Music, to Pause, to Catch One's Breath

The story begins with Courtney's diagnosis of multiple myeloma, when our Allegro paced life suddenly halted—we had no idea what the next bars of music would sound like. I became not only Courtney's primary caregiver, but also the main contact person for our friends and family during this time. I initially started writing not for myself, but because I knew everyone was in shock about Courtney's diagnosis—they needed information and support, and I could not talk to all of them individually. I did not have the time or the energy to repeat the story of what was happening, and truthfully, I could not cope with their pain. In some sense, they were struggling more than we were because they were at a distance, worrying, and they did not have information or help to deal with their feelings.

Courtney had been in physical rehab for several months when he called a friend from the hospital. She then asked me what she could tell other colleagues so I enlisted her help:

> I am starting to let other people know what is happening—I figure it will be too much of a shock for them later—so better sooner. I just don't want to have to talk to a lot of people … I know everyone wants to support me but it is harder to have to put out that energy—I know you understand. So tell anyone you think should know … just no phone calls please. I know people are sending their love and that is all we need at the moment. I'm so glad he called you and he is reaching out to others. Today is the first day in more than two months that I have had time for myself at home. Whew! It was a beautiful spring day, good for raking leaves, hauling out the hoses, and reading a good book.

My emotional experience is evident throughout the prose, woven into sometimes very practical emails updating loved ones about our challenges and Courtney's health. An early email demonstrated a resolution to be hopeful:

> We don't know what this disease will bring—but it is not a 'war on cancer'. Our vision is that Courtney not only maintains his current energy, but also improves his strength and abilities and becomes involved in his creative projects again. Last year I added Deepak Chopra's comment: *'what would be possible in your life if you were able to see the world with new eyes'* to my email signature, thinking it was an endorsement of the Pool of Possibilities. It has also become a personal daily meditation on miracles, trying to find that place inside 'where nothing is impossible' [5].

The Pool of Possibilities project was Courtney's focus in his last 10 years of photography, exploring the interplay of light, wind and nature on the water in our swimming pool. In this body of images he saw the whole world, and all its opportunities—hence the name, *The Pool of Possibilities*.

I referred to being thrust into the palliative care journey as 'a left hand turn', which was a metaphor for the mystical 'dark night of the soul', and the death of our life as we knew it. It was a time of grace, an opportunity to flow in our own rhythm. It made the vast unpredictability of life very real and tangible. I shared some of our early insights:

> Perhaps the greatest lesson here is to know we are not invincible, so if you have things you want to do in your life, don't wait—one never knows where the next left hand turn will be. Wayne Dyer said it well: "don't die with your music still inside you" [6].
>
> We are learning lessons about really living in the moment, about truly loving oneself, each other and everything around us and being grateful for every moment of every day, and particularly right now, for the glorious spring greens and smells of summer on the prairie.

This optimistic passage captured our thankfulness for each mindful moment, but I have recently discovered it also helped others. One friend and colleague who advised us on alternative health options wrote not only of how my emails helped her cope with her own feelings, but also how they helped her to assist us:

> It seemed no matter how bleak the circumstances would have looked to most people, there was always an aura of hope and expectant miracles woven in the lines. So when I could spend time with both of you, I didn't feel like I needed to waste precious time 'catching up.' I could walk right in and know exactly what was happening and carry on the best I could. [MK]

2.2.2 Entering Rubato: Stealing Time

The emails also served to document the journey of caring for Courtney and offered an expanded understanding of my own and Courtney's lived experience of his illness, both at the time, and retrospectively. Psychology calls this an experience of 'meaning making':

> The other day the host on CBC radio's *Tempo* said that Chopin's brilliance as a composer was due to his great understanding of the piano. She gave an example of a solo section in a concerto, explaining that Rubato means 'stolen time'. This allows the soloist flexibility to take some liberties with his interpretation of the music. I told Courtney that I am practising Rubato ... and we are going to 'steal time'.

Despite starting as a means of staying in contact to support our friends and family, my email message writing unexpectedly evolved as a tool for many of us to process the grief experience in real time, and to further enhance my understanding of it in hindsight. The emails, thus, had a therapeutic effect. One friend recently reinforced this with a very poignant comment:

> It was important because I was so far away—it made me feel closer to you all. I remember weeping at times when I read the emails and I wanted to delete them, to make my grief go away.... too bad I'm a therapist and know better! [JG]

I think the emails also gave the recipients time to ponder, to absorb information at their own rate, and to gradually process their own feelings. Phone calls had a more informative nature and were more difficult to absorb because of the immediacy and even shock value, not allowing the same opportunity for emotional processing that re-reading an email could provide. It was dealing with this emotional upheaval that I feared I could not offer to others as I was in the midst of similar and constant processing for myself, and with Courtney. Many people said in retrospect the emails reassured them that we were being supported:

> Courtney had a huge community generating heartfelt encouragement/support. But that was also influencing YOU supportively. And we also know that those who only witness (are not direct recipients but hear or see some of the stories or pictures, etc.) are positively impacted AS WELL. [LS]
>
> When you hear that a friend is ill, the internal struggle of how best to help begins. Should you jump right in or step back respectfully waiting to be asked? Your emails felt like a guide showing us how to proceed, when to step forward and when to step back. [JL]

Because Courtney was well known and there was a lot of communication between friends and colleagues, one friend observed that the emails helped others to know what was really happening, rather than what they might have heard as second hand information or repeats on social media:

> The emails provided the 'official story' to a select audience, rather than through social media where you might lose the truth, and the intimacy of a personal connection. [LN]

Courtney and I also had the day-to-day rhythm and ability to make adjustments, so in some strange sense it was easier for us, a gradual moving forward, one step in front of the other into Rubato time. I also realized that writing helped me clarify my feelings and to be more transparent than I might have been in person—I just put it 'out there', and also tried to portray how we were adjusting to whatever came along. Writing became a creative act, allowing me to draw from my experience, intuition, spiritual beliefs and positivity … it became a rather poetic way of portraying our life. Most of the writing was my own impressions, but sometimes I included comments from Courtney. It was like a journal … a diary of our life … a record of his medical situation … and a way of being intimate at a distance:

> Courtney came home from the hospital (on a weekend trial visit) last night and is feeling very perky—we have set up our big king bed in the dining room, looking out the big picture window onto the trees and pool … last night the stars were awesome! (for those of you who haven't been here, we do not have any curtains to impede the view!) He is managing well and loving basking in the sun through the window … our duvet is like a spring garden of flowers, so it feels like a Monet experience!

2.2.3 Largo and Staccato: The Slow Bumpy Journey

Our palliative care journey continued over a period of 18 months, portraying the setbacks and successes as Courtney's illness improved, then the losses as his health dramatically declined. One of Courtney's favourite teachings in his *Seeing with New Eyes* photography workshops was "telling your story makes who you are more tangible". He had always been pretty emotionally transparent, and that continued, and deepened at times, as he/we were called to delve into our feelings. I know the emails helped people to feel more connected to us and to be part of the process, making their (and our) grieving easier, while facing the new realities of our life in a more gradual and genuine way. For example:

> They provided a wonderful sense of inclusion and closeness, to keep involved and somewhat aware of the circumstances of your lives, and also gave us opportunity to respond with wee notes of caring. [LH]
> The emails made us feel more closely connected with both you and Court during this most sacred time and helped us psychologically and spiritually journey with you in a more intimate way. [JGE]
> We were hungry for information but very aware that the demand for updates was taxing for you. We thus tried to hang back and wait. There were times when messages came in so often that I felt overloaded in spite of having my head full of [thinking of] Courtney every day. [AC].

This witnessing and modelling effect of the emails helped several friends in subsequent years to cope with sudden family illnesses and meet their need to keep family and friends informed. One wrote about her own email saga:

> It allowed me to be thoughtful, sensitive, and concerned about others, but not overly engaged—with time to think, record thoughts and feelings … to deal with queries, but also protect myself from the barrage of opinions from my family. [EP]

Even with an excellent Home Care nursing team, a major part of my role was being Courtney's advocate, interfacing with the many services he needed. We were able to borrow a hospital bed from the Saskatchewan Abilities Council. Pain management was a big problem that required medical assessment in the city. I had a prolonged debate with the provincial medical plan to cover a new prescription drug for pain—they finally approved it, but ultimately it was not very effective. We lived in the country so every time a problem surfaced, such as a bladder infection (which can be life threatening to a paraplegic), we had to go into town for medical assessment. Radiation and other ancillary treatments and evaluations resulted in more trips. That required me to help Courtney make 8 transfers each trip which were exhausting for him (and me): bed to wheelchair, in/out of the car, wheelchair to hospital bed (and reverse on the way home), and a bumpy ride that activated every pain neuron. Even in a wheelchair taxi in his own cushioned power wheelchair, he felt every rock on our country roads and dips in the city pavement. Sometimes infections resulted in treatment with intravenous antibiotics that I had to learn how to administer at home. This advocacy and organizational role was familiar to me, and despite the added stress, in some way it allowed me to retain and reclaim a sense of my previously efficient self, and to have a small sense of control. Falling into the nursing role was surprisingly easy and I recognized how I enjoyed the familiarity of my expertise, being able to help Courtney and establish a routine that would ease the discomfort of his days as much as possible—but there was still much for me to learn and to manage. The palliative care journey had many twists and turns, and, like a traditional maze, no clear path to exit.

Despite the ever-present pain, a year later Courtney was much stronger and he yearned for freedom. On his instigation, I packed up both his manual and power wheelchairs and supplies for a month, and with the help of Westjet Airlines we flew to California and stayed with cousins in Palm Springs:

> We have been able to adjust, jerry-rig, and figure out the flow of Courtney's care quite easily. The big question, 'The Bed', was easily solved with a queen-sized bed with memory foam that has treated his skin well, and there is room enough for me—we have both been sleeping very well. The head elevates so it makes it easier for him as well.
>
> Courtney is loving it here ... sunny, warm, colourful flowers, a house with a beautiful patio overlooking the golf course—and he has discovered he can easily 'motor' in his power chair over to the clubhouse, about 10 min from here, and take his friends out for lunch. He is glorying in the freedom and ease of moving around in this temperature and with these facilities. Our cousin has taken over most of the shopping and cooking, which has been a great blessing for me!

This was the ultimate Rubato experience. I was also able to enjoy this holiday from the medical regimen, to relish my own solitary 'stolen' time. My early back spasms diminished and I played tennis in the sunshine. Late at night, I could turn to my writing to clarify my feelings and process the events of the day in this neutral setting. It was a time to breathe, to reflect, to think, feel, understand and integrate—more meaning making.

2.2.4 Nocturne: The Night Journey

We returned in good spirits but later in the spring faced a recurrence of infections requiring hospitalization followed by the need for more intense care at home, as well as the ongoing difficulty in the management of pain. He had a series of palliative radiation treatments requiring numerous 8-transfer trips to the city. It was a challenge to accept the limits of the health care situation and my inability to 'fix' things, focusing instead on the things I could do to keep him comfortable and safe.

Courtney had been doing well; he was stronger, we were in the process of buying a wheelchair van, he passed his driving test using hand controls, and he was excited about the independence that would give him. Suddenly an unexpected and drastic complication occurred. Courtney developed seizures that resulted in two traumatic 911 emergency calls and ambulance trips to the hospital. He developed speech and coordination problems which became worse … it was not clear if this was the disease process or if he was overmedicated (to stop the seizures), and I had trouble getting clear medical advice (on a holiday weekend, which was also our 20th wedding anniversary). The daily visit from our Home Care nurse was an anchor for both of us, giving us a sense of constancy and support during this tremulous and extremely upsetting and confusing time.

At this time I wrote less, mostly because of time and energy constraints, but it was just as important because I knew people would be in shock. I needed to prepare others—and perhaps myself—for this ominous turn. Speaking the words and putting them in writing also made it more real for me. Other emotions that came through in the emails a few weeks before Courtney died are a sense of disbelief at the reality of his declining health, as well as gratitude for things for which I found to be thankful. For example:

> It is day by day, hoping he will perk up and get stronger again … I just keep being grateful that he is still here, and can't believe he might not be.

This was my way of acknowledging the possibility of Courtney's death—to speak it out loud, preparing both others and myself for that possibility. Looking back on it now, I realize I was being 'realistic' with this statement, but not giving in. In fact, I continued to feel hopeful almost to the end, saying to Courtney 'we can handle this—we can learn to live with it'. Some people may have seen this as denial—but for me, it was possibility:

> Courtney is not doing well … he is having more tremors this morning at 0530 … he is resting now, at 0700, but we need to be prepared for the worst. I just wanted to let you know—I know you will be pretty shocked and upset … there seems no way around this. Maybe he will settle down, but even if we sedate him heavily, which we don't want to do, this is the likely scenario. I slept beside his bed last night and he was quite peaceful till this happened. So my friends, prepare yourselves - and hope that it will not be imminent. I am just in the moment, knowing I have no control over this.

Even though I was eternally positive and felt we could manage anything, I finally let go of that hope when, after a month of struggling and becoming weaker, Courtney decided to stop eating and drinking. He clearly said he did not want to live this way—it was "time to go". His last words to us were "from now on the heart is in charge".

My emails again offered me the vehicle to direct how others could best support us, explaining what would be helpful and what would only cause difficulty, and an email update as circumstances continued to change:

I know you will all be saddened and shocked, and I also know you are sending us much love and support. Please do not feel the need to reply to this. I'll keep you posted as to his progress.

A few days ago Courtney said he did not want any more visitors or phone calls. I have passed on all your messages to him, but the phone is quite disruptive and takes our energy away from him. He knows how much everyone loves him, and he is basking in that.

He did, however, allow one last visit with some special friends and their 6-year-old twin granddaughters who had loved playing and joking with Courtney. One said to him: "Courtney, I don't want you to die" and he responded: "remember I will always love you". The depth of their bond was revealed years later when their mother reported:

> You may be surprised to hear how many times his name comes up around here. Just the other day when S. (age 13) was posing for a picture, all of a sudden she decided to reposition into a 'Courtney pose' … one leg up, arms in the air, and a big grin—you know the one! We smiled, remembered, got a bit teary, and were grateful once again for the influence of childlike fun he infused into so many interactions. [JB]

This Nocturne space was a sacred time of gratitude and connection. As Courtney gazed out at the pool from his bed, we continued to read his daily e-calendar as a reminder of the impact of his work. Near the end I wrote:

> Courtney said he has fulfilled his purpose, and that his work is done. Yesterday morning, with great clarity and directness, he repeated this, saying he was "ready to go" … and "I have been on the other side a long time". I know many of you have seen that 'other side' through his images. We can feel the change in energy in this space. So once again, ever the gentle man, Courtney has made it easier for us. We now know exactly where he is at, and do not have to guess. That has been the hardest part for all of us, to not know. He has gifted us with his certainty.

I don't know where those words of insight came from … the words just seemed to flow into my fingers on the computer. Courtney died at home, surrounded by the beauty and peace he had always known. A friend who was a shamanic practitioner accompanied him energetically at a distance. Two close friends were in the house with us, holding the space with me—I called us the Guardians at the Doorway. On the day he died, I spoke to immediate family, and then turned again to my email entitled *Courtney Milne Oct. 3, 1943 - Aug. 29, 2010* (Fig. 2.3):

> On the Pool of Possibilities e-calendar this is the day of *Appreciation*, where Courtney invites readers to *Observe how the day brightens around you when you share with others what you appreciate about them, with no strings attached, and what you appreciate about yourself, without qualifying your statement.*
>
> I appreciate the outpouring of grief and love that is happening near and far. I'm sorry I can't talk to all of you but it is too difficult. Please don't try to phone or send flowers. Instead, I would encourage you to follow Courtney's invitation at the end of his Sacred Earth Concerts—to *find your own sacred place in nature where you feel a connection with the Divine Mystery …a place that you care for and feel connected to, whether in your own back yard, in the park down the street, or a piece of wilderness.* Do that in honour of him, and imprint his inspiration in your heart.

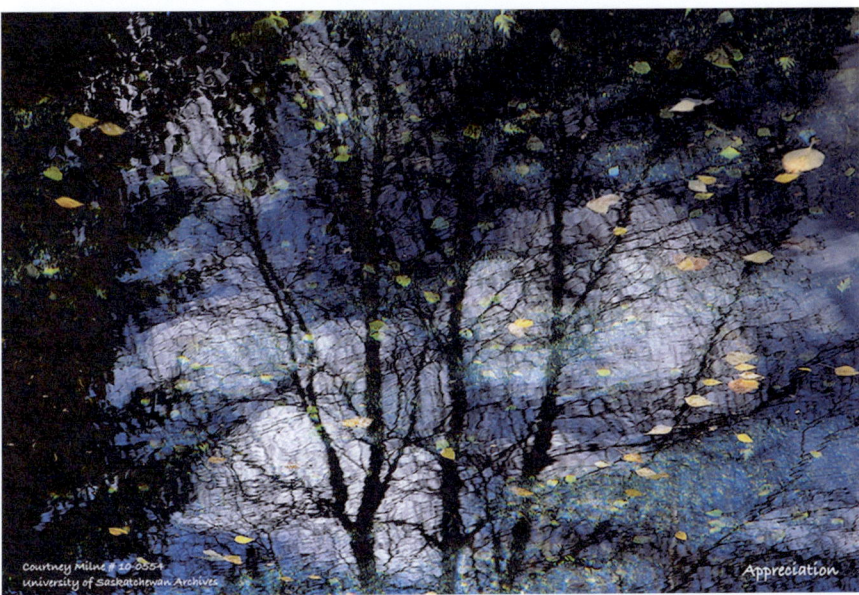

Fig. 2.3 'Appreciation' # 10-0554. Image source: Courtney Milne Fonds, University of Saskatchewan Library, University Archives and Special Collections

We kept him home for a day before calling the funeral home—this allowed us to take in the reality of his death on a deeper level. Our Home Care nursing team was invaluable in these final days, walking with us every step of the way. Looking back, I realize I was—and still am—being led by Courtney's Vision Statement for his work: *to reveal the unfolding Mystery, not to try to solve it.*

2.2.5 Recapitulation: A Retrospective Synthesis

On reflection, I think email was the perfect vehicle for me as I already had an extensive list of people who were accustomed to communicating with me in this way. This process may not be for everyone, but it helped me go deeper into my own intuitive wisdom. It also helped me find refuge in the sanctuary we created on our private acreage (10 miles from town). Others might have preferred to gather more people around them, but for us it was important to retreat and become more introspective. We spoke to close family and friends, but too many phone calls or personal visits would have exhausted me (as well as Courtney) because of the emotional outlay I felt would have been required of me. Our Home Care nurses were vital at this time, giving me a break from caregiving, and giving Courtney another person to relate to. His favourite daily nurse not only matched his sense of humour, but also had a great interest in him as a person, and he loved sharing his work with her. Her visits lifted his spirits immensely, even at the toughest times, and seeing this also helped me feel encouraged.

Being able to write these emails was a relief—for me to portray what was happening, clarify my understanding, share my thoughts and feelings, and not have to put out more energy to talk and repeat the same information to many different people. Even more importantly, I recognized the depth of grieving in so many friends, so this writing gave me the most intimate connection I could offer, but protected me in not having to deal directly with the grief of others. I knew I could not handle that. I don't think it was a selfish reaction, but one of self-preservation and containment—I needed my energy for myself and for Courtney. Writing was sometimes a celebration, and other times it was finding a way through the chaos.

A blog may be an option for some people but would have been harder for me to set up and monitor, and I feel, less intimate. The email chronicle became my personal journal. In the years after Courtney died, as my brain fog, exhaustion, and confusion gradually waned, re-reading this writing has helped me to further understand our journey. Part of my continuing work in various educational settings allowed me to share my story and to integrate the deeper meaning of my losses. Stroebe and Schut's Dual Model of Coping with Bereavement (2007) portrays the concept of an alternating focus between experiences of loss and activities of restoration [7]. For me, teaching and retelling my story helped me to discern what I needed to let go of and what I could bring forward into my new life. Looking back on my writing, I am amazed that my perceptions were so clear—this seemed to crack me open and allow me to share at a deeper level, more than I would have thought possible before. It may have been partly due to less editing of my feelings because of ongoing fatigue. Almost without thinking the words seemed to flow from a deep well of knowing. This often surprised me as I sat at the computer, asking myself 'where did that come from?', but this has continued to serve me in my writing today. It was like a veil was lifted and it was easier to access my thoughts and feelings, as well as Courtney's—he had always been very passionate and emotionally transparent, so I just tried to honestly convey his feelings to others (he did not use email so this protected him from having to put out the energy to account to others on the phone). We felt grateful we were not alone in our journey, knowing others were holding us in this space. I now see this opening as an example of Leonard Cohen's invitation in his song *Anthem*, to *ring the bells that still can ring, forget your perfect offering, there is a crack in everything, that's how the light gets in* [8].

As I look back 9 years later, I'm often amazed at my words and the profound intuitive knowing they delivered. What began as a way of connecting started me on a creative journey I could not have anticipated. It has become the foundation of the *Gift of Change* multimedia show that I created as an opportunity to keep Courtney's photography alive, and also to inspire others who are seeking to reinvent a life after a major change.

In musical notation, *recapitulation* is a repetition of the major themes; for me, this 'recap' is the opportunity to 'see again', to experience, and perhaps understand in a new way. Through subsequent years of presenting lectures and my *Gift of Change* show, I have discovered unfamiliar grooves on the spiral of grief. Even now as I write this chapter, I am again re-living the losses, and entering another turn of grief and growth. Despite the sorrow, I actually welcome these dives into sadness as I know they hit pockets of unseen feelings that are important to move out of my body—it reminds me I am alive. It is the rhythm of Appassionato, for myself, and for others. A few of those dear friends on my email list have since died, while others have lost partners or close friends or family. My experience has also helped me cope with their grief, and ease my own new grief. I feel my heart is more open, and I do not need to ask what I call the 'default' question: 'how are you doing?'; I can sit with the sadness more easily. I understand now that time itself does not heal, but healing does take time.

In the first years after Courtney died, many events were held to honour his life. Over those intervening years, I continued to write email updates about my changing life and these celebrations such as the posthumous award of the Saskatchewan Order of Merit, the transfer of his work to the University of Saskatchewan Library and Archives, and annual memorial notices in the newspaper. I spent 3 years creating a catalogue for the Archive, which was both a labour of love and a tool of bereavement for me, providing an opportunity to re-live our life's projects and tell the stories surrounding them. At the time I didn't realize that writing this catalogue was a vehicle for grieving—I thought I was just 'helping them' to make sense of 35 years of work captured in hundreds of files on multiple projects, a collection of more than 500,000 images, and 12 books. The process allowed me to laugh, to cry, to reminisce, to review, to put our life into context, to conclude our life together, and to celebrate all our accomplishments and reach a kind of completion. This life review brought back many personal memories, and indeed, I joke that if I were to be cheeky, I would say it gave me the 'last word'—but it was also a reminder that I had often served in an arm's length role that is so important to artists, not to 'interpret' their work, but to step back and see it in a way that others might better understand.

In 2016, I suddenly realized that my work was done and it was time for me to sell our property and move back to the west coast of Canada where I had grown up. This move brought an amazing insight: I needed to literally move away from my 'Courtney and Sherrill' identity to find out who I really was at this point in my life. It has been a time to treasure as well as a struggle to establish this new identity of 'Sherrill', to forge new relationships and make new meaning in this new period of my life. When I sometimes complain about how hard it can be to start over, I try to remember my own advice in my *Gift of Change* show: the only thing in life that is really predictable is that change *will* happen, and adjusting to that change revolves around three interwoven tasks: to *reclaim* oneself, discerning and keeping the parts of one's life that are still valid and useful today; to *reinvent* a life with new meaning and purpose; and then to challenge one's creativity to find ways to *re-enchant* and enliven that new life that is emerging … and as we respond to the gifts that flow from the changes in our life, we need to discover the wonder, the promise, and the enchantment in our *own* 'Pool of Possibilities'.

2.2.6 Reprise: An Elegy for the Ongoing Journey

A character from a favourite novel advises: 'each person's heart breaks in its own way—and each has a different cure' [9]. That is such a good observation.

I have come to see bereavement as the process of coping not only with loss of **the Other**, but equally—and at times *more* profoundly—is a recognition of the **loss of**

oneself and **one's life as it had been with the Other.** It involves mourning this loss of possibility, frequently circling back to the past to what was seemingly lost, sifting through, picking up the pieces and bringing forward what is still useful in the present—establishing what the Buddhists call a Right Relationship with the past … and with the present. The healing of bereavement is about finding that new version of self, and re-weaving the texture of that new life.

One major recent insight is that the palliative care journey never ends. Once initiated, it continues to inform one's sense of the fragility of life … and that is good … and keeps me moving forward. Anniversaries are difficult, prompting old feelings to surface. For the first time this year, instead of writing a memoriam on the anniversary of Courtney's death, I felt happy to write one to celebrate his birthday. I suddenly realized that the musical form of an Elegy fits here: a sad lament that expresses a feeling. The ongoing journey is about recognizing how grief thrusts us into a keener sense of death, seducing us into the deeper questions of the meaning of life, when one is so aware of the exquisite uncertainty of one's own mortality. It is about learning how to soften, to ameliorate that fear, and practising how to live again. And as time continues to pass, while aging deepens that search for understanding and meaning, we must find a way to say 'yes' to life, to find our own joy.

Now, 9 years later, many friends responded to my invitation to comment on how their life was impacted by my emails. I felt honoured as many expressed gratitude for how our situation thrust them into confronting their feelings about their own mortality, and that my emails were a model of strength and hope that helped them cope with their own grief and fears. One friend, herself a medical doctor, shared several profound comments after going through the recent deaths of several family members:

> I do fondly remember your eloquently tender emails. I have been the recipient of such from others undergoing similar situations and it has always felt like a most intimate privilege. My life's work involved the excavation of the most intimate aspects and events in people's lives and because of that, I have little tolerance for small talk. There was no small talk in your emails. It was the laying bare the hard facts and lining them up for the purpose of processing. And then heart wrenching examination of the implications and impacts.
>
> … I believe the power of this approach dually benefits the recipients and the writer. The writer's courage is called upon, banishing denial and temerity. It all becomes part of the current and preparatory grief, though my belief is that the latter is just the broth compared to the elaborate stew that is full grief. And it serves the same purpose, though of a very different nature, for the recipients. The greater benefit to them becomes the teaching about suffering. A wise witness can acquire encyclopaedic knowledge! Just knowing that someone you care about CAN walk the minefield, with individuated style, and survive, gives hope. [LS]

This model of courage and suffering was echoed by another friend who remembered our journey as she faced the recent death of her own husband:

> Seeing, feeling, sensing your quiet dignity and peace in the face of death are for me a model of how I would hope to face death. Being with Courtney through email contacts was a special privilege and blessing. It maintained a connection that had developed over more than three decades, beginning with Courtney as photography instructor, then mentor, and eventu-

ally valued and special friend. Over the years, as I photographed or pursued other art endeavours I always had a sense of Courtney 'being' with me. Journeying with Courtney through emails in his final weeks remains a daily reminder for me to never neglect the journey. [MW]

So the long-term effect on others was profound, helpful, and comforting as time went on and they were called to confront new rounds of grief and loss in their lives. Another friend could not remember the details of the emails, but she still remembered the feelings they evoked. When I commented that her response shows that 'memory' is not the only way to embed experiences, she replied:

> Feelings last longer than details … I felt like I was a part of the letting go, of the loving circle, of the focused attention on your Highest Good. [DH]

Numerous people recognized how the email conversations pushed them into exploring and expressing their own spiritual questions about life and death. One friend who lives in a religious community wrote:

> My reading of your mailing was continued inspiration, peace, and a touch of the Almighty that BOTH you and Courtney could never avoid in whatever you did and said. When someone shows God to me I know for certain that we are indeed created in that image and likeness of God, and that our epilogue will be that moment of recognition and true fullness of life. [MS]

Another long-time friend, photography student, and colleague wrote:

> Your writing encouraged me to access deeper, more meaningful and spiritual aspects of myself, for which I was very grateful. On a more basic level, it was much gentler to accompany the loving progress of his dying than to suddenly have the shock of an email notification that he had died. Courtney created much beauty in his lifetime, and played a much bigger role in my life than he probably realized; your beautiful writing was a fitting tribute to all that he stood for. [KA]

Another recognized how the continued email conversation over recent years has had a deep impact on how she now views life—and death:

> Parts of our stories continue to be woven together and that fabric provides a comfort, a warmth and a security reminding me that this whole journey through life is a Great Mystery to be embraced—there is a bridge from the mundane world to the Sacred that lives both in our hearts and our minds. It is our connections with one another that matter most. Every time you reach out I see it as a blessing and an opportunity to keep alive the magic that is our story. You have always stirred me to look more deeply into myself and see more clearly things I might have otherwise missed. [CC]

This palliative care journey is continuing through my life, taking different forms and turns as the years go by. As I write this chapter, I am still cycling through Recapitulation and Reprise, as the path creates a different composition, perhaps like Shubert's Unfinished Symphony.

Many books helped me navigate the melodies of the repeating themes in this Reprise movement. Anne Michaels offered a powerful allegory of the process:

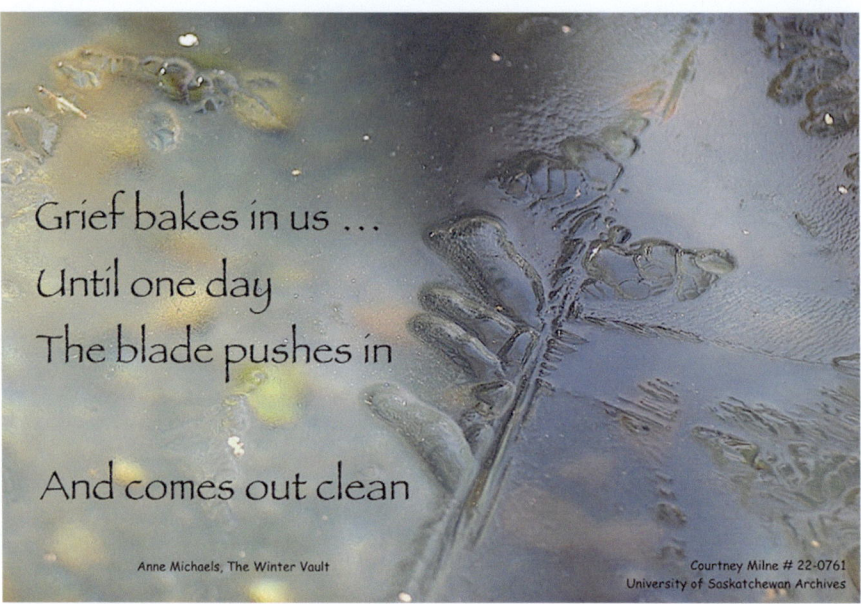

Fig. 2.4 # 22-0761 Image source: Courtney Milne Fonds, University of Saskatchewan Library, University Archives and Special Collections

"Grief bakes in us … until one day the blade pushes in, and comes out clean" [10] (Fig. 2.4). My blade may be almost clean but I think the scars will always be there as a reminder to live my life to the fullest. This is Kairos time, where I seek to live with a more sacred awareness of the world, through the portals of meandering, pondering, sauntering, recognizing, and re-cognizing, while being aware of the underlying mythic patterns that are playing out in my life. It is a life structured more around sensory awareness of the world and the resonance that is embedded within us—our inner landscape—that interior personal mirror that I explore in the techniques of inner awareness work that I call *Landscapes of Consciousness*. I resonate with poet Rainer Maria Rilke's suggestion that "work of the eyes is done … now go and do heart work on all the images imprisoned within you" [11]. I also remember Courtney's certainty that "the presence of your being is the greatest gift you can give". And, finally, I remind myself of Mark Nepo's wise words: "there is a sliver of beginning in each of us … you need to lean in softly, with a willingness to be changed by what you hear" [12]. My new symphony has a variety of themes and variations still being created. I think, perhaps, it will never be finished.

Acknowledgements Telling this story was prompted through sharing my experience of the Palliative Care Journey with Professor Lorraine Holtslander at the University of Saskatchewan College of Nursing.

I would like to acknowledge her continued support, the assistance of her students Sarah Bocking MSc RN and Kelly Mills MEd who provided background reference material, and Derek Tannis, PhD, for introducing me to the philosophy of phenomenology.

References

1. Pennebaker JW, Beall SK. Confronting a traumatic event: toward an understanding of inhibition and disease. J Abnorm Psychol. 1986;95(3):274–81. https://doi.org/10.1037/0021-843X.95.3.274.
2. Dames, Michael. Mythic Ireland. London: Thames and Hudson; 1992. p. 71.
3. The Estate of John O'Donohue. Four elements: reflections on nature. New York: Random House; 2010. p. 5–6.
4. Devine, Megan. https://refugeingrief.com.
5. Chopra, Deepak. The seven spiritual laws of success: a practical guide to the fulfillment of your dreams. San Rafael: Amber-Allen Publishing; 1994.
6. Dyer, Wayne. Your sacred self. New York: William Morrow; 2001.
7. Stroebe MS, Hansson RO, Stroebe W, Schut H. Introduction: concepts and issues in contemporary research on bereavement. In: Stroebe MS, Hansson RO, Stroebe W, Schut H, editors. Handbook of bereavement research: consequences, coping, and care. Washington, DC: American Psychological Association; 2007. p. 3–22.
8. Cohen, Leonard. "Anthem" from *The Future*. Sony music Canada; 1992.
9. Baumeister, Erica. The school of essential ingredients. New York: Putnam and Sons; 2009.
10. Michaels, Anne. The winter vault. Toronto: McClelland & Stewart; 2009.
11. Rilke, Rainer Maria. *Turning Point*, poem translated by Stephen Mitchell; 1914.
12. Nepo, Mark. Seven thousand ways to listen: staying close to what is sacred. New York: Atria/Simon & Shuster; 2012.

Other Helpful Resources

Canadian Hospice and Palliative Care Association. "Reinventing a life after loss—a bereaved caregiver's path through the palliative care journey and beyond." Webinar, Sherrill Miller, 2016. https://vimeo.com/161823653.

Contact the author for more information on *The Gift of Change* inspirational multimedia presentation and workshops on *Landscapes of Consciousness* techniques for inner awareness.

Didion, Joan. The year of magical thinking. New York: Knopf; 2005.

Extence, Gavin. The Universe Versus Alex Woods. New York, NY: Red Hook; 2013.

Fraser, Antonia. Must you go? DOUBLEHYPHEN my life with Harold Pinter. Toronto: Bond Street Books; 2010.

Gawande, Atul. Being mortal: medicine and what matters in the end: Thorndike Press; 2014.

Jenkinson, Stephen. Die wise: a manifesto for sanity and soul. Berkeley CA: North Atlantic Books; 2015.

Kagan, Annie. The afterlife of Billy Fingers: how my bad-boy brother proved to me there's life after death: Hampton Roads Publishing; 2013.

Kalanathi, Paul. When breath becomes air: Random House Canada; 2016.

Pearson, Patricia. Opening heaven's door – what the dying may be trying to tell us about where they're going: Random House Canada; 2015.

Psilocybin treatment to relieve death anxiety. http://video.newyorker.com/watch/a-reporter-at-large-magic-mushrooms-and-the-healing-trip-2015-02-02.

The Pool of Possibilities background story. http://library.usask.ca/courtneymilne/ecal/poolstory. Information and registration for free daily e-calendar. http://library.usask.ca/courtneymilne/ecal.

Global Perspectives on Palliative Care: Nigerian Context

Agatha Ogunkorode

Contents

3.1	Introduction	35
3.2	Palliative Care	36
3.3	Palliative Care in Nigeria	37
3.4	Challenges to Palliative Care Provision in Nigeria	37
3.5	Prospects and the Way Forward	38
3.6	Integration of Palliative Care into the Mainstream Healthcare Delivery System in Nigeria	39
3.7	Education and Training of Healthcare Professionals	39
3.8	Home-Based Care	39
	3.8.1 Research	40
	3.8.2 Culture	40
	3.8.3 Spiritual Care	40
3.9	Psychosocial Care	41
3.10	Making Available and Improving Access to Opioid Medication	41
3.11	The Role of the Nurse	41
3.12	Palliative Care for Women with Advanced Breast Cancer	42
3.13	Conclusions	42
References		43

3.1 Introduction

Palliative care is an approach that improves the quality of life of patients (adults and children) and their families as they face issues associated with life-threatening illness [1]. The World Health Organization statistics worldwide indicate that breast

A. Ogunkorode (✉)
College of Nursing, University of Saskatchewan, Saskatoon, SK, Canada
e-mail: aoo121@usask.ca

cancer is the leading cause of malignancy-related mortality in women [2, 3]. Also, breast cancer is the most common cause of cancer-related death in Nigerian women [4]. In Nigeria, empirical literature indicate that about 70–80% of breast cancer patients present with the advanced stages of the illness [4–7]. The advanced stages of breast cancer bring untold hardship, misery, and pain to the afflicted and their families, resulting in social isolation as a result of abandonment, and destruction of family system as a result of its physical, huge emotional burden and distress, and socioeconomic demands on the family [8]. The reasons for the late presentation include misinterpretation of the initial breast cancer symptoms, preferential use of alternative treatment modalities, misconception of the etiology of breast cancer, poverty, and fear [9]. The presentation at the advanced and metastatic stages of the illness emphasizes the need for palliative care measures.

Because the women have severe pains with some other distressing symptoms, palliative care and services are essential for both the women and their families in order to manage pain, suffering, provide information, and support. Also, the traditional extended family system where support and care are usually provided to ill family members is being gradually lost to changes in population values. Some families now focus on their nuclear family while neglecting the distant relations. This trend of diminishing extended family support is resulting in the neglect of some terminally ill patients. Therefore, organized palliative care seems to be the last hope of this group of patients. Palliative care can have a beneficial impact on the course of an illness by improving the quality of life of patients through timely identification of deteriorating health, holistic assessment and management of pain and other physical, psychosocial, and spiritual needs, and individualized planning of care [10].

3.2 Palliative Care

Palliative care is a comprehensive, integrated, and total care approach provided to patients and their families as they handle problems related to life-threatening illness and end of life by providing care that (a) relieves patient's pain and other distressing symptoms, (b) regards dying as a normal process and affirms life, (c) neither intends to hasten nor postpone death, (d) provides support to enable patients to live as actively as possible until death, and (e) provides holistic care that amalgamates the psychological and spiritual aspects of patient's care. Palliative care helps patients to live as fully as possible until death by facilitating effective communication and enabling patients and their families make informed decisions about the goals of care. It offers a system to help patients' families cope during the patient's illness and their bereavement [10].

Palliative care involves early assessment, identification, and treatment of pain and other physical, psychosocial, and spiritual problems [1, 10]. It is meant to be initiated from the point of diagnosis of any life-threatening illness until the end of life [11]. Palliative care is applicable according to patient's needs throughout the cause of an illness [10]. Palliative care can be provided wherever a person's care takes place, whether it is in the patient's own home, a care facility, hospice, inpatient unit, hospital or outpatient or day care service [1, 10]. It employs a team approach to address the needs of patients and their families [1]. Palliative care can be provided by professionals with basic palliative care training. However, referral to specialist palliative care with multi-professional team may be necessary in complex cases [10].

The palliative care team usually comprises of nurses, medical doctors, pharmacists, social workers, spiritual leaders, and psychologists [12]. Palliative care can be applicable in conjunction with other therapies that are intended to prolong life such as chemotherapy, radiotherapy, and other investigations needed to understand and manage distressing illness manifestations and complications. Palliative care promotes holistic patient-centered care, as it addresses the totality of the patient's physical, psychological, social, and spiritual dimensions [11]. Palliative care improves the quality of life of both patients and their families by providing relief from unnecessary suffering and pain throughout the illness trajectory [13]. Although the definition of palliative care is globally relevant, what constitutes palliative care and services need to be country-specific in the light of cultural, economic, and political structures.

3.3   Palliative Care in Nigeria

Palliative care is an emerging specialty and a new addition to the Nigerian healthcare delivery system, with only a few units established in a few tertiary healthcare institutions located in major cities [12, 14–18]. The first public palliative care unit was opened in 2007 at the University College Hospital Ibadan, Nigeria [19]. Thereafter, five other palliative care centers have been established, one in each of the five the geopolitical zones of the country. For a Country with a population of about 190 million people, more palliative care centers are needed to attend to the needs of the people. Findings from a cross-sectional study of the level of awareness of palliative care among seminarians and religious leaders in Southwestern Nigeria indicated that there is a low level of awareness of palliative care among the study respondents [19]. According to the authors, this observation was probably due to the fact that palliative care is a relatively new area in the Nigerian healthcare delivery system and little efforts have been made to enhance the public awareness of the specialty.

3.4   Challenges to Palliative Care Provision in Nigeria

The introduction of palliative care into the Nigerian healthcare delivery system has its challenges which are shared with other West African countries and beyond [20]. However, a few that appear to be peculiar to the Nigerian society include: (a) national and policy challenges, which involve limited national policy, needs for funds allocation for palliative care, lack of strategic planning, and institutional policy to promote palliative care services; (b) social and economic challenges, which comprise of poverty, difficulties in reaching rural communities, and social and economic instability; and (c) home-based care challenges which consist of lack of adequately trained caregivers, lack of access to essential drugs, and limited access to patients in inaccessible geographical areas [20]. Despite these challenges, palliative care seems to be a way forward in improving the quality of life of patients presenting with the advanced stages of life-threatening illnesses like cancer in Nigeria. This is so because at the advanced stages, cure is no longer an option. Therefore, non-governmental organizations, faith-based organizations, and inspirited individuals could be encouraged to collaborate with the government in providing palliative care centers and hospices for patients who are in need of such services.

3.5 Prospects and the Way Forward

The International Association for Hospice and Palliative Care [10] and World Health Organization [1] recommend essential approaches to improve access to palliative care by governments in low-income countries. Three of those approaches are: (a) integrating palliative care into the mainstream healthcare delivery system facilitated by appropriate national policies and norms; (b) training of healthcare professionals, education of the public and policy makers, and undertaking research; and (c) making available and improving access to opioid and other essential medications and technologies for pain relief including pediatric formulations [1, 10]. These approaches would go a long way to ensure that patients and their families have timely and effective access to and benefit from holistic care, support, and effective palliative care services.

The incorporation of palliative care into the Nigerian healthcare delivery system will involve building the capacity of healthcare providers and all palliative care stakeholders. Hospital administrators need to identify dedicated wards and units to accommodate patients in need of palliative care. These units should focus on providing a conducive and peaceful environment for the patients and their families [21]. Policy makers and healthcare administrators need to ensure that there are necessary equipment and supplies to care for patient's needs adequately. Healthcare administrators should create a system that not only identifies patients in need of specialist palliative care, but also facilitates interfacility, intrafacility, and community transfers to palliative care units.

Governments and healthcare administrators are to ensure that palliative care is part of all health services (from community health-based programs to hospitals), that everyone is assessed, and that all staff can provide basic palliative care with specialist teams available for referral and consultation. Frontline healthcare providers such as nurses and physicians, therefore, need to be educated regarding issues relevant to palliative care and be empowered to develop standardized order sheets and protocols for symptom management and end-of-life care [21]. There is also the need to involve other allied healthcare providers such as social workers and spiritual care specialists to provide psychosocial support, grief, and bereavement counseling [21].

3.6 Integration of Palliative Care into the Mainstream Healthcare Delivery System in Nigeria

The integration of palliative care services into the mainstream healthcare delivery system in Nigeria will require the creation of a national palliative care policy, which will provide a framework for the implementation of palliative care services at all levels of patient healthcare delivery [22]. In order to be successful, the policy needs to outline the objectives of palliative care and how to achieve the stated objectives. The policy also needs to specify strategic areas such as the availability of services, essential medication, education and training, community participation, and research. Palliative care for patients with cancer may be straightforwardly implemented when it is incorporated into the national cancer control policy as a fourth pillar of cancer control strategy with primary prevention, early detection, and curative treatment [13]. A community approach may be initiated to identify community leaders for palliative care advocacy, increase public awareness, and empower the community to participate and offer services as volunteers so that more people may make use of the services [13, 15]. A community approach will also allow the community to take ownership of the program to ensure its sustainability and continuity.

3.7 Education and Training of Healthcare Professionals

The education and training in issues relevant to palliative care should involve policy makers, nurses, and physicians [22]. The education needs to include training in the identification of the palliative care needs of patients and their families, communication skills, assessment of pain and other symptoms, supportive care, prescribing and dispensing of medication at an appropriate level [23]. Incorporating issues relating to palliative care into the education preparation of nurses, physicians, and other allied healthcare professionals will empower these healthcare providers to provide palliative care for the patients in need of the services [13]. Moreover, incorporating palliative care into the education curricular of healthcare professionals could facilitate its incorporation into the mainstream healthcare system. At the basic level, palliative care training could involve a set of essential components in the undergraduate education preparation which should lead the student to acquire the minimum competencies that are expected of all health and social care professionals [10]. The education should not stop at the basic level, rather, it should be a continuing process of acquiring knowledge and skills throughout the healthcare provider's professional life [10]. Continuous education will also ensure the incorporation of evidence-based strategies and techniques from current research studies into the care of the patients and that of their families.

3.8 Home-Based Care

In Nigeria, caring for older members of the family at home is a social expectation. Older people prefer to remain at home, where they are cared for by their family, usually women [18]. Older people prefer home-based care that promotes a person's maximum level of comfort and healthcare, including care toward a dignified death. As such, others that should be trained in basic palliative care should include family members, community volunteer workers, spiritual caregivers, traditional healers, and social workers. Training of family members and community volunteers in palliative care will assist in delivering comprehensive and holistic home-based palliative care to patients who prefer to receive care in the home setting where they are surrounded by their family and friends. In Nigeria, healthcare is paid for *out-of-pocket* by patients. Therefore, the financial requirements of providing home-based palliative care should be discussed with the patient, and his or her other family members and adequate arrangements should be made to ensure that family caregivers receive adequate financial support to carry out this essential role.

3.8.1 Research

Research in palliative care in Nigeria will make available evidence-based strategies which will serve as the bedrock of high-quality palliative and end-of-life care [22]. Collaborating with universities, academia, and teaching hospitals to include palliative care research as well as training as an integral component of ongoing education at the basic, intermediate, specialist, and continuing levels will lead to creating available experts in palliative care [10]. Integrating individual clinical expertise with the best available clinical evidence from systematic research into the decision-making process for palliative care will ensure that evidence-based quality care is provided for patients and their families [10]. Knowledge of evidence-based palliative care needs through research studies within the country may be essential to guide budgeting for infrastructure, training of personnel, and practice [24].

3.8.2 Culture

Culture shapes how individuals make meaning out of illness, suffering, and dying. It also influences an individual's response to diagnosis and treatment preferences. Therefore, in planning to provide palliative care, careful consideration needs to be given to the patient and his or her family's culture. For instance, traditional healers form a unique part of the healthcare delivery system in Nigeria. In some instances, overreliance on these healers has been associated with unrealistic hope for a cure, and delayed presentation for medical attention, leading to advanced stage illness. Therefore, better healthcare outcomes may result when mainstream healthcare providers work in collaboration with traditional healers, whose system of belief and practices may be more culturally acceptable to patients and their families [24].

3.8.3 Spiritual Care

Faith in the healing power of God, hope, and spirituality are critical components of the average Nigerian's coping mechanism in the context of ill-health. When possible, spiritual care providers should be part of the interdisciplinary team of palliative care providers. Early involvement of spiritual care providers may help patients and their families to cope with grief and receive support to make informed decisions. Spiritual care must be provided by an appropriately trained provider, who should be available in all care settings either locally or by referral. However, nurses or counselors who have been trained in a spiritual capacity could assess and provide the spiritual needs of patients and their families. All healthcare providers should be observant and sensitive to the religious norms of patients and that of their families [23]. Individuals providing spiritual care should endeavor to be available to know the patient and his or her family, asking them what might be necessary and relevant to their situations and respecting their stated wishes and preferences.

3.9 Psychosocial Care

Patients' psychosocial needs and those of their families should be addressed across the illness trajectory. This role can be undertaken by social workers, mental health professionals, or community health workers who have received appropriate training in palliative care. In situations where specialized counselors are not available, nurses and physicians who have received training in this domain can perform this role. Such professionals should be given enough time to be with patients and their families to allow them to perform the necessary activities and functions [23]. This is important because explanations about unexpected and uncontrollable events, as well as explanations about emotional and existential issues, may help to empower patients and provide hope and treat distress in the presence of uncertainties.

3.10 Making Available and Improving Access to Opioid Medication

Many of the patients needing palliative care live with severe pain and other distressing symptoms. Improving access to pain-relieving medication is an essential component of palliative care. The WHO's [1] global resolution on palliative care included pain relief medications for adults and children in the list of essential medications and called on all member states to improve access to pain relief medications. The assembly [1] emphasized its readiness to support member states in improving access to palliative care medications through improved national regulations and delivery systems. Also, policy makers and hospital administrators are called on to not only provide opioids including pediatric preparations, but further, they should ensure that the supply is readily and continually available for dispensing by trained professionals to the patients to meet their needs [23].

3.11 The Role of the Nurse

Nurses can play essential roles in building and maintaining an interdisciplinary team by promoting coordinated care in the context of palliative care. Nurses must assess, treat, and maintain adequate symptomatic control for their patients. Nurses would benefit from being trained to assess patients' palliative care needs including, but not limited to, pain assessment, control, and evaluation, spiritual and other psychological needs, as well as make recommendations, and communicate the patients' needs to appropriately trained healthcare personnel for necessary actions [23]. Nurses are in the right position to integrate palliative care practices into their patients' care plans throughout the disease trajectory and ensure that the palliative care needs of the patients and those of their families are appropriately met. Appropriately trained nurses such as nurse practitioners may prescribe pain relief medications and other essential drugs for patients as the need arise [23].

Nurses' roles should not be limited to the hospital environment alone. Their roles as coordinators and care providers must be extended to the community and home-based care level. They could serve as linkages among the patients' caregivers, physicians, and other members of the interdisciplinary and interprofessional palliative care team [23]. Nurses, because of their unique roles and relationships with patients, are well suited to identify patients' essential needs and provide suitable interventions for the patients.

3.12 Palliative Care for Women with Advanced Breast Cancer

Although some support is available for women with breast cancer in Nigeria, more remains to be done to create and sustain appropriate community palliative care in the country. There is the need to create more palliative and home-based care centers closer to the patient's homes, so that the patients will not have to travel long distances to access the services. When considering the experiences of Nigerian women dying with advanced breast cancer palliative care for them may include an interdisciplinary team of care providers comprising of doctors, nurses, social workers, community volunteers who would provide physical care, and religious groups, who would provide emotional, and spiritual support for psychosocial issues. The involvement of trained chaplains, alfas, and other religious leaders would enhance providing a more comprehensive and holistic service. Issues around financial support, care of family, and income would have to be discussed with the patients and their family members.

3.13 Conclusions

Palliative care alleviates and reduces suffering, as well as improves the quality of life for both patients and their families. To ensure that the needs of Nigerian patients afflicted with advanced cancer and other life-threatening illness, and their caregivers are adequately met, it will be essential to incorporate palliative care into the mainstream healthcare delivery system. Nigerians need a system of palliative care delivery that is suited to their sociocultural context. Therefore, it will be essential to engage the family system as well as, the community, cultural, and spiritual systems in planning and providing palliative care. However, nurses and other healthcare providers also need to be well informed about the cultural perceptions and experiences of their patients. This is essential because lack of sensitivity to and lack of respect for cultural differences may compromise end-of-life care. Nurses and other palliative healthcare providers need to create opportunities to listen to what their patients think is important and offer ongoing support.

Like most other people, many Nigerians prefer to die at home, it is essential to empower relatives and community volunteers to adequately care for patients who prefer to have palliative care at home. As much as possible, the cultural beliefs that underpin health, sickness and the societal responses to health, ill-health and their interpretations need to be identified and incorporated into palliative care services. Provision of guidelines on the policies and strategies to guide palliative care will go a long way to ensure the provision of standardized care. Provision of palliative care can prevent an unnecessary suffering, including painful, lonely, and disrespectful death. An inclusive approach to palliative, hospice, and home-based care is essential to capture the variety of specialized services relevant to the holistic care of persons with the advanced stages of life-threatening illness and those of their families who are bereaved.

Relieving patients' pain and suffering as a result of advanced breast cancer provides the foundation to the discussion of palliative care in Nigeria for this chapter. However, these strategies can be valid and could benefit other terminally ill patients and all those living with other chronic conditions. In a vast country like Nigeria, the management of patients with advanced and end-staged cancer and other life-threatening chronic illness should be centered on providing evidence-based and quality palliative and home-based care.

References

1. World Health Organziation. Global action plan on noncommunicable diseases 2013–2020. Lyon: International Agency for Research on Cancer; 2014.
2. Ferlay J, Soerjomataram I, Dikshit R, Eser S, Mathers C, Rebelo M, et al. Cancer incidence and mortality worldwide: sources, methods and major patterns in GLOBOCAN 2012. Int J Cancer. 2015;136(5):E359–86.
3. World Health Organization. GLOBOCAN 2012 (IARC). Estimated cancer incidence, mortality, and prevalence worldwide in 2012. Lyon: International Agency for Research in Cancer; 2016.
4. Jedy-Agba E, McCormack V, Adebamowo C, dos-Santos-Silva I. Stage at diagnosis of breast cancer in sub-Saharan Africa: a systematic review and meta-analysis. Lancet Glob Health. 2016;4(12):e923–e35.
5. Okobia MN, Bunker CH, Okonofua FE, Osime U. Knowledge, attitude and practice of Nigerian women towards breast cancer: a cross-sectional study. World J Surg Oncol. 2006;4:11.
6. Ogunkorode A, Holtslander L, Anonson J, Maree J. An integrative review of the literature on the determinants of health outcomes of women living with breast cancer in Canada and Nigeria from 1990 to 2014: a comparative study. Int J Africa Nur Sci. 2017;6:52–73.
7. Ajekigbe AT. Fear of mastectomy: the most common factor responsible for late presentation of carcinoma of the breast in Nigeria. Clin Oncol. 1991;3(2):78–80.
8. Agodirin SO, Rahman GA, Olatoke SA, Durojaiye AO. Patterns of breast cancer referal to palliative care and the complementary role of a palliative care unit in a resource-limited country. Postgrad Med J Ghana. 2017;6(1):42–7.

9. Ogunkorode A. Health-seeking behaviors of women with advanced breast cancer in southwestern Nigeria. [Unpublished Manuscript]. Saskatchewan: University of Saskatchewan; 2019.
10. The International Association for Hospice and Palliative Care. Global consensus- based palliative care definition. Houston, TX: The International Association for Hospice and Palliative Care; 2018. https://hospicecare.com/what-we-do/projectsconsensus-based-definition-of-palliative-care/definition/.
11. Shambe HI. Palliative care in Nigeria: challenges and prospects. Jos J Med. 2014;8(3):53–5.
12. Fadare JO, Obimakinde AM, Olaogun DO, Afolayan JM, Ogundipe KO. Perception of nurses about palliative care: experience from South-West Nigeria. Ann Med Health Sci Res. 2014;4:723–7.
13. Stjernswärd J. Palliative care: the public health strategy. J Public Health Policy. 2007;28(1):42–55.
14. Olaitan S, Oladayo A, Ololade M. Palliative care: supporting adult cancer patients in Ibadan, Nigeria. J Palliat Care Med. 2016;06(03):258.
15. El Saghir NS, Adebamowo CA, Anderson BO, Carlson RW, Bird PA, Corbex M, et al. Breast cancer management in low resource countries (LRCs): consensus statement from the breast health global initiative. Breast. 2011;20(Suppl 2):S3–11.
16. Eke G, Ndukwu G, Chukwuma N, Diepiri B. Knowledge and perception of healthcare providers towards palliative care in Rivers State, Nigeria. Port Harcourt Med J. 2017;11(3):156–60.
17. Oyebola F. Palliative care trends and challenges in Nigeria-the journey so far. J Emerg Int Med. 2017;1(2):1–5.
18. Omoyeni N, Soyannwo O, Aikomo O, Iken O. Home-based palliative care for adult cancer patients in Ibadan-a three year review. Ecancermedicalscience. 2014;8:490.
19. Badru AI, Kanmodi KK. Palliative care awareness amongst religious leaders and seminarians: a Nigerian study. Pan Afr Med J. 2017;28:259.
20. Inem V. Palliative care in West Africa-Educational imperatives. Department of Community Health and Primary Care, College of Medicine, University of Lagos, Nigeria 2013:1–31.
21. Downar J, Seccareccia D. Associated medical services Inc. Educational fellows in care at the end of L. Palliating a pandemic: "all patients must be cared for". J Pain Symptom Manag. 2010;39(2):291–5.
22. Fraser BA, Powell RA, Mwangi-Powell FN, Namisango E, Hannon B, Zimmermann C, et al. Palliative care development in Africa: lessons from Uganda and Kenya. J Glob Oncol. 2017;(4):1–10.
23. Osman H, Shrestha S, Temin S, Ali ZV, Corvera RA, Ddungu HD, et al. Palliative vare in the global setting: ASCO resource-stratified practice guideline. J Glob Oncol. 2018;4:1–24.
24. Hannon B, Zimmermann C, Knaul FM, Powell RA, Mwangi-Powell FN, Rodin G. Provision of palliative care in low- and middle-income countries: overcoming obstacles for effective treatment delivery. J Clin Oncol. 2016;34(1):62–8.

Home Palliative Care in the United Kingdom and Europe

Elaine Stevens and Stuart Milligan

Contents

- 4.1 Hospice Palliative Home Care in the United Kingdom 46
  - 4.1.1 Introduction 46
  - 4.1.2 Background 46
  - 4.1.3 Identifying People Who Have Palliative Care Needs 47
  - 4.1.4 Integrated and Coordinated Palliative Home Care Services 48
  - 4.1.5 Community Specialist Palliative Care Services 49
  - 4.1.6 Specialist Palliative Day Services 50
  - 4.1.7 Hospice at Home Services 51
  - 4.1.8 Palliative Care Education 51
- 4.2 Hospice Palliative Home Care in Europe 53
  - 4.2.1 Introduction 53
  - 4.2.2 History of Palliative Home Care in Europe 54
  - 4.2.3 The Current Situation With Regard to Palliative Home Care Services in Europe 55
  - 4.2.4 Palliative Home Care Services in Three Countries: France; Turkey; Romania 56
  - 4.2.5 International Initiatives and Current Priorities for Palliative Home Care 58
- 4.3 Implications for Home Palliative Care 59
- 4.4 Conclusion 59
- References 60

E. Stevens (✉)
School of Health and Life Sciences, University of the West of Scotland, Paisley, Scotland
e-mail: elaine.stevens@uws.ac.uk

S. Milligan
Ardgowan Hospice, Greenock, Scotland
e-mail: stuart.milligan@ardhosp.co.uk

© Springer Nature Switzerland AG 2019
L. Holtslander et al. (eds.), *Hospice Palliative Home Care and Bereavement Support*, https://doi.org/10.1007/978-3-030-19535-9_4

4.1 Hospice Palliative Home Care in the United Kingdom

4.1.1 Introduction

The United Kingdom (UK) is considered the birthplace of the modern hospice movement. However, UK hospice care has evolved significantly since its inception in the middle of the twentieth century. One of the most significant developments to influence service delivery is the division of palliative care into two levels. The first is general palliative care, or the **palliative care approach**, and should be available to all people with advanced illness when they require it. This level of palliative care is provided by the ill person's day-to-day care team. The second is **specialist palliative care** which is required by a smaller, but significant number of people with far advanced illness who have more complex needs that may not be fully managed by their day-to-day care team. Specialist palliative care (SPC) is provided by an expert multi-professional team who have received additional education to meet the needs of this patient group. Consequently, the majority of UK palliative home care is provided by General Practitioners (GPs), Community Nurses (CNs) and Social Services' employees, supported by specialists in palliative care for people who have additional care and support needs.

4.1.2 Background

With an estimated population of sixty-six million the United Kingdom (UK) consists of four countries: England with 84% of the population, Scotland with 8%, Wales with 5% and Northern Ireland with 3% [1]. Similar to other developed countries, the UK has an aging population and the most common causes of death are ischaemic heart disease, cancer, dementia and non-malignant respiratory illnesses. There is a single UK Parliament which oversees UK wide issues such as the defence of the nation; however, the responsibility for the National Health Service and healthcare provision is devolved to the Government of each country. Consequently, each country develops its own healthcare strategies, including those that provide direction for the delivery of palliative and end-of-life care [2–5]. Not surprisingly, and despite country-specific differences in the quantity and ranking of their priorities, there is significant overlap in the four strategies as each was developed from contemporary research and international palliative care strategies and policies. The outcome of all four strategies is the sustainable delivery of high-quality palliative and end-of-life care which is based on need not age, diagnosis, geographical location or place of care. The aim of such care is to improve the quality of life of people with advanced illness and their families through a proactive approach to whole-person assessment and management of needs. Table 4.1 identifies the main priorities found within every UK palliative care strategy.

As the focus of this text is palliative home care, the remainder of this section will discuss and provide examples of approaches to service delivery, developed to support these core priorities. This will give a flavour of how palliative home care services in

Table 4.1 Core priorities in UK palliative care delivery strategies [2–5]

1	Identification of people who have palliative care needs is crucial
2	A 24/7 integrated and coordinated palliative care service, which includes health and social care services and palliative care specialists, is essential
3	An accurate primary care register of people with advanced illness is a necessity
4	Palliative care providers should use evidence-based tools to aid care delivery and to evidence improvements in quality of life and service provision
5	Professionals providing palliative and end-of-life care should have the requisite knowledge and skills to do so

the UK are organised and the importance palliative care education has within this. However, as services are developed regionally or locally to meet the outcomes of national strategies, what is provided in one area may not work in another due to culture heritage, geographical location and levels of deprivation. The use of specific tools will be integrated into the approaches to palliative home care considered here as many utilise these within their approach to palliative home care provision.

4.1.3 Identifying People Who Have Palliative Care Needs

Recognising decline in people with advanced illness is key to them accessing palliative care services. However, while people with advanced cancer are more likely to be referred for palliative care this is less likely for people with non-malignant illnesses as their illness trajectory is more difficult to predict. To rectify this inequity *The Gold Standards Framework* (GSF) was designed to enhance access to palliative home care services across the UK and includes a number of guidelines. The first of these focuses on identifying people who may benefit from palliative care [6]. The Proactive Identification Guidance (PIG) includes the 'surprise question' to trigger professional thinking in terms of whether or not they would be surprised if the person died within a specific time frame, e.g. a year. To complement this and to trigger a more in-depth assessment of the person's health status the PIG also provides clinical indicators that signal decline in frailty and common non-malignant conditions. Working through the PIG algorithm, consequently informs professional decision making and supports the initiation of palliative care.

A second tool, which aims to improve the identification of the deteriorating person, is the Supportive and Palliative Care Indicators Tool (SPICT) [7]. SPICT also recommends the use of the 'surprise question' to initiate the process of identifying deterioration and provides condition-specific clinical indicators as well as a range of prompts to aid professional decision making. These are much in keeping with those used in GSF PIG; however, additional SPICT guidance, for palliative home care, suggests that assessment of deterioration should be undertaken at specific times, which includes:

- following a hospital admission,
- where there are poorly controlled symptoms,
- when the person is becoming more reliant on others for their activities of daily living.

SPICT also provides professionals with a concise action plan when deterioration is identified. This enables a palliative care approach is initiated and individual needs are addressed.

4.1.4 Integrated and Coordinated Palliative Home Care Services

High-quality palliative home care hinges on an integrated approach to service delivery, provided by jointly managed health and social care services [2–5]. However, the integration of such services differs considerably across the UK in terms of budgetary and role responsibilities which prevent professionals and service users from determining which service would be best placed to meet peoples' palliative care needs. For example, in some parts of the UK social care services, managed by the local authority, provide assistance with washing, bathing, dressing, medication administration and meal times while in others areas such services are provided by NHS-funded community nursing service. To add further complexity, some English primary care services are contracted out to the private sector which challenges integration and in turn may impede the delivery of effective primary palliative care.

Northern Ireland has the most established integrated health and social care system in the UK and has endeavoured to improve integrated palliative care through their 'Transforming Your Palliative and End of Life Care' programme. However, by the end of the programme, while some system-level approaches had improved, further work was required to improve access to and coordination of palliative home care delivery outside of normal working of hours [8]. Consequently, while all four UK palliative care strategies aspire to have an integrated approach to palliative care at systems level, the experience of Northern Ireland suggests this may take many years to achieve and may be impractical for some services to fully deliver. However, there is evidence within the other countries of the UK that the development of integrated health and social care is ongoing. For example, within Scotland the recently developed regional Integrated Health and Social Care Partnership's specific guidance has been developed to enable them to meet the outcomes of the national palliative care strategy [9].

Despite a lack of integrated services at systems level, progress has been made in the delivery of coordinated palliative home care at regional and local levels. One significant improvement in providing a coordinated approach to 24/7 primary palliative care has been the development of a community palliative care register, originally conceived as part of the GSF programme [6]. Many GPs subsequently developed and continue to maintain a register which enables the multi-professional home care team to regularly review the small minority people with advanced illness on their caseload and to be proactive in their approach to care planning based on changing health status. This practice also maximises opportunities to improve future care and treatment decisions; however, this can only happen if these are disseminated to all members of the palliative home care team. Across the UK, there are a number of approaches to advance care planning which include the completion of both hard copy and electronic documents.

An example of a hard copy document utilised in some areas of England and Wales is the Advance Decisions to Refuse Treatment (ADRT) [10]. This provides a statement of advance care planning wishes, which the patient usually completes with someone from their care team and in conjunction with their family where possible. The statement may include the patient's wishes around 'do not attempt cardiopulmonary resuscitation' (DNACPR). ADRT enables advance decisions to be taken into account at a time when the patient cannot make these for themselves. If the ADRT statement satisfies the legal requirements of the Mental Capacity Act 2005, then its content may be legally binding. This allows people with advanced illness to be more confident that their wishes will be upheld at a time when they cannot make decisions for themselves.

An electronic approach, utilised in Scotland, focuses on the dissemination of the patient's current health status and medications as well as any future care planning decisions that have been made. GPs and CNs add significant information into a specific part of the patient's electronic GP record over time which can be accessed via the NHS intranet [11]. The Key Information Summary (KIS) is then made available to a range of services such as out of hours GPs, the ambulance service, acute hospitals and hospices. Accordingly, should the patient require assistance out of hours or in an emergency, the most up to date information is available to allow a clinical decision to be made based what is already known. To complement KIS, the patient usually holds a hard copy of the national DNACPR form, so the clinicians treating them in crisis situations have evidence they have made this decision.

Such proactive approaches to ensuring that all agencies have information about the patient's current position and the advanced decisions that have been made support whole-person conversations with people with advanced illness about their future treatment and care preferences. This in turn promotes a coordinated palliative home care approach which can enable the person to lives as well as they can within the confines of their illness and to die the most appropriate death for them and their families.

While the bulk of palliative home care is provided by GPs, CNs and social care services, a significant number of patients also require more specialist care to support their needs. The next part of this section therefore offers a summary of what SPC can add to the delivery of high-quality palliative home care within the UK to further enhance the quality of life.

4.1.5 Community Specialist Palliative Care Services

Community specialist palliative care (CSPC) professionals are an integral part of the palliative home care team and may be provided by the NHS as well as third sector charities such as hospices and Macmillan Cancer Support. The CSPC team usually consists of a Consultant in Palliative Medicine and one or more Clinical Nurse Specialists with Allied Health Professionals' expertise being utilised to meet specific patients' needs. Research on community specialist palliative care (CSPC) has shown that services reduce symptom burden and increase the probability of people with advanced illness dying at home [12]. Many CSPC services have a single point of referral and as such referrals from primary care teams will be

Table 4.2 Levels of specialist palliative care support and advice

Level of intervention	Advice and support provided
1	Advice and support would be offered by the CSPC team to the primary care team. This is usually conducted by telephone or video conferencing
2	The CSPC team will make an initial advisory visit to the patient, either on their own or with a member of the primary care team. This is usually for a single visit and further communication for advice and support will be between the professionals in primary care and CSPC teams
3	The CSPC team will provide a short-term intervention for the patient or family when specific problems need several visits. Following this the patient or family member would be discharged from the service. Future referrals would be re-triaged as required
4	The CSPC team provides a range of interventions when there are ongoing problems that require ongoing assessment and management visits. Close liaison with the primary care team is ongoing to maintain coordinated care

triaged to determine the level of CSPC advice and support required. Table 4.2 provides a summary of the different levels of advice and support that may be offered by a CSPC team.

This tiered approach to managing individual palliative care needs not only promotes the efficient use of the CSPC team but also enhances the knowledge and skills of the primary care team so if a similar patient presents in the future they would feel more confident to manage their issues. In addition, most CSPC services also offer a 24-h advice line which supports both primary care professionals working out of hours and patients and their families, as this improves patient outcomes through increased access to SPC beds out of hours and reduction on emergency admissions to hospital [13].

4.1.6 Specialist Palliative Day Services

Many SPC services in the UK provide specialist palliative day services (SPDS) which employ a rehabilitative approach to living with advanced illness. This approach supports people to remain as well as they can within the confines of their advancing illness and enables them to live independently at home, while under the surveillance of the SPC team [14]. Most SPDS attendees visit the service for around 6 h a day, once per week, which enables them to come together with others in similar circumstances for peer support as well as gaining access to a range of SPC individual or group interventions. Interventions include symptom management, functional ability improvement classes, complementary therapies, acupuncture, psychological and spiritual support and art and music therapy. SPDS also supports families by providing dedicated education and relaxation sessions as well providing time off from their caring role and bereavement support [14]. Most SPDS are managed by a Clinical Nurse Specialist who is supported by a core team of registered nurses, support workers, allied health professionals and volunteers. In most SPDS, there is access to a Consultant in Palliative Medicine should specialist medical interventions be required. To maintain a coordinated approach to care, the SPDS team will also, with the attendees' permission, keep their family, General Practitioner and other members of the palliative home care team up to date with any changes in their condition or treatment changes. The care support provided by SPDS is less medically orientated than other SPC community services and as such not only manage symptom burden but also improve quality of life through improved self-esteem and psychological, spiritual and functional well-being [15].

4.1.7 Hospice at Home Services

Although Marie Curie Cancer Care has been providing specialist palliative and end-of-life nursing care to people in their own home for around 60 years, the UK has recently seen the rapid development of other home care services called 'Hospice at Home' (HAH). While HAH services vary widely in their approach across the UK, their overall aim is to enable people with advanced illness to be cared for and to die at home if this is their wish [16]. HAH assists the home care team by providing practical care and support to people and their families when this is not available by their day-to-day care team. HAH services are usually managed by a Clinical Nurse Specialist with the practical care and support being provided by a team of registered nurses and support workers who have received specialist training in palliative and end-of-life care. Some HAH services also utilise the expertise of specially trained volunteers to provide respite for family carers or to provide complementary therapies to the patient and/or family member. In contrast to CSPC services, the practical support provided by HAH occurs over a number of hours during the day or overnight, depending on need. However, there is conflicting evidence of the effectiveness of individual services in enabling people to die at home and as such further research to explore the effective components of such services in allowing people to die in their preferred place [16].

From this discussion, it is obvious that approaches to palliative home care in the UK vary widely but have the ability to improve patient and family outcomes when these take a proactive stance. However, all four UK strategies emphasise that high-quality palliative care cannot exist without a workforce that have the knowledge and skills to do so [3–6]. Consequently, the final part of this section on UK palliative home care will outline examples of initiatives that have been developed to improve the knowledge and skills of both generalist and specialist palliative care providers.

4.1.8 Palliative Care Education

It is recognised that high-quality palliative care can only be provided by professionals who have the knowledge and skills to do so [2–5]. Consequently, national and regional approaches to palliative care education and training have emerged across the UK in response to the strategies. However, many initiatives have been designed to teach specific palliative care topics such as symptom management and end-of-life care, while others have been developed for a specific professional discipline or are related to the care of people with a specific diagnosis. For example, in England, there is a national approach to training healthcare professionals on how to communicate effectively with patients and families in complex situations [17]. This training is currently delivered by a multitude of education organisations, including universities and local hospices, although it is mainly directed at healthcare professionals who work in SPC. Another example is the delivery of education on best practice symptom management, which is based on regional or local guidance and is available to professionals who provide palliative care in that specific locality. For example, The Yorkshire and Humber Palliative and End of Life Care Groups [18] have developed a symptom guidance manual and training associated with this provided by local education providers to upskill the workforce. However, such focussed approaches to education may only impact on one aspect of palliative care and upskill particular groups of professionals within a specific location. This may go some way to explaining why there are ongoing reports of people with advanced illness receiving poor quality of palliative care, as the team looking after them does not have the requisite knowledge and skills.

To address the shortfall in the quality of palliative care provision, a pioneering national education framework, for all members of the palliative care workforce, has been developed by NHS Education Scotland and the Scottish Social Services Council [19]. The framework is divided into two distinct components. The first identifies the four levels of knowledge and skill required by professional carers. The levels are dependent on the role the professional has in palliative care provision rather than their specific job title. These are:

1. Informed level: outlines the knowledge and skills required by all health and social service workers in relation to palliative and end-of-life care.
2. Skilled level: outlines the knowledge and skills required by health and social service workers who by virtue of their role and level of responsibility regularly provide care and support to people with palliative and end-of-life care needs, their families and carers.
3. Enhanced level: outlines the knowledge and skills required by health and social service workers who by virtue of their role and level of responsibility provide, co-ordinate and manage the care and support of people with palliative and end-of-life care needs, their families and carers.
4. Expert level: outlines the knowledge and skills required by health and social service workers who by virtue of their role and level of responsibility play an expert specialist role in the care and support of people with palliative and end-of-life care needs.

The second component of the framework identifies the five core domains of palliative care which the professional needs to understand to enable them to provide high-quality palliative care within their role. The domains are:

1. Fundamentals of palliative care,
2. Communication and conversations,
3. Loss, grief and bereavement,
4. Care planning and delivery,
5. Care in the last day of life.

The two components of the framework are subsequently dovetailed to identify the level of knowledge and skills required by the professional providing palliative care within each domain. This information is then utilised in workforce planning and in the development of palliative care educational initiatives. Early indications are that this novel approach is having a specific impact in upskilling social care professionals and those providing generalist palliative care. Consequently, it is envisaged that the provision of high-quality palliative care across Scotland will improve.

In summary, while palliative care in the UK is a devolved issue, all four countries have similar strategic priorities to ensure that the delivery of high-quality palliative care is based on the needs of individual patients and their family. However, it would appear easier to develop a national approach to ameliorate the challenges that may hamper the optimal provision of palliative home care in less populous countries. Nonetheless, dedicated regional approaches would appear as effective, where a national approach may not be sustainable. Such initiatives have been evidenced through examples to show how they have been utilised to improve the provision of coordinated and person-centred palliative home care.

This chapter will now go on to review palliative care in Europe and how it is organised to meet the needs for people with advanced illness and those peoples' families.

4.2 Hospice Palliative Home Care in Europe

4.2.1 Introduction

The previous section touched on the crucial role that the hospice movement played in the development of palliative care in the UK, but has also shown how subsequent advances have reflected regional and national priorities, leading to a considerable diversity of provision between the different countries. A similar trend can be seen across the continent of Europe, with palliative care services, and particularly palliative home care services developing in response to a wide variety of local needs, circumstances and, in some cases, constraints. The result is a complex array of provision, ranging from fully integrated to predominantly ad hoc and from comprehensive to sporadic. It is in response to this variability that international bodies including the European Association of Palliative Care, the Council of Europe and the World Health Organisation (European Region) are working to standardise provision and ensure that anyone across Europe can access the palliative care he or she needs, including care provided in his or her home or place of residence.

4.2.2 History of Palliative Home Care in Europe

No other European country can lay claim to the broad and enduring influence on palliative care that the UK has had; nevertheless, several countries have a long and proud history of organised care for the dying and continue to do so.

In France in 1842, Mme Jeanne Garnier established L'Asociacion de Dames du Calvaire, a group of women dedicated to the care of the dying poor [20]. The association opened a home for dying people in Lyons that year, which was subsequently acknowledged by Cicely Saunders as the first hospice in Europe. Further homes were to follow as the appropriateness of organised care for the dying became more accepted. However, for a number of reasons, palliative home care was slow to develop in France. Those reasons included the poor availability of morphine outside institutional care and the perception that an institutional setting would entail a more comfortable and dignified death. As a result, the first informal palliative home care services were not established in France until the early 1980s, with organised projects only emerging later that decade [21].

In Ireland, the Irish Sisters of Charity, a religious order established by Mary Aikenhead in 1787, opened Our Lady's Hospice for the Dying in Dublin in 1879 [22]. Similar institutions followed in the early 1900s and thereafter, creating the network of hospices that can be traced today. The Sisters of Charity and other groups had strong traditions of visiting the dying poor in their own homes, but again it was not until 1985 that the first formal palliative home care service in Ireland was established.

For several European countries, the British hospice movement can be seen to have had a significant role in the development of their palliative care provision. The German Association for Palliative Medicine traces the origins of the practice in that country to an encounter between a group of German chaplains and Cicely Saunders in 1969 [23]. Similarly, other countries across the continent have benefitted from the formative influence of clinicians and academics from countries with already established palliative care services.

Broadly speaking, the countries of Eastern Europe have tended to be slower to develop palliative care services than those of the West. This difference is probably due to a number of factors including less contact with those countries where thinking on palliative care was most advanced, less of a tradition of organised healthcare generally, a correspondingly greater dependence on family care at times of illness and poorer socio-economic circumstances [24]. Nevertheless, for some countries, the lack of a long history of organic growth of hospice and palliative care services has meant that services can be planned on the basis of demand, need and government priority [25]. This appears to have been the case in countries such as Romania and Turkey where very different service profiles have been developed, the former with a strong home care element but the latter oriented much more towards hospital services [26–28].

4.2.3 The Current Situation With Regard to Palliative Home Care Services in Europe

One of the most important events in the development of palliative care across Europe was the establishment, in 1988, of the European Association of Palliative Care (EAPC). The aim of the association was to promote palliative care across the continent and to act as a hub for individuals and organisations working in the field of palliative care [25]. Helpfully, the EAPC provides a typology of the palliative care services it recognises. Under the heading of 'Patient care provided at home' are two categories:

1. Resources and services providing a basic level of palliative care and
2. Specialised palliative care.

The former is defined as 'assistance provided by general or family physician and nurses in primary care teams' while the latter encompasses:

- Specialized palliative care services or supportive palliative care services,
- Home care support team (where the GP has primary responsibility for the patient),
- Other specialized palliative care services,
- Palliative care unit in an inpatient hospice,
- Day hospice or day-care centre for palliative care,
- Home palliative care team (where primary responsibility for the patient rests with the palliative care team) [29].

In practice, when referring to palliative care services available at home, the EAPC distinguishes principally between general palliative care (provided by community practitioners) and specialist palliative home care (provided by palliative care specialists who might be variously referred to as 'Home palliative care support teams' or 'Home support Teams').

In 2013, the EAPC published its Atlas of Palliative Care in Europe [29]. This document gathers together the best available statistics on the palliative care services available across Europe at the beginning and end of the 7-year period covered. It provides a snapshot of palliative care developments and enables Europe-wide and individual, national trends to be identified.

Looking at services as a whole, the atlas reveals considerable variation with some countries having a high level of provision (such as Sweden and Belgium with more than 16 services per million inhabitants), but also some (such as Azerbaijan and Estonia) having none at all. Although the trend across Europe is towards greater provision and sophistication, the fact that several countries (especially in central and Eastern Europe) are showing little or no expansion should give cause for concern [28].

In terms of specialist palliative home care services, the 2013 atlas demonstrates that coverage (i.e. the proportion of a country's population who have access to those services) increased to 52% (from 39% in 2005) in Western European countries but to only 3% (from 2%) in Central and Eastern European countries. Overall, this means that Western Europe has 31% of the specialist home care services it needs (based on the EAPC recommendation of one service per 100,000 inhabitants) while Central and Eastern Europe has only 14%.

The reasons for this inadequacy of provision are numerous and complex, but are likely to include resource constraints, competing priorities and lack of integration with mainstream services. However, the Council of Europe [30] has highlighted some less obvious but potentially more-easily addressed reasons such as lack of government policies, shortcomings in training (especially in pain management) and issues around the regulation and availability of opioids. The particular disparity shown between the progress being made in Western Europe and in central and Eastern Europe has led the EAPC to formulate a vision of excellence focussed on the latter region and the former Soviet Union countries [25].

4.2.4 Palliative Home Care Services in Three Countries: France; Turkey; Romania

France has already been highlighted as a country that has a long history of organised care for the dying, although it is also one where palliative home care services were initially slow to develop. Today, palliative care is an important theme in French government health policy with four national action plans published since 1999 [29, 31].

The model of palliative home care most widely utilised in France is 'hospital at home'. According to the 2013 atlas, 188 specialist palliative home care teams were in existence in France [29, 31]. This total equates to 19% of the number required on the basis of EAPC calculations, a fact recognised by the most recent French National Plan for palliative care. That document has recommended considerable expansion of the 'Hospital at home' network as well as the upskilling of generic community professionals [31].

Wider French government policy has also assisted the development of palliative home care with initiatives such as paid carers' leave making caring for the dying at home more affordable for some families [32]. Such policy measures are increasingly being used by Western European countries to encourage the uptake of palliative care at home, thus reducing the considerable financial and human costs associated with hospital admissions near the end of life. France is ranked tenth in the Economist 2015 Quality of Death Index (sixth in Europe).

Turkey has a much shorter history of organised palliative care than France, with the first evidence of concerted progress towards the adoption of palliative care principles not seen until the 1990s. Nevertheless, the country has made considerable strides since then. By 2009, palliative care was identified as one of the five key elements of the country's national cancer control programme and in 2011, a national palliative care programme ('Pallia-Turk') was introduced. The latter has been implemented at primary, secondary and tertiary levels of the Turkish health system [27].

Palliative home care, like all health care in Turkey, is strongly influenced by cultural beliefs which regard family members and especially adult children as having a central role to play in the care of sick and elderly relatives [27]. Organised palliative home care is delivered primarily by non-specialist home care teams. There were over 400 of these teams in 2010, increasing to over 800 by 2014. On this evidence, it would appear that availability is increasing, but funding of these services is complicated and reimbursement may be problematic for some potential users. Specialist home care teams are fewer in number with the 2013 atlas only identifying five of these [29]. In spite of what appears to be progress in this area, the majority of Turkish people continue to die in hospital [33].

Unlike several other countries in Europe, Turkey has only a small hospice movement, and therefore most of its progress in palliative care has been government-led. Turkey is proud of its achievements and hosted a large international palliative care conference in 2018. The country is ranked forty-seventh in the Economist 2015 Quality of Death Index (20th in Europe) [24].

Whereas Turkey's is an example of a largely government-led palliative care system, Romania has a strong history of initiatives predominantly established by non-governmental institutions and often funded by external partners. Amongst these, Hospice Casa Sperantai in Brasov, Hospice Emanuel in Oradea and Hospice Sf. Irina in Bucharest have been particularly influential [29]. The impetus created by these pioneering organisations has gradually influenced Romanian government policy to the extent that a range of services providing home care, day care, outpatient care and inpatient care is increasing [26].

In terms of palliative home care, the 2013 atlas recognised 15 palliative home care services in Romania whereas a 2015 survey identified 24 palliative home care services, five palliative care outpatient services, four palliative care day centres and four mobile specialist hospital teams [26, 29]. Nevertheless, the EAPC estimated that only 7% of the national requirement for palliative home care was being met and many Romanian counties had no or very few palliative home care services. This partly explains why Romania is ranked only sixty-fourth in the Economist 2015 Quality of Death Index (24th in Europe).

According to Mosoiu, Mitrea and Dumitrescu [26], the Romanian government has committed to establish an additional ninety home care teams and the same number of outpatient clinics as well as providing training for primary care professionals in the delivery of general palliative care. These developments will further contribute to the integration of palliative care into the Romanian national health care system.

Volunteering was not, traditionally, a common occurrence in Romanian healthcare. However, in 2014, the Romanian government set up a recruitment and training scheme to encourage volunteers in palliative care. The aim is to emulate countries like Germany where there is a well-established volunteer population of around 100,000 [23].

4.2.5 International Initiatives and Current Priorities for Palliative Home Care

In spite of the advances highlighted in the previous paragraphs, a report from the Council of Europe in 2018 contained the damning statement: 'In Europe, hundreds of thousands of people do not have access to appropriate palliative care services, including, in particular, access to appropriate pain relief' [30]. This statement was prompted by the observation that few of the recommendations of a previous report (by the Council of Ministers in 2003) had been adequately addressed. The 2018 report presents strong economic, legal, moral and social arguments in support of increasing palliative care provision across Europe. Not only that, but there is a stipulation that community and home care should be particularly prioritised.

Demographic changes have created an unprecedented crisis in European health care with more and more people living longer and developing life-limiting and chronic conditions, potentially requiring palliative care. As the Council of Europe report argues, it is simply unsustainable to care for that growing, terminally ill population in hospital. Instead, additional provision must be made for these people in or close to their places of residence, and additional support must be provided to those who find themselves providing care for them at home. In these ways, patient choice over preferred place of care and preferred place of death is more likely to be respected. Other expected benefits will be financial savings and better equity of access for those groups who may otherwise find themselves excluded from services [12, 30].

There is also a need for even greater integration of palliative care into all healthcare systems and settings. That means that people should have access to the palliative care they need, irrespective of diagnosis, location or care setting. In other words, access to palliative care should be regarded as a fundamental human right [34].

Several other aspects of palliative care practice need to be reviewed in order to optimise the environment for effective palliative home care. Additional education may be required, and should be tailored to the needs of both groups likely to access this education (palliative care specialists and primary care professionals). Where a particular patient group has complex or unique care needs, these may have to be covered by specifically focused education packages such as the 'Palliaire' programme covering prudent dementia care [35].

Effective palliative home care practice should be promoted both at the level of service delivery and at the level of individual care delivery. An understanding of the keys to successful home care (namely a relationship of trust between patient and care team; a satisfactory level of co-operation between the care team and the patient's family; an effective multi-disciplinary team and effective leadership) [21] is vital. It is also essential to recognise the practical barriers to successful palliative home care including family exhaustion, lack of time and resources, and a change of mind on the part of the patient about his or her preferred place of death.

Another consideration determining the effectiveness of palliative home care must be the ease of access to palliative care for certain patient groups. There is evidence that people with non-malignant diseases are repeatedly discriminated against in terms of the palliative care services available to them [30]. Homeless people and prisoners are examples of other groups who may face additional barriers. However, a newly recognised group of people having difficulty accessing the palliative home care that they need is the growing number of people in Europe with a migration background [36].

4.3 Implications for Home Palliative Care

This chapter has outlined a number of approaches that promote the provision of high-quality palliative home care that is based on individual need, rather than age, diagnosis, geographical location or place of care. For service providers an organisational approach identifying people living at home who have palliative care needs is essential. Once people are identified service providers need to provide a coordinated, 24/7 multi-agency service to ensure a range of palliative care needs are assessed and managed continually over the illness period. Depending on the country service developments may be delivered by the healthcare system, but also by the charitable and third sectors. It is therefore incumbent on commissioners to develop services that have the ability to provide high-quality home palliative care.

For professional carers, the key to high-quality palliative care provision is open and honest communication with the ill person, their family and other care providers to ensure current and future care needs are identified and managed. Professionals need to understand the types of palliative care that exist to meet individual palliative care needs and work as part of a cohesive team within resource constraints. Such an approach will help ensure the person and their family are well as they can be within the confines of advanced illness. Creative approaches to care and support within poorly resourced areas can have a huge impact on the quality of life of those who have advanced illness and local professionals have a key role in these. It is essential that all professionals have access to high-quality palliative care education; however, it is understood that working and networking with specialists can promote knowledge and skill and such opportunities should be made available to the professional team to work alongside specialist palliative care providers.

Finally, while there is sound evidence that early palliative care has a positive impact on the quality of life further research is required to investigate how this can be made available to all citizens of the world. Further research on how to identify those living at home with advanced illness is therefore imperative. In addition, palliative care provision could be improved through further research which investigates the outcomes on quality of life of different models of integrated and coordinated home palliative care.

4.4 Conclusion

There are complex differences in the history, organisation and delivery of palliative care between the UK and Europe (and indeed between individual European countries); nevertheless, many of the issues faced are similar across the continent. An ageing population, rising rates of chronic, progressive and life-limiting diseases, changing family structures with an increase in single person households and the rising cost of hospital care are all placing tremendous strain on health and social care systems. The human cost is substantial too, with the number of people missing out on the palliative care they need running into hundreds of thousands.

Shifting the balance of care from acute to community settings offers some cause for optimism that these challenges can be addressed. However, national governments and international bodies will require to continue to improve availability and drive up standards of palliative care through legislation and funding decisions. Increasingly sophisticated and responsive community-based service delivery models and public health initiatives that raise public awareness and build social capital are both essential if the ambition of providing palliative home care for all who need it is to be realised.

References

1. Office of National Statistics. Overview of the UK population. London: ONS; 2018. https://www.ons.gov.uk/peoplepopulationandcommunity/populationandmigration/populationestimates/articles/overviewoftheukpopulation/november2018.
2. National Palliative and End of Life Care Partnership. Ambitions for palliative and end of life care. 2015. http://endoflifecareambitions.org.uk/.
3. Scottish Government. Strategic framework for palliative and end of life care. 2015. https://www.gov.scot/publications/strategic-framework-action-palliative-end-life-care/.
4. Department of Health. Living matters, dying matters strategy. 2010. https://www.health-ni.gov.uk/publications/living-matters-dying-matters-strategy-2010.
5. Welsh Government. Palliative and end of life care delivery plan. 2017. https://gov.wales/docs/dhss/publications/170327end-of-lifeen.pdf.
6. Thomas K, Wilson JA And the GSF team. The gold standards framework proactive identification guidance. 6th ed. 2016. https://www.goldstandardsframework.org.uk/cd-content/uploads/files/PIG/NEW%20PIG%20-%20%20%202020.1.17%20KT%20vs17.pdf.
7. The University of Edinburgh. Supportive and palliative care indicators tool (SPICT). 2018. https://www.spict.org.uk/.
8. The Regulation and Quality Improvement Authority. Review of the implementation of the palliative and end of life care strategy. 2016. https://www.rqia.org.uk/RQIA/files/1c/1c349f45-1c38-49bb-aeeb-e6a363f4c5ad.pdf.
9. Scottish Government. Strategic commissioning of palliative and end of life care by integration authorities. 2018. https://www.gov.scot/binaries/content/documents/govscot/publications/guidance/2018/05/strategic-commissioning-palliative-end-life-care-integration-authorities/documents/00535146-pdf/00535146-pdf/govscot%3Adocument.
10. National Council for Palliative Care. Advance decisions to refuse treatment: a guide for health and social care professionals. 2013. http://www.ncpc.org.uk/publication/advance-decisions-refuse-treatment-guide-health-and-social-care-professionals.
11. Mason B, Boyd K, Steyn J, Kendall M, Macpherson S, Murray SA. Computer screening for palliative care needs. Br J Gen Pract. 2018; https://doi.org/10.3399/bjgp18X695729.
12. Gomes B, Calanzani N, Curiale V, McCrone P, Higginson IJ. Effectiveness and cost-effectiveness of home palliative care services for adults with advanced illness and their caregivers. Cochrane Database Syst Rev. 2013;(6):Art. No.: CD007760. https://doi.org/10.1002/14651858.CD007760.pub2.
13. Joint Specialist Committee for Palliative Medicine for the Royal College of Physicians, the Specialty Advisory Committee for Palliative Medicine from the JRCPTB and the Association of

Palliative Medicine. Night, weekend and bank holiday specialist palliative care services. 2017. https://apmonline.org/wp-content/uploads/2018/02/Specialist-Palliative-Care-night-weekend-and-bank-holiday-working.pdf.
14. Stevens E, Martin CR, White CA. The outcomes of palliative day services: a systematic review. Palliat Med. 2011;25:153–69. https://doi.org/10.1177/0269216310381796.
15. Stevens, E. A critical investigation of the outcomes of the traditional model of specialist palliative day services on specific components of attendee quality of life, wellbeing and mood: a mixed methods study. 2018. University of the West of Scotland, PhD thesis.
16. Butler C, Brigden C, Gage H, Williams P, Holdsworth L, Greene K, Wee B, Barclay S, Wilson P. Optimum hospice at home services for end-of-life care: protocol of a mixed methods study employing realist evaluation. BMJ Open. 2018;8:e021192. https://doi.org/10.1136/bmjopen-2017-021192.
17. Wilkinson S, Perry R, Blanchard K, Linsell L. Effectiveness of a three-day communication skills course in changing nurses' communication with cancer/palliative care patients: a randomised controlled trial. Palliat Med. 2008;22:365–75. https://doi.org/10.1177/0269216308090770.
18. Yorkshire and Humber Palliative and End of Life Care Groups. A guide to symptom management in palliative care. 2016. https://www.yorkhospitals.nhs.uk/seecmsfile/?id=819.
19. NHS Education Scotland. Palliative and end of life care: a framework to support the learning and development needs of the health and social service workforce in Scotland: enriching and improving experience. 2017. https://learn.nes.nhs.scot/2452/palliative-and-end-of-life-care-enriching-and-improving-experience/palliative-and-end-of-life-care-enriching-and-improving-experience.
20. Richard M-S. Jeanne Garnier - a pioneer of palliative care. In: Salamagne M-H, Thominet P, editors. Accompaniment: thirty years of palliative care in France. Paris: Demopolis Quaero; 2016. p. 47–56.
21. Palliative GJ-M. Home care - from first experiences to conceptualization. In: Salamagne M-H, Thominet P, editors. Accompaniment: thirty years of palliative care in France. Paris: Demopolis Quaero; 2016. p. 47–56.
22. O'Brien T, Clark D. A national plan for palliative care – the Irish experience. In: Ling J, O'Síoráin L, editors. Palliative care in Ireland. Maidenhead: Open University Press; 2005. p. 3–18.
23. Deutsche Gesellschaft für Palliativmedizin (German Association for Palliative Medicine) Focussing on patients and families. Berlin. Deutsche Gesellschaft für Palliativmedizin. 2018. https://www.dgpalliativmedizin.de/images/170530_FlyerMadrid_engl_online.pdf. Accessed 1 Mar 2019.
24. The Economist Intelligence Unit. The 2015 quality of death index - ranking palliative care across the world. A report by The economist intelligence unit, commissioned by the Lien foundation. London: The Economist Intelligence Unit Ltd; 2015.
25. Radbruch L, Ling J, Hegedus K, Larkin P. European association for palliative care: forging a vision of excellence in palliative care in central and eastern European and former Soviet Union countries. J Pain Symptom Mgmt. 2018:55(2S) S117–S120. https://www.jpsmjournal.com/article/S0885-3924(17)30363-9/pdf. Accessed 1 Mar 2019.
26. Mosoiu D, Mitrea N, Dumitrescu M. Palliative care in Romania. J Pain Symptom Mgmt. 2018:55(2S) S67-S75. https://www.jpsmjournal.com/article/S0885-3924%2817%2930384-6/pdf. Accessed 1 Mar 2019.
27. Emuk Y, Naz I. The current situation of palliative care in turkey. J Can. Policy. 2017;13(9):33–7.
28. Centeno C, Lynch T, Garralda E, Carrasco JM, Guillen-Grima F, Clark D. Coverage and development of specialist palliative care services across the World Health Organisation European region (2005-2012): results from a European Association for Palliative Care Task Force survey of 53 countries. Palliat Med. 2016;30(4):351–62.
29. Centeno C, Lynch T, Donea O, Rocafort J, Clark D. EAPC atlas of palliative care in Europe 2013. Full edition. Milan: EAPC Press; 2013.

30. Council of Europe. The provision of palliative care in Europe. Council of Europe parliamentary assembly. Committee on social affairs, health and sustainable development. 2018. Document number 14657. https://barnepalliasjon.no/wp-content/uploads/2018/12/Rapport-fra-Europar%C3%A5det.pdf. Accessed 1 Mar 2019.
31. Poulalhon C, Rotelli-Bihet L, Moine S, Fagot-Campagna A, Aubry R, Tuppin P. Use of hospital palliative care according to the place of death and disease one year before death in 2013: a French national observational study. BMC Pal Care. 2018;17(75). https://www.ncbi.nlm.nih.gov/pmc/articles/PMC5954461/pdf/12904_2018_Article_327.pdf. Accessed 1 Mar 2019.
32. Maetens A, Beernaert K, Deliens L, Aubry R, Radbruch L, Cohen J. Policy measures to support palliative care at home: a cross-country case comparison in three European countries. J Pain Symptom Mgmt. 2017;54(4):523–9.
33. Özsezgin S. A journey into palliative care in Turkey: everyone has the right to live without pain. EAPC Blog - the blog of the European Association for Palliative Care. 2017. https://eapcnet.wordpress.com/2017/08/28/a-journey-into-palliative-care-in-turkey-everyone-has-the-right-to-live-without-pain/. Accessed 1 Mar 2019.
34. Open Society Foundations. Palliative care as a human right: a fact sheet. 2016. https://www.opensocietyfoundations.org/sites/default/files/palliative-care-human-right-fact-sheet-20160218.pdf. Accessed 1 Mar 2019.
35. Tolson D, Fleming A, Hanson E, Abreu W, Crespo ML, MacRae R, Jackson G, Hvalič Touzery S, Routasalo P, Holmerová I. Achieving prudent dementia care (palliare): an international policy and practice imperative. Intl J Int Care. 2016;16(4). https://www.ijic.org/articles/10.5334/ijic.2497/. Accessed 1 Mar 2019.
36. Janksy M., Owusu-Boakye S, Nauck F. 'An odyssey without receiving proper care' – experts' views on palliative care for patients with migration background in Germany. BMC Pal Care. 2019:18(8). https://pdfs.semanticscholar.org/056c/a20ef89a83cf066dca0b9a984df0048cc628.pdf. Accessed 1 Mar 2019.

Mapping a New Philosophy of Care: The State and Future of Implementing a Palliative Approach Across Canada

5

Chad Hammond and Sharon Baxter

Contents

5.1	What Is a Palliative Approach to Care?...	63
5.2	The Way Forward: A National Initiative to Promote a Palliative Approach................	66
	5.2.1 The Way Forward Goals and Process..	66
	5.2.2 Public and Health Professional Support for a Palliative Approach to Care.........	67
	5.2.3 Recommendations for Implementing an Integrated Palliative Approach..........	68
	5.2.4 Integrated Palliative Approach Models...	70
5.3	CHPCA Stakeholder Surveys on Implementing a Palliative Approach.....................	73
	5.3.1 Surveys of National Health Stakeholders and Provincial/Territorial Governments..	73
	5.3.2 National Health Stakeholders: QELCCC Survey Results.............................	74
	5.3.3 Provincial/Territorial Governments Survey Results....................................	76
	5.3.4 QELCCC & P/T Governments: Shared Priorities to Advance a Palliative Approach..	78
5.4	The Way Forward, Phase II: We Know the Way, Now Let's Walk It Together.............	82
5.5	Conclusions...	83
References...		83

5.1 What Is a Palliative Approach to Care?

Hospice palliative care is a philosophy of care that aims to relieve suffering and improve the quality of living and dying. It is an approach that supports patients and their families facing the problems associated with life-threatening illness, through the prevention and relief of suffering by means of early identification, assessment

---

C. Hammond (✉) · S. Baxter
Canadian Hospice Palliative Care Association, Ottawa, ON, Canada
e-mail: CHammond@cphca.net; SBaxter@chpca.net

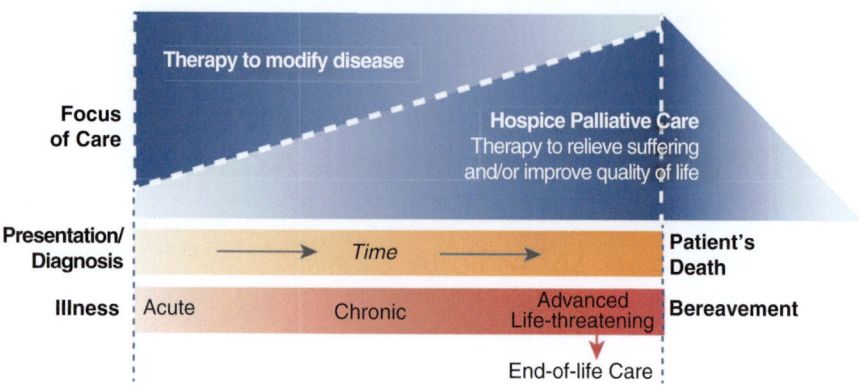

Fig. 5.1 The role of hospice palliative care during illness [1] Source: Canadian Hospice Palliative Care Association

and treatment of pain and various other forms of distress (Fig. 5.1). The World Health Organization [2] describes hospice palliative care as having the following features:

- provides relief from pain and other distressing symptoms,
- affirms life and regards dying as a normal process,
- intends neither to hasten nor postpone death,
- integrates the psychological and spiritual aspects of patient care,
- offers a support system to help patients live as actively as possible until death and help the family cope before and after a person's death,
- uses a team approach to address the needs of patients and their families, including bereavement counseling, if indicated,
- enhances quality of life and may also positively influence the course of illness,
- applies early in the course of illness, in conjunction with other therapies that are intended to prolong life, such as chemotherapy or radiation therapy.

The way hospice palliative care is practiced globally is evolving with momentous demographic changes. Populations across Canada and around the world are aging. Canada recently reported—for the first time—more people retiring than people entering the workforce. Hospice palliative care services in all jurisdictions are facing similar pressures from the aging population and from changing needs and expectations.

In the past, hospice palliative care was provided only in the last 6 months of life. With advances in treatment, time of death is less predictable and people with a wide range of chronic life-limiting illnesses now need hospice palliative care services over a longer period of time. These drastic changes have placed increasing pressures on healthcare systems across the globe, especially in Canada. Compared to other developed nations, Canada has higher mean per capita hospital expenditures—much of which is for care during people's final weeks of life—and the highest proportion of people dying in acute care hospital settings [3].

Those involved in hospice palliative care are calling for systemic changes in order to accommodate their needs in this emerging milieu. Patients and families desire hospice palliative care provided at home—wherever home may be—by their family physician or care team. Healthcare systems want to reduce inappropriate and costly hospital and emergency admissions by providing more cost-effective care in the community. The specialized palliative care workforce is not large enough to meet the growing demand and changing needs. There is growing pressure for other providers to care for people who do not have complex medical needs, and hence, specialized providers can concentrate on those who need their skills.

The high need for improved hospice palliative care in Canada demands an innovative approach that addresses the complexities of quality of life, patient-centered care, and healthcare cost efficiencies. One such approach that has gained traction in recent years is a model that shifts hospice palliative care from being a specialized service available to the few to a more general integrated service available to people with life-limiting conditions in their homes and communities [4, 5]. An **integrated palliative approach to care** focuses on meeting a person's and family's full range of needs—physical, psychosocial, and spiritual—at all stages of illness or frailty (not just the final weeks), and in all settings where they live and receive care [6].

An integrated palliative approach to care addresses the needs and goals of people impacted by serious illness and/or frailty by promoting best practices in pain and symptom management, timely referrals to specialist hospice palliative care, open communication about patient prognosis and illness trajectory, psychosocial and spiritual support, advance care planning and goals of care discussions, and integration of patient goals and preferences into the treatments they receive [7–9]. What an integrated palliative approach looks like may change over time and the trajectory of a person's illness. After diagnosis and in the early stages of the illness, the focus may be primarily on advance care planning and the management of pain, symptoms, and psychological and spiritual distress. At later stages of the illness, the focus may shift toward reviewing the person's goals of care and adjusting care strategies to reflect any changes in those goals, as well as identifying if and when to engage specialized palliative care providers.

There are many proven benefits to the early and sustained integration of palliative care into the care of seriously ill and frail people. Research has shown that the above practices of an integrated palliative approach improve the quality of patient care [10–12], reduce unnecessary hospital visits and deaths [13, 14], and minimize costs associated with care at the end of life [10, 15, 16]. There is strong and growing evidence that a palliative care approach—when combined with treatment—leads to better outcomes for persons and their family caregivers, including: improvement in symptoms, quality of life and patient satisfaction; less burden on caregivers; more appropriate referral to and use of hospice; and less use of futile intensive care [10, 14, 17, 18]. Advance care planning also promotes choice and improves quality of care [19].

A few examples demonstrate the major impact a palliative approach can have on patient and family suffering and healthcare utilization:

- Housebound terminally ill people with cancer who received in-home palliative care (e.g., coordinating and managing care and discussing goals of care, expected course of the disease, expected outcomes, and success of treatment options) as well as usual care reported greater satisfaction with care, had fewer emergency room visits and hospital days, and had lower costs of care. They were also more likely to die at home [20].
- Caregivers of people with cancer who have access to a palliative care approach early in their loved one's treatment reported significantly less decline in their psychological, social, and spiritual quality of life scores [17].
- Comprehensive curative and palliative care of people with congestive heart failure reduced hospitalizations by at least a half—reducing utilization of health services and avoiding suffering [21].
- Nursing home residents with advanced dementia were less likely to undergo a burdensome intervention such as hospitalization, an emergency room visit, parenteral therapy, or tube feeding when their substitute decision makers had a better understanding of the poor prognosis from these interventions [13].

Implementation of an integrated palliative approach reinforces patient autonomy and the right to be actively involved in their own care—and strives to give patients and families a greater sense of control. An integrated approach sees palliative care as less of a discrete service offered to dying persons when treatment is no longer effective and more of an approach to care that can enhance quality of life throughout their illness. It also recognizes that, in a healthcare system focused on cure and treatment, people may not be given the opportunity to talk about dying or be truly informed about their illness and prognosis. They may not be asked about their care goals.

5.2 The Way Forward: A National Initiative to Promote a Palliative Approach

5.2.1 The Way Forward Goals and Process

Between 2012 and 2015, the Government of Canada provided funding for a 3-year initiative called *The Way Forward: An Integrated Palliative Approach to Care* that culminated in the development and dissemination of practical resources and tools to help governments and policymakers, regional planners, health service organizations and healthcare providers adopt a palliative approach to care. The initiative was led by the Quality End-of-Life Care Coalition of Canada (QELCCC) and managed by the Canadian Hospice Palliative Care Association (CHPCA). The goals of *The Way Forward* (TWF) project were: (1) to change the understanding and approaches to aging, living with chronic diseases and "living well until dying", and (2) to promote a palliative approach across all settings of care, and encourage advance care planning conversations.

TWF was intended to be a catalyst for action in Canada by raising the awareness and understanding of a palliative approach to care. Traditionally, the last days or weeks of life were the most common time for referral to hospice palliative care programs or services, if at all, and most often reserved for individuals designated as dying. The overarching goal of the initiative was to ensure more Canadians could live well until dying by enhancing their quality of life throughout the course of illness or through the process of aging, not just at the end of life.

The CHPCA and QELCCC members engaged in 3 years of consultations with federal, provincial, and territorial governments, policymakers, healthcare professionals, home care, primary/acute care and long-term care associations, patients and their caregivers and families, and organizations representing Canada's First Peoples (i.e., First Nations, Inuit, and Métis). As a result of these consultations, TWF identified a number of practical steps toward implementation of a palliative approach.

5.2.2 Public and Health Professional Support for a Palliative Approach to Care

The first phase of TWF commissioned Harris/Decima to conduct a public opinion survey of 3000 Canadians. The survey found that most Canadians support the concept of early initiation and integration of palliative care into ongoing chronic disease management across settings [22]. Of those surveyed, 96% supported hospice palliative care and 87% believed a palliative approach to care should be available earlier in the course of a life-limiting illness. Additionally, 93% felt that palliative care services and programs should be available in the setting of their choice; 96% supported hospice palliative care after being provided with information about the services entailed within a palliative approach.

The majority also found it important to discuss care near the end of life [22]: 97% with family, 81% with healthcare providers, and 75% with friends. Lawyers and financial advisors were also considered important people to talk to, by 67% and 63% of respondents, respectively. Canadians, however, are at an early stage of awareness and knowledge of both hospice palliative care and advance care planning. For example, in the TWF poll, only 58% of Canadians had heard of advance care planning and 49% were aware of the hospice palliative care services offered within the home.

Survey participants speculated that people die in hospital (despite their wishes) because of three determinants [22]: (1) people need certain treatments only accessible in hospital (81%), (2) dying at home is too much of a burden on families (75%), and (3) hospitals offer superior pain and symptom management (71%). They expressed concern that palliative care does not receive sufficient attention and funding by governments relative to other healthcare issues; 35% stated that governments place far too little priority on hospice palliative care. They expected healthcare practitioners to be a key source of information about what services are available across care settings; however, while most said that they would go to healthcare providers for information on advance care planning (60%), very few (5%) actually had conversations with their own providers.

For their part, healthcare providers seem to know the benefits of a palliative approach but need to become more comfortable. TWF commissioned Ipsos Reid to conduct a second survey [23], this time with primary care nurses and general practitioners/family physicians (GP/FPs). Among them, 61% of nurses and 41% of GP/FPs believed people should start advance care planning when they are healthy. However, only 18% of nurses and 26% of GP/FPs reported feeling very comfortable initiating ACP discussions. In addition, 32% of nurses and 36% of GP/FPs reported feeling very comfortable initiating discussions about palliative care. In terms of how they go about closing these gaps in their comfort level, many identified needing resources to help facilitate these conversations and expressed an interest in tapping into the expertise of palliative care specialists.

These survey results indicate strong support for an integrated palliative approach to care but identify several gaps on the part of the public and providers in terms of feeling prepared and readied to have conversations about palliative care and advance care planning.

5.2.3 Recommendations for Implementing an Integrated Palliative Approach

TWF released a series of reports and recommendations as a result of the extensive consultation process.[1] Most notable among them were: (1) an environmental scan of [inter]national indicators and frameworks, (2) six discussion documents describing an integrated palliative approach, different models of a palliative care, the cost effectiveness of a palliative approach, the role of family caregivers, and other key topics, and (3) the survey results with Canadians and primary care providers. These reports collectively summarize a breadth of international experience and knowledge about the impacts of a palliative approach on health, quality of life, reduction of suffering, and cost minimization.

In addition to these reports, TWF produced a National Framework outlining a roadmap for implementing a palliative approach in Canada. The roadmap identified 7 key steps forward [6]:

1. *Promote a culture shift in healthcare toward increased acceptance of death as part of life:* To integrate the palliative approach into routine care for people who are aging or have chronic illnesses, we must shift attitudes. Loss and death are part of life, yet we continue to be a death-denying society. Culture shifts are needed among healthcare professionals to adopt a palliative approach. This can start with initiation of conversations about advance care planning and integrating a palliative approach into usual medical care. In all parts of the healthcare system

---

[1] Available via: www.hcpintegration.ca. Accessed 1 Mar 2019.

and all parts of society, we must start the conversation about how loss, dying, and death are part of life.

2. *Establish a common language around palliative care*: Words are important. For many people—including many healthcare providers—the word "palliative" is associated with the last days or weeks of life. The words we use must embody dignity, compassion and empathy, as well as respect for different cultural attitudes toward dying. TWF created a Lexicon of Terms that can form the basis for more discussion about a common language.

3. *Educate and support health professionals*: To achieve our goals, practitioners in all care settings—including primary care practices, chronic disease programs, home care, long-term care, hospitals, prisons, and shelters—must have the skills and competencies to integrate the palliative approach into routine care. To reach healthcare providers, we must leverage existing training initiatives, such as the Canadian Society for Palliative Care Physicians' *Educating Future Physicians in Palliative and End-of-Life Care* (EFPPEC) program, the BC Centre for Palliative Care's training program for clinicians to use the *Serious Illness Conversations Guide* (developed by Ariadne Labs, Harvard Medical School), and Pallium Canada's *Learning Essential Approaches to Palliative and End-of-Life Care* (LEAP) program for healthcare professionals.

4. *Engage Canadians in ongoing advance care planning*: A truly integrated palliative approach to care should start much earlier—before people become frail or ill—with a strong focus on having conversations about what people value and the kind of care they want when they become ill. In those conversations, we must reinforce that advance care planning is an ongoing process—not a one-time discussion. Advance care planning initiatives like *Speak Up*[2] offer resources to facilitate more open and supported communication about death, dying, and living well until the end.

5. *Create caring communities that can better support patients, families, and caregivers*: Only a small proportion of people with complex needs require expert hospice palliative care services. For the majority of people who are ill, they can receive their care within their own communities. In order for that to be possible we need to cultivate communities that are prepared and supported by health systems to provide such palliative services as advance care planning, psychosocial and spiritual support, and pain or symptom management. Health and social services need to adopt a palliative approach to care to ensure that Canadians are aware of choices along the illness trajectory (not just treatments), resources available, and preferences for where individuals can receive care until death. The *Compassionate Communities*[3] movement is working toward strengthening communities' capacity to support and care for people where they live and receive care.

---

[2] More information about the national Speak Up initiative is available via: www.advancecareplanning.ca. Accessed 1 Mar 2019.

[3] Information about Compassionate Communities in Canada is available via: https://pallium.ca/work-with-us/launch-a-compassionate-community/. Accessed 1 Mar 2019.

6. *Ensure culturally safe practices are integrated into palliative care with First Nations, Inuit, and Métis*: In implementing the integrated palliative approach to care, we must include approaches that reflect the unique needs, diversity, and jurisdictional realities of Canada's First Peoples, particularly in the rural, remote, and isolated regions of Canada where most reside. In order to adapt an integrated palliative approach within these communities, it is essential to engage local leaders and community resources (e.g., Elders, cultural advisors) as true partners in the development and delivery of their care, enhance local capacity based on needs and community strengths, and develop culturally safe approaches and resources that address the physical, mental, emotional, and spiritual components of well-being within a family and community context.[4]
7. *Develop outcome measures and monitor system changes*: We need specific measurable goals to drive the system-wide shift in practice, as well as ways to monitor changes, report on impact, and identify barriers and challenges. Some of these measures can eventually be used to set standards for the integrated palliative approach to care. We need to identify targets and quality indicators that go beyond location of death and may include among others: whether an individual has an ACP, whether the ACP was followed, acknowledges where the individual received the bulk of their care until death, and if the location of death matched the patient's preference. This work should be enabled nationally with provincial adaptation/prioritization.

This roadmap describes concrete steps that can be taken at the federal and provincial/territorial levels, the regional health planning level, and in each sector or setting to help the system make the shift.

5.2.4 Integrated Palliative Approach Models

TWF also provided a general overview of the factors and key ingredients to success of implementing a palliative approach, based on the results of an environmental scan of models used around the world [24]. A total of 11 innovative models were reviewed from Canada, England, New Zealand, and Australia, to see how they delivered an integrated palliative approach to care (Fig. 5.2).

The models were chosen based on reports in the literature and recommendations from key informants. They were also chosen because they served a mix of urban, suburban, rural and remote populations, and several delivered hospice palliative care services to a significant Indigenous population. The innovative models varied by care setting (e.g., primary care, long-term care homes) and geographical focus (e.g., urban, rural, etc.), yet all shared common elements that made them successful and transferrable to the Canadian context (Table 5.1).

---

[4] A resource toolkit for implementing palliative care programs in First Nations communities is available via: http://eolfn.lakeheadu.ca/. Accessed 1 Mar 2019.

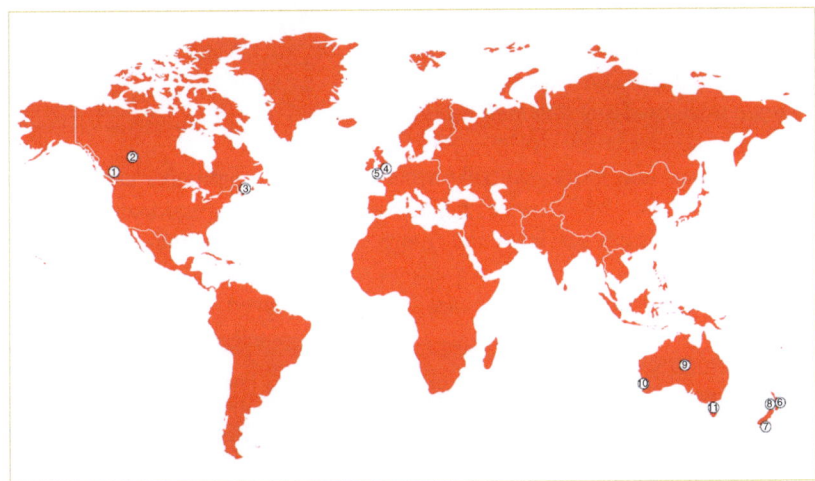

Fig. 5.2 Innovative models reviewed in The Way Forward Project. 1. Fraser Health End-of-Life Care Program in British Columbia, Canada; 2.Edmonton Zone Palliative Care in Alberta, Canada; 3. Colchester East Hants Health Authority Palliative Home Care Model in Nova Scotia, Canada; 4. St Christopher's Hospice Comprehensive Model in England; 5. Dorset Primary Care Trust Model in southwest England; 6. Arohanui Hospice Regional Program in New Zealand; 7. Otago Community Hospice Model in New Zealand; 8. North Haven Hospice Hub and Spoke Model in New Zealand; 9. Palliative Care Northern Territory in central Australia; 10. The Silver Chain Group that provides a range of health and social support services including comprehensive palliative care in Perth, Western Australia; 11. Living Well and Dying Well Aged Care Homes Model in Tasmania, Australia. Source: Canadian Hospice Palliative Care Association

Table 5.1 Shared elements of integrated palliative care models

Component	Factor
Vision	1. Commitment to person-centered care
	2. Focus on building capacity in the community
	3. Focus on changing organizational culture
	4. Senior management support
People	5. Dedicated coordinators
	6. Interprofessional teams
	7. Strong role and more support for family physicians
	8. Support for providers in long-term care facilities
	9. Key roles for nurses
	10. Relationships, partnerships, and networks
Delivery of care	11. Integration of primary–secondary–tertiary care
	12. Cultural sensitivity
	13. Single access point and case management
	14. 24/7 community support and care
	15. Advance care planning
Supportive tools	16. Common frameworks, standards, and assessment tools
	17. Flexible approaches to education
	18. Shared records
	19. Research, evaluation, and quality improvement

Source: Canadian Hospice Palliative Care Association

In a synthesis of the 11 models under review, TWF listed several demonstrated impacts the implementation of these models had on patients and families, healthcare providers, and the health system in general [24]:

On people who are dying and their families

- Easier, faster, and more equitable access to hospice palliative care through a single-entry point, 24/7 service and support from interprofessional teams.
- Better coordinated services and more seamless transitions between care settings.
- Higher quality hospice palliative care services, improved after-hours service, and better access to medications.
- More culturally sensitive care.
- More respect for their wishes and preferences in all care settings, more recognition of their dignity and voice, and more influence and control over their care—even when people are cognitively impaired.
- Ongoing involvement of their family physician throughout the disease trajectory.
- More confidence in community-based hospice palliative care and fewer requests for hospital admissions.
- Fewer—and more appropriate—hospital admissions.
- Fewer crises and fewer unneeded or unwanted interventions.
- More people able to die at "home" (wherever they define "home") or in their communities.
- More people receiving the palliative approach to care regardless of their disease.
- Less stress and burden on families, more meaningful time with the person who is dying and more support for family members.

On healthcare providers

- More skills for primary care providers, allied healthcare professionals (e.g., social workers, pharmacists) and care workers (e.g., licensed practical nurses, home care support workers).
- More confidence in their ability to provide hospice palliative care because of the strong system of education, support, consultation, and good communication.
- Greater sense of being valued for their work.
- Better working relationships between primary and specialist providers.
- Better, more respectful working relationships between physicians and nurses.
- Better communication between primary care providers and other services in the system, and the ability to work within a coordinated system providing high-quality hospice palliative care.
- Access to ongoing training and professional education.
- Ability to remain involved in patients' care across different care settings.
- Less distress, burnout, and turnover.

On the healthcare system

- Practice innovations that improve quality, timeliness, care transitions, and integration of hospice palliative care.
- Fewer unplanned hospitalizations and lower acute care costs.
- A more skilled workforce.
- Advances in policies for advance care planning and after-hour services.
- More effective use of resources with generalists providing primary palliative care and specialists providing consultation, advice, coordination, and inpatient care.
- Progress in making high-quality hospice palliative care available to more people with a wider range of diagnoses.

The results of the environmental scan show that through interprofessional/intersectoral integration, leadership support and buy-in, advance care planning mechanisms, and standardized assessments and evaluations, a palliative approach to care may transform for the better the experiences of patients, families, healthcare providers, and health administrators in the provision of care.

5.3 CHPCA Stakeholder Surveys on Implementing a Palliative Approach

5.3.1 Surveys of National Health Stakeholders and Provincial/Territorial Governments

TWF ended in early 2015, and then in 2017 the CHPCA conducted a pan-Canadian assessment of how far the palliative approach to care had been advanced in Canada. The survey was distributed to provincial and territorial governments and the QELCCC members (all of whom are national stakeholders in palliative care), asking to what degree a palliative approach remained a priority and what more could be done to increase implementation. The surveys also sought to gain information on how existing enablers, such as advance care planning strategies and healthcare provider education and training, were facilitating adoption efforts.

Information was gathered through two online surveys using Survey Monkey® between December 2016 and January 2017. The provincial/territorial government survey was completed by 12 jurisdictions, including nine provinces and all three territories. Quebec did not complete the survey, but provided a website link to the government's palliative care program for information only. Their program details are not represented in this report. The QELCCC survey was completed by 19 of 39 national members.[5]

---

[5] The QELCCC included 35 full national members and four associate members as of February 2017. The list of current members is available via: http://www.qelccc.ca/about-us/coalition-members.aspx. Accessed 1 Mar 2019.

Overall results from both surveys demonstrated that the integration of a palliative approach to care is an ongoing and pressing issue across jurisdictions and among national healthcare stakeholders (Table 5.2). According to the two surveys, 83 percent of P/T governments and 89 percent of QELCCC members said that advancing a palliative approach is a high priority. Let us look more closely at each survey in turn to understand where their particular priorities reside.

5.3.2 National Health Stakeholders: QELCCC Survey Results

The QELCCC membership includes a varied group of national patient/disease-based associations, professional associations, non-government healthcare organizations, and population-based entities. Given the different mandates of QELCCC members, there are differing degrees of adoption of the palliative approach; however, some consistent themes and priorities emerged through the survey.

There are some over-arching drivers of adoption of a palliative approach over the last 3 years (Table 5.3). These reflect a collective move in the health system toward more patient-centered care that is informed by patient and family preferences, values, quality of life, access to services, and satisfaction with care.

Ongoing advocacy to raise awareness about the palliative approach to care and encouraging Canadians to complete advance care plans through promotion of "Speak Up" ACP materials and resources were supported by the majority of

Table 5.2 Survey results from both CHPCA surveys

Question	Prov/Terr	QELCCC members
The palliative approach is a high priority	83%	89%
Used The Way Forward's National Framework for guidance	92%	84%
Have ongoing programs to encourage advance care planning	90%	84%
Limited resources are a major barrier toward integration	67%	72%
There is a lack of healthcare provider training and competence in providing a palliative approach to care	83%	44%
Healthcare provider education is a major enabler toward integration of the palliative approach to care	75%	74%

Source: Canadian Hospice Palliative Care Association

Table 5.3 QELCCC's top identified drivers of adopting a palliative approach

What are the main drivers of adoption of the palliative approach in your organization?	
Reducing unnecessary burden on patients, families, healthcare providers by enabling primary and home and community care to provide palliative care in the patient's preferred setting	14
Recognizing patient preferences for location of death (e.g., home, hospice, hospital, long-term care)	12
Providing greater access to palliative care at an earlier stage in the illness trajectory	12
Policy priority of the organization	11

Source: Canadian Hospice Palliative Care Association

Table 5.4 QELCCC's top identified enablers and barriers to implementing a palliative approach

Enablers facilitating a palliative approach		Barriers to adoption of a palliative approach	
Public awareness efforts about advance care planning	13	Limited resources to advance a palliative approach to care	13
Public awareness efforts about a palliative approach to care	12	Healthcare providers are reluctant to talk about death or advance care planning unless a patient is near death	8
A policy framework or organizational strategy	7	Healthcare providers lack training to build confidence/competence in adopting a palliative approach	8
Continuing medical education/continuing professional development of healthcare providers for palliative care	7	Not an organizational priority	6

Source: Canadian Hospice Palliative Care Association

QELCCC members. There were several enablers and barriers to adoption of the palliative approach from the perspective of these national organizations (Table 5.4).

Top priorities to accelerate the adoption of a palliative approach to care identified by QELCCC members included:

- **Advance Care Planning**: More national public and healthcare provider awareness of the palliative approach and ACP.
- **Education and Competency**: Education and national curriculum for healthcare providers, continued push to train more providers.
- **HealthCare Provider Training**: Continuing Medical Education/Continuing Professional Development for healthcare professionals to have ongoing goals of care conversations to inform and integrate a palliative approach to care early and often throughout illness trajectories.
- **Integration**: Adopting a palliative approach to care as part of ongoing person-centered disease management and not seen as a separate or referral-based program.
- **Practical Frontline Resources**: Tools and materials for healthcare systems and professionals to adopt and modify current care pathways to include a palliative approach.
- **Awareness and Access**: Ongoing advocacy efforts for high-quality hospice palliative care that is accessible to all Canadians, provided in the setting of their choice and meeting their care needs.
- **Adequate Resources**: Ensuring resources are available and dedicated to advancing a palliative approach to care.

The prioritization survey with QELCCC members marked a shared concern among stakeholders that Canadians are not well informed about the choices and services available to them in support of a palliative approach to their care, including a lack of awareness around advance care planning and resources to facilitate public discussion and action. We will see below that although these are not the top priorities among the provinces and territories, the two groups of stakeholders share some key concerns and recommendations for better integrating a palliative approach to care.

5.3.3 Provincial/Territorial Governments Survey Results

This survey indicated that all provincial and territorial governments have regional or local hospice palliative care programs. In 9 of the 12 jurisdictions who responded, there is a provincial policy framework for hospice palliative care, supported by strategies for training and skills development of healthcare providers.[6] The results of this survey are reported below.

There are several important drivers of adoption of the palliative approach to care identified across jurisdictions (Table 5.5). It was unanimously agreed that it was essential to reduce unnecessary burdens on patients, caregivers, and healthcare providers by ensuring that primary care and home and community care can provide palliative care. This is followed closely by a recognized need to ensure that patient preference for location of care and ultimately death–whether home, hospital, hospice, long-term care, or other–is supported by a person-centered approach. While the demand from the public to adopt a palliative approach was only identified by half of the P/T respondents, all jurisdictions confirmed that enhancing public and health-professional awareness about a palliative approach to care would improve adoption. This is supported by the findings from the Harris/Decima public survey that highlighted the gap in public awareness of where hospice and palliative care is provided (only 49% of Canadians are aware of palliative care services outside of hospitals or residential hospices), and a further gap in access to programs and services.

The P/T survey also explored enablers and barriers to the adoption of the palliative approach. The primary enablers included interprofessional palliative care teams in community care, palliative care competency training, policy development, and funded working groups to lead developments (Table 5.6). Other enablers cited by respondents included: (1) palliative care strategy that engages stakeholders, (2) primary care teams providing palliative care and use of telehealth, (3) funding

Table 5.5 P/T top identified drivers of adopting a palliative approach

What are the main drivers of adoption of the palliative approach in your jurisdiction?	
Provinces/territories	# of jurisdictions ($n = 12$)
Reducing unnecessary burden on patients, families, healthcare providers by enabling primary and home and community care to provide palliative care in the patient's preferred setting	12
Recognizing patient preferences for location of death (e.g., home, hospice, hospital, long-term care)	11
Providing greater access to palliative care at an earlier stage in the illness trajectory	10
Health system utilization challenges	9
Growing public awareness of and demand for a palliative approach to care	6

Source: Canadian Hospice Palliative Care Association

---

[6] P/T jurisdictions who noted a provincial or policy framework included: BC, AB, SK, MB, ON, NS, PEI, NWT, YK.

Table 5.6 P/T top identified enablers and barriers to implementing a palliative approach

Enablers facilitating a palliative approach		Barriers to adoption of a palliative approach	
Inter-disciplinary teams in primary care or home and community care focused on palliative care	10	Healthcare providers lack training to build confidence/competence in adopting a palliative approach	11
Continuing medical education/continuing professional development or small group-based learning for improving competence and confidence of healthcare provider for palliative care	10	Healthcare providers are reluctant to talk about death or advance care planning unless a patient is near death	10
Provincial/territorial policy framework or strategy	8	Lack of incentives/funding to provide palliative care other than at the end of life	9
Provincial/territorial or regional working groups with dedicated funding to develop clinical pathways, tools and resources	6	Lack of culturally relevant programs and services for specific populations	7

Source: Canadian Hospice Palliative Care Association

received by the Canadian Partnership Against Cancer to support the adoption of advance care planning, (4) health authorities with standardized medical orders, and (5) standardized service delivery models. Other barriers cited by respondents included: (1) a need for a provincial clinical information system, (2) many competing healthcare priorities (e.g., home care alone addresses many client needs including dealing with the frail elderly living alone, dementia, Acquired Brain Injury [ABI], post-surgical care, among others), (3) mitigation strategies and plans to address identified barriers are needed, and (4) dedicated funding must also be flexible in terms of meeting local needs.

Several important priority areas were identified by the jurisdictions as opportunities to accelerate the adoption of a palliative approach to care.

- **Home Care**: Increased/dedicated and flexible funding for expanded home care services to enable a palliative approach in primary, home, and community care based on provincial/territorial population health needs.
- **Education and Competency**: Undergraduate education and postgraduate training of healthcare providers about the palliative approach to care. In particular, postgraduate training should focus on improving the competence and confidence of healthcare professionals in discussing and providing a palliative approach to care throughout illness trajectories and not just at end of life.
- **Culture Shift and Change Management**: Practice support and change management activities to move from disease and cure-focused care to person-centered care that includes a palliative approach.
- **Public Engagement**: Public awareness about the palliative approach to care and advance care planning is needed. This includes understanding how and where hospice palliative care programs and services are provided and that a palliative approach is about living well until dying, and not just about end-of-life care.

- **Advance Care Planning**: Funding/incentives (or ensuring no disincentive) to provide comprehensive palliative care and support for ACP discussions.
- **Measurement and Accountability**: Quality indicators and a minimum dataset to ensure meaningful outcome measures.

Below is a brief snapshot of each P/T in terms of their identified key activities and priorities toward integrating a palliative approach into their health systems (Table 5.7). This snapshot is not intended to be comprehensive, but to highlight major movements in a palliative approach implementation across Canada.[7]

In summary, the reported priorities for many provinces and territories were increased training and education for health professionals with interprofessional and policy support for implementing a palliative approach across care settings. With 90% of P/Ts using TWF's National Framework to guide implementation, these priorities draw from a strong evidence base on the key ingredients and impacts of integrating a palliative approach across care settings.

5.3.4 QELCCC & P/T Governments: Shared Priorities to Advance a Palliative Approach

In survey questions about what would help to advance a palliative approach to care, it was unanimously identified by the provinces and territories and QELCCC member organizations that there was a need for three key priorities:

1. **Engage Canadians and healthcare providers**—Across the two surveys, respondents noted a lack of understanding and awareness about what a palliative approach is and offers to improve patient and family outcomes, delivery of care, and health system functioning. Both the QELCCC and P/T recommended a national awareness campaign about a palliative approach to care and its benefits with targeted messaging for the Canadian public as well as for healthcare providers.
2. **Facilitate Advance Care Planning**–Advance care planning was seen as a cross-cutting factor to support a palliative approach. QELCCC members recommended making ACP part of healthcare visits for everyone over 50, for people with life-limiting illnesses, integrated into electronic health records, and having earlier discussions could support better choices along illness trajectories and at end of life. The P/Ts consistently identified select ways to encourage ACP, including through sustained awareness campaigns and by supporting education and training of healthcare providers to initiate discussions.
3. **Measurement**—QELCCC respondents raised the issue of poor data on palliative care across the country, precipitating the conclusion of a recent national report on palliative care by the Canadian Partnership Against Cancer [25]. Most P/T have or are developing quality indicators and outcome measures to help

---

[7] Snapshots from Quebec and Nunavut were not provided and therefore are not included.

Table 5.7 Provincial and territorial snapshots of implementing a palliative approach

Prov/Terr	Activities	Priorities
Alberta	• A PEOLC Alberta provincial framework (2014), overseen by the palliative and end of life innovations steering committee • Amendment of continuing care health service standards to increase emphasis on PEOLC training, patient/family information, and advance care planning • Evaluating uptake of provincial policy on ACP/GOC designation and EMS PEOLC assess, treat, and refer program	1. Ongoing operational support for the PEOLC provincial framework and recommended initiatives 2. Increasing public awareness of the benefits of advance care planning and earlier referral to palliative care 3. Capacity planning to identify program and infrastructure needs and direct appropriate investments in PEOLC 4. A provincial clinical information system with the ability to share goals of care between sectors and providers
British Columbia	• A provincial end-of-life care action plan (2013) • Ministry of Health funding for the BC Centre of palliative care to support PEOLC practices and programs • Implementation direction from a provincial palliative care advisory committee • Physicians provided with fee codes related to advance care planning and palliative care planning	1. Education, awareness, and support for healthcare providers on the benefits of a palliative approach to care 2. Incorporate a palliative approach to care into redesign of enhanced integrated primary and community care services 3. Enhance public awareness and resources for advance care planning
Manitoba	• Dedicated funding to health authorities to provide direct palliative care services • A provincial palliative care drug access program offering deductible-free coverage for registrants • A provincial palliative care program specialist to develop, coordinate and deliver education and support program planning • With funding from CPAC, Cancer care Manitoba launched a project to encourage ACP/GOC discussions	1. Provincial coordination of palliative education and training for healthcare providers and volunteers 2. Encourage uptake of advance care planning and goals of care discussions 3. Building a provincial measurement framework
New Brunswick	• Royal assent of a provincial advance health care directives act (2016) • The New Brunswick Cancer network, a branch of the Department of Health, is the provincial lead for palliative care	1. Releasing a provincial palliative care strategy 2. End-of-life care inclusion of all life-limiting diseases and prioritization based on hospital utilization 3. An awareness campaign on the palliative approach to care aimed at the general public and healthcare providers

(continued)

Table 5.7 (continued)

Prov/Terr	Activities	Priorities
Newfoundland and Labrador	• Legislation, regional programs and policies, and public forms to promote ACP across sectors • Care coordination supported through case conferences, patient navigators, and palliative care consult teams	1. Public awareness and understanding of a palliative approach including engaging people and families 2. Healthcare provider education and training. 3. Provincial policies and standards
Northwest Territories	• Professional development initiative funding, which may be used for palliative care training • The seniors and continuing care division, which oversees palliative care provincially, is engaging with the transitions in care initiative to improve care coordination	1. Finalize a palliative care service model for the territory 2. Consistent assessment and care planning where healthcare providers identify frail elderly clients who would benefit from a palliative approach to care 3. Coordinated approach to education and training for health professionals
Nova Scotia	• A provincial palliative care strategy (2014), with implementation assigned to the Nova Scotia Health Authority (2016). • Working groups to support the strategy, including one on identifying quality indicators • Involvement with the Canadian Foundation for Healthcare Improvement EXTRA project to develop an operational framework to support integration of a palliative approach in primary care	1. Establish benchmarks for staffing, location of death/care, number of days in hospital 2. Identify solutions for the "fee code" issues that would support appropriate compensation for primary care providers to provide advance care planning, home visits, and after-hours and on-call care 3. Ensure that palliative care is integrated across settings of care, including a shared accountability framework
Ontario	• Created the Ontario palliative care network (2016), a partnership between Cancer Care Ontario, health quality Ontario, hospice palliative care Ontario, and the 14 local health integration networks • The network's activities are determined by a provincial vision outlined in a collaboratively developed declaration of partnership and commitment to action	The declaration addresses three core system goals: 1. Quality: To improve client/family, caregiver, and provider experience by delivering high quality, seamless care and support 2. Population health: To improve, maintain, and support the quality of life and health of people with progressive life-limiting illnesses 3. Sustainability: To improve system performance by delivering better care more cost-effectively and creating a continuously self-improving system

Table 5.7 (continued)

Prov/Terr	Activities	Priorities
Prince Edward Island	• A provincial policy to support ACP • Health PEI, the provincial health authority, collects data on palliative care indicators • Funding from the Canadian partnership against Cancer facilitated the development of resources around ACP and goals of care	1. Dedicated funding for continuing education focused on palliative care 2. A commitment by the government to support the adoption of a palliative approach to care 3. Increased education around palliative care in school curricula
Saskatchewan	• A partnership between the provincial cancer agency and the health regions to provide clinics for pain/symptom management, ACP/GOC, and early integrated care services • A provincial palliative care steering committee to review policies, best practices, resources, and education	1. Education for healthcare professionals, including innovative training options such as online education modules 2. Improved access to palliative care services through innovations within existing programs 3. Developing provincial standards to ensure service consistency across the province 4. Focusing on support for families through provision of palliative care at home
Yukon	• A palliative care consult team that is part of the continuing care division of the Department of Health and Social Services • A fee code for counseling time associating with completing advance directives with patients	1. Better identification of transitions in health status to identify individuals who would benefit from a palliative approach earlier in their illness trajectory 2. Education and awareness of a palliative approach by the public and healthcare professionals, including the benefit of advance care planning discussions and changes in goals of care 3. A territorial palliative care strategy that includes support for caregivers

Source: Canadian Hospice Palliative Care Association

manage and monitor progress and assist with ongoing planning. However, a lack of standards and minimum datasets creates a barrier for improving the provision of a palliative care within and across jurisdictions.

The message is clear from P/T governments and healthcare stakeholders that Canada is ready to implement a palliative approach to care, consistent with the action steps from *The Way Forward's National Framework*. The surveys provided important information about what has helped to drive adoption of the palliative approach over the last few years, and what more needs to be done to ensure all Canadians have access to high-quality hospice palliative care. In summary, the two surveys offered the following insights:

- While **public awareness** is one driver of adoption of a palliative approach, there is more to do to enhance the understanding of a palliative approach to care and advance care planning with the public and healthcare providers.
- **National education curriculum, and ongoing continuing professional development** through enhanced skills and training are needed for all healthcare providers across all settings of care to improve competence and confidence to deliver a palliative approach to care.
- **Conversations about a palliative approach** need to be better integrated with usual medical care. This would help to make a palliative approach part of ongoing treatment and not seen as a separate, specialized, or referral-based program.
- Ongoing **advocacy efforts for a palliative approach to care** must continue, particularly in light of the introduction of Medical Assistance in Dying (MAiD) in Canada, which has created a need to clarify what hospice palliative is and isn't about, and what more needs to be done to ensure it is accessible to all Canadians, provided in the setting of their choice, and meeting their care needs.
- Current care pathways need to include a palliative approach, and **tools and materials** for healthcare systems and professionals must enable adoption.
- **Ensuring resources are available** and dedicated to hospice palliative care, and flexible to meet population health needs, including for Canadians who are members of indigenous, cultural, or vulnerable groups.

5.4 The Way Forward, Phase II: We Know the Way, Now Let's Walk It Together

So much progress has been made across Canada and internationally toward identifying, implementing, and monitoring an integrated palliative approach to care. Through evidence-based practices and approaches, adopting a palliative approach to care would better integrate aspects of hospice palliative care with usual medical care or treatment services, enabled by advance care planning, and supported in community settings where most people receive their care—primary care, home care, long-term care, and hospitals.

In Canada, we see palliative care leadership in the P/T development of provincial palliative care and advance care planning policies; the consultations, reviews, and policy recommendations conducted by national health organizations like the CHPCA, QELCCC, and CPAC; and in the strong public support for earlier conversations about their wishes and values for future care and better access to hospice palliative care services. In late 2017, the federal department Health Canada put forth a national Framework on Palliative Care in Canada that sets out guiding principles, best practices, and priorities for short, medium, and long-term action.[8] These actions, from community-based stakeholders to regional authorities to federal governments, collectively move the country closer to the goal of enabling all Canadians with life-limiting illnesses to live well until the very end of their lives.

---

[8] Available via: https://www.canada.ca/en/health-canada/services/health-care-system/reports-publications/palliative-care/framework-palliative-care-canada.html. Accessed 1 Mar 2019.

5.5 Conclusions

While there has been significant progress made by several healthcare leaders and P/T governments—including more education and training, more policy and program development, and more monitoring and evaluation of relevant outcomes—more needs to be done to enable the change process so that more Canadians have access to high-quality hospice palliative care in the setting of their choice [6]. TWF project and follow-up surveys on implementing a palliative approach provide a map of both what has been accomplished and where to go from here. Now that the way forward has been paved, together let us follow the roadmap toward a better future for everyone impacted by illness.

References

1. Canadian Hospice Palliative Care Association. A model to guide hospice palliative care: based on national principles and norms of practice. Ottawa, CHPCA. 2013. http://www.chpca.net/professionals/norms.aspx. Accessed 1 Mar 2019.
2. World Health Organization. Strengthening of palliative care as a component of integrated treatment throughout the life course. J Pain Palliat Care Pharmacother. 2014;28(2):130–4.
3. Bekelman JE, Halpern SD, Blankart CR, et al. Comparison of site of death, health care utilization, and hospital expenditures for patients dying with cancer in 7 developed countries. JAMA. 2016;315(3):272–83.
4. Glare PA, Virik K. Can we do better in end-of-life care? The mixed management model and palliative care. Med J Aust. 2005;175(10):530–3.
5. Hawley P. The bow tie model of 21st century palliative care. J Pain Symptom Manag. 2014;47(1):2–5.
6. Canadian Hospice Palliative Care Association. The Way Forward National Framework: a roadmap for an integrated palliative approach to care. 2015. Ottawa, ON: CHPCA. http://hpcintegration.ca/resources/the-national-framework.aspx. Accessed 1 Mar 2019.
7. iPANEL. Initiative for a palliative approach in nursing: Evidence and leadership. 2012. http://www.ipanel.ca. Accessed 15 Feb 2019.
8. Quill TE, Abernethy AP. Generalist plus specialist palliative care – creating a more sustainable model. N Engl J Med. 2013;368(13):1173–5.
9. World Health Organization. Cancer control: knowledge into action. WHO guide for effective programs. Module 5: palliative care. 2007 Geneva WHO. https://www.ncbi.nlm.nih.gov/books/NBK195248/. Accessed 15 Feb 2019.
10. Bakitas M, Lyons KD, Hegel MT, et al. Effects of a palliative care intervention on clinical outcomes in patients with advanced cancer: the project ENABLE II randomized controlled trial. JAMA. 2009;302(7):741–9.
11. Detering KM, Hancock AD, Reade MC, Silvester W. The impact of advance care planning on end of life care in elderly patients: randomised controlled trial. BMJ 2010;340:c1345. https://doi.org/10.1136/bmj.c1345. Accessed 1 Mar 2019.
12. Wright AA, Zhang B, Ray A, et al. Associations between end-of-life discussions, patient mental health, medical care near death, and caregiver bereavement adjustment. JAMA. 2008;300(14):1665–73.
13. Lussier D, Bruneau MA, Villalpando JM. Management of end-stage dementia. Prim Care. 2011;38(2):247–64.
14. Temel JS, Greer JA, Muzikansky A, et al. Early palliative care for patients with metastatic non–small-cell lung cancer. N Engl J Med. 2010;363(8):733–42.
15. Fowler R, Hammer M. End-of-life care in Canada. Clin Invest Med. 2013;36(3):127–32.

16. Klinger CA, Howell D, Marshall D, et al. Resource utilization and cost analyses of home-based palliative care service provision: the Niagara west end-of-life shared-care project. Palliat Med. 2013;27(2):115–22.
17. Meyers FJ, Linder J, Beckett L, et al. Simultaneous care: a model approach to the perceived conflict between investigational therapy and palliative care. J Pain Symptom Manage. 2004;28(6):548–56.
18. Smith TJ, Temin S, Erin R, et al. American Society of Clinical Oncology provisional clinical opinion: the integration of palliative care into standard oncology care. J Clin Oncol. 2012;30(8):880–7.
19. Sanders C, Rogers A, Gately C, et al. Planning for end of life care within lay-led chronic illness self-management training: the significance of 'death awareness' and biographical context in participant accounts. Soc Sci Med. 2012;66(4):982–93.
20. Brumley R, Enguidanos S, Jamison P, et al. Increased satisfaction with care and lower costs: results of a randomized trial of in-home palliative care. J Am Geriatr Soc. 2007;55(7):993–100.
21. Lynn J, Forlini JH. "serious and complex illness" in quality improvement and policy reform for end-of-life care. J Gen Intern Med. 2001;16(5):315–9.
22. Canadian Hospice Palliative Care Association (CHPCA). What Canadians say: the way forward survey report. 2013. Ottawa, CHPCA. http://hpcintegration.ca/resources/what-canadians-say.aspx. Accessed 1 Mar 2019.
23. Canadian Hospice Palliative Care Association. The way forward survey: general/family practitioners and nurses in primary care. 2014. Ottawa: CHPCA. http://hpcintegration.ca/resources/health-care-professional-research/primary-care-research.aspx. Accessed 1 Mar 2019.
24. Canadian Hospice Palliative Care Association. Innovative models of integrated hospice palliative care, the way forward initiative: an integrated palliative approach to care. 2013. Ottawa: CHPCA. http://hpcintegration.ca/resources/discussion-papers/innovative-models.aspx. Accessed 1 Mar 2019.
25. Canadian Partnership Against Cancer. Palliative and end-of-life care. 2017. Toronto, CPAC. https://www.systemperformance.ca/report/palliative-end-of-life-care/. Accessed 1 Mar 2019.

Global Perspectives of Paediatric Palliative Care in the Home in Aotearoa, New Zealand

6

Karyn Bycroft and Rachel Teulon

Contents

6.1	Introduction to New Zealand (Aotearoa)...	86
	6.1.1 History..	86
6.2	Children's Palliative Care in New Zealand...	87
	6.2.1 Epidemiology..	87
	6.2.2 Place of Death...	88
	6.2.3 Definition..	88
	6.2.4 Philosophy of Care..	89
	6.2.5 Model of Care...	89
	6.2.6 Development of Children's Palliative Care...	90
	6.2.7 Funding..	91
	6.2.8 Respite..	91
6.3	Provision of Care for Children..	92
	6.3.1 Specialist Care..	92
	6.3.2 Children's Community Nursing..	92
	6.3.3 Remote Services and Technology...	93
	6.3.4 Hospices...	93
	6.3.5 Case Example 1...	94
6.4	Implications for Nursing Practice...	95
	6.4.1 Hope...	95
	6.4.2 Communication..	95
	6.4.3 Advance Care Planning/Te Wa Aroha..	96
	6.4.4 Case Example 2: Te Wa Aroha...	97
	6.4.5 Cultural Support..	98

K. Bycroft (✉)
Paediatric Palliative Care, Starship Child Health, Auckland District Health Board, Auckland, New Zealand
e-mail: Karynb@adhb.govt.nz

R. Teulon
Paediatric Palliative Care, Hospice Palliative Care Service, Nurse Maude, Christchurch, New Zealand
e-mail: Rachel.Teulon@nursemaude.org.nz

© Springer Nature Switzerland AG 2019
L. Holtslander et al. (eds.), *Hospice Palliative Home Care and Bereavement Support*, https://doi.org/10.1007/978-3-030-19535-9_6

	6.4.6 Case Example 3: Communication End-of-Life Care for Baby at Home	98
	6.4.7 Discharge Planning/Symptom Management Plan	99
	6.4.8 Siblings	99
	6.4.9 After a Child Has Died	99
	6.4.10 Grief and Bereavement	100
6.5	Implications for Nursing Education	101
6.6	Implications for Nursing Research	101
6.7	Conclusion	102
References		102

6.1 Introduction to New Zealand (Aotearoa)

Sitting in the South Pacific Ocean lies a relatively small country, Aotearoa, New Zealand (NZ). By both size and population, it is small in comparison to Australia, Canada, the USA, or Europe. NZ is an independent commonwealth country with a growing population of over five million people. It is made up of three main islands: the North Island (Te Ika-a Maui), South Island (Te Waipounamu) and Stewart Island (Rakiura), with the largest population in the North Island and approximately one million people living in the South Island. Although Wellington is the capital city, Auckland has the greatest population with around 1.5 million people. Both these cities are in the North Island. Distances between major cities require significant time for travel as roads are often single-lane, with extensive farmland, bush-clad hills and mountain passes between towns.

6.1.1 History

NZ's history as a small nation stems from its beginnings around the 1250–1300s when Polynesians settled the two main islands and the distinct Māori people, with their unique culture, grew and inhabited the country, each group of Māori identifying with an iwi (tribe). European settlers first arrived in 1642 and over the next 200 years, there was a growth in European and Pacific Island settlers. The Treaty of Waitangi was signed in 1840 by over 550 Māori cultural leaders and the British Crown; this treaty was a statement of principles to found a nation state and build a government in NZ. In more recent years, it became apparent that there had been a different interpretation and understanding between the Māori and English version of the Treaty, leading to misinterpretation and losses to the Māori people. This resulted in social, health, education, financial and other inequities. Since the 1970s, there has been redress to acknowledge the transgressions of the past that have had an impact the Māori people [1]. This has led to ongoing change, with a deeper understanding for Māori and the need to build a strong bicultural backbone, utilising the three key concepts of the Treaty: protection, participation and partnership which now informs the cultural basis of our country.

Over the last 100 years, there has been additional immigration from different regions and the population is now approximately 75% European, 15% Māori, 11% Asian, 8% Pacific and 1% Middle Eastern/Latin and American/African [2]. Healthcare and disability services are funded by the government; eligible people (NZ citizens and those with a permanent resident visa) receive free inpatient and outpatient public hospital services. This also includes subsides on medicines and support services for those with disabilities in the community [3]. There has been limited need for reliance on private healthcare in paediatric services in NZ. As with other publicly funded first world health services, with a small population, there are limited resources and not all health treatments are freely available.

Regional and local health services are provided at differing levels by 20 district health boards (DHBs) throughout the country. The DHBs set the strategic direction and monitor performance, with four members of the board being government appointed. Local services are predominantly population based, with limited paediatric services in towns smaller than 25,000. Auckland has the only children's hospital (Starship) with many specialist services, including palliative, cardiology, metabolic and paediatric intensive care. Complex paediatric healthcare services are centred in bigger cities, with tertiary centres, including Christchurch and Wellington. In the South Island, tertiary services are based in Christchurch, including neurology and oncology services.

6.2 Children's Palliative Care in New Zealand

6.2.1 Epidemiology

Identifying numbers of children and young people requiring paediatric palliative care (PPC) in NZ has challenges; however, they are likely to be similar to data from the UK: approximately 32 per 10,000 [4, 5]. An assessment of palliative care need in NZ in 2006 revealed approximately 2.3 per 10,000 children died from a life-limiting/serious illness [6], while a review of deaths over a period of 4 years in 2006–2009 estimated 125 children aged between 28 days and 18 years died each year and would have benefitted from palliative care involvement [7]. The lack of clear figures is due to a number of factors including prognostic uncertainty, the wide range and long-term nature of health conditions and the lack of consistent recording of conditions in NZ's small population.

Recent data provided to the PPC National Clinical Reference Group revealed an increasing number of children and young people with congenital anomalies who are surviving longer [8]. With advances in care provision and technology, this is not unexpected but indicates an increasing need for paediatric palliative care services that potentially have longer involvement in care with many requiring transition into adult services.

6.2.2 Place of Death

A recent New Zealand retrospective review of paediatric palliative deaths aged 28 days to 18 years identified that around 54% died in hospital, 42% at home and 1% in hospice, similar to the UK, Australia and Canada [7]. Furthermore, there was a decreased likelihood of a hospital death for children with cancer, as well as those referred to the specialist PPC team [7]. Differences were also identified for those of Asian and Pacific ethnicity, who were found to be more likely to die in the hospital setting. Where possible, every effort is made to accommodate those families who prefer care at home.

6.2.3 Definition

PPC in NZ utilises and adheres to the definition provided in the New Zealand Palliative Care Council Glossary [9]. This closely aligns with the definition provided by the World Health Organisation [10]. It identifies that palliative care for children is the active and total care of the child's body, mind and spirit and it is a support for the whole family.

- PPC begins when the illness is diagnosed and continues regardless of whether or not a child receives treatment directed at the disease.
- Health providers must evaluate and alleviate a child's physical, psychological and social distress.
- Effective palliative care requires a broad multidisciplinary approach that includes the family and makes use of available community resources; it can be successfully implemented even if resources are limited.
- It can be provided in children's homes, in community health centres and in tertiary facilities [9, 11].

Palliative care for children is distinct from their adult counterparts due to the diverse range of diagnoses or disease groups involved, the differing cognitive and physical developmental stages and the illness trajectory these children will follow [12, 13]. Four distinct groups of children have been identified by Goldman [13], where palliative care will be required in their lifetime. These relate to the type of trajectory a condition or illness is likely to follow:

- Diseases for which curative treatment may be feasible but may fail.
- Diseases in which premature death is anticipated but intensive treatment may prolong with a good quality of life.
- Progressive diseases for which treatment is exclusively palliative and may extend over many years.
- Conditions with severe neurological disability that, although not progressive, may lead to vulnerability and complications which are likely to cause a premature death [12, 13].

6.2.4 Philosophy of Care

PPC is for all children with serious illness, from infants to young people who may require transition to adult services. The aim is to achieve the best quality of life for children until they die, whenever that may be, preferably in a place of the child's and family's choosing [14].

PPC in New Zealand utilises a collaborative approach which intertwines a family centred, culturally sensitive approach to care, with seamless links between hospital, community and home. It aims to do this by:

- ensuring the child is comfortable and in the best possible condition so that they can go about doing things that are important and fun (such as going to school or kindergarten),
- helping families with difficult decisions,
- supporting parents,
- helping parents to support their child around any worries or questions they might have,
- helping parents support the brothers and sisters of the sick child,
- providing practical help with equipment, medications and respite care,
- ensuring families are able to access support in bereavement [14].

Palliative care can be provided alongside other active treatments by other specialist clinical teams, with PPC an active participant in care, particularly for those who have challenging healthcare needs and serious illness [12].

6.2.5 Model of Care

Our people's history brings a rich and unique cultural essence to each person's individual heritage. However, it is the unique beliefs, values and cultural heritage of the indigenous Māori that guides and informs our present and future healthcare. Several models relating to Māori healthcare exist to enable appropriate care and respect. While not wanting to be presumptive and suggest one model over another, or over simplify these needs, it is important to listen and acknowledge how best to support each individual child and family.

One model, Te Whare Tapa Whā (Fig. 6.1), relates to health and well-being [15]. Te Whare Tapa Whā demonstrates and describes the holistic nature of health and well-being. This acknowledges how unique Māori customs, beliefs and culture are very much an integral part of and influence daily life. The four cornerstones of this model encompass taha whānau (family), taha tinana (physical health), taha hinengaro (mental health) and taha wairua (spiritual health). Te Whare Tapa Whā recognises the interconnected nature of each of these domains, as well as the importance of addressing each to ensure the care of the whole person. The strength of the metaphorical whare (house) is based on the balance and support of the interconnecting cornerstones or domains which are supportive to daily life, health and well-being.

Fig. 6.1 Te Whare Tapa Wha Māori Health Model in Ministry of Health. Maori health models. Te Whare Tapa Whā: Mason Durie, 2015. Wellington, New Zealand, 2015. https://www.health.govt.nz/our-work/populations/maori-health/maori-health-models (accessed 26 January 2019)

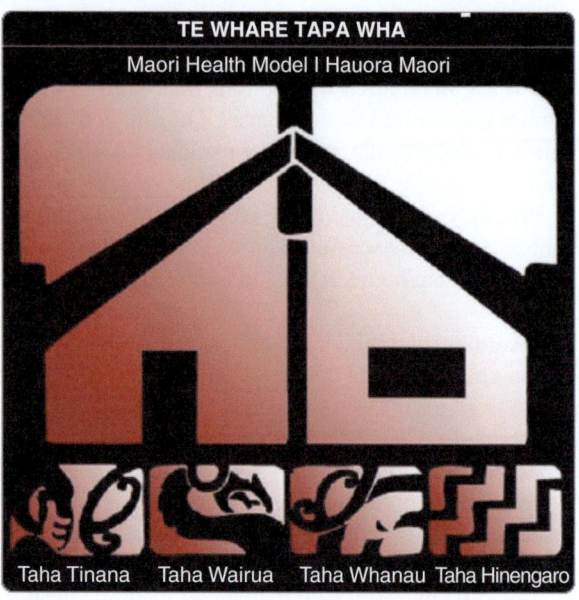

Culture and spirituality must influence how specific healthcare is provided and this is at the core of PPC provided in NZ.

Family-centred care, with a focus on the child and family, is an international model and philosophy of nursing care which began to have an influence in NZ in the 1980s [16]. Family-centred care is a holistic approach to care, recognising that the care for the child sits at the centre and includes the whole family as recipients of care [17]. 'Through the Eyes of the Child' is a document that addresses this and identifies that specialist services must be firmly focused on the child and family; this has become the guiding principle for paediatric services in NZ [18]. Family-centred care acknowledges parents as experts in their child's care and uses the guiding principles of partnership and collaboration, negotiation, respect and honouring as well as information sharing [19].

Palliative care and family-centred care embrace Te Whare Tapa Whā with the strong bond of Taha whanau, as core requirements to meeting a child and family's individual and unique needs. An additional model 'Comfort as a Model of Care or Whakamarietia rite ki te tauira o te tiaki' recognises the specific and unique palliative care needs for neonatal infants [20]. This model supports holistic end-of-life care in either the hospital or home and gives practical information and guidance.

6.2.6 Development of Children's Palliative Care

A review of paediatric tertiary services in NZ in 1998 resulted in the first PPC Service being established at Starship Child Health in Auckland in 1999 [18]. The PPC service initially covered the northern region of NZ with the first position filled by a nurse specialist closely followed by social worker and child psychotherapy roles. A medical specialist was appointed 3 years later. This service is now recognised as the national PPC service for NZ. In 2011, the Paediatric Society of NZ partnered with the Ministry of Health to form the New Zealand Paediatric Palliative Care Clinical Network. The *Guidance for Integrated Paediatric Palliative Care Services in New Zealand* was published in 2012 [11]. This document has been instrumental in shaping and guiding a model of care that can be delivered nationally.

The guidance document identified the need to develop evidence-based clinical guidelines to support NZ's health professionals throughout a child's palliative care trajectory. Guidelines to support end-of-life care for children have been completed and implemented via website access [21]. These were developed using a rigorous and evidence-based process and can be freely accessed through the Starship Child Health website.

Advocacy and lobbying to the Ministry of Health, key health leaders and government officials continue to be a focus of the NZ PPC Clinical Network. One of the key recommendations was to have coordinators with advanced skills to improve provision and more equitable palliative care to children throughout NZ in all paediatric centres; however, funding has not been forthcoming as children's palliative care has not been prioritised, given the many competing health needs.

6.2.7 Funding

Funding, specifically for children's palliative care, is very limited, notwithstanding the national service at Starship; there is no other service in NZ that meets specialist criteria. There are some small charitable services providing additional care for children and their families with palliative care needs, such as *@heart, Child Cancer Foundation, Canteen and the Muscular Dystrophy Association New Zealand*. These organisations are disease-specific support groups which mean many children and young people and their families with rare conditions do not have the same level of support. *Guardian Angels*, a charitable organisation, provides practical support, including grocery, petrol and clothing vouchers and funeral grants to children and young people under the Starship PPC national service.

A child and their family in their last months of life receive no additional funding, in fact financial support can be less, when compared to a child with a long-term health condition or disability. DHBs provide variable financial assistance to adult hospices as well as full funding for community nursing services, so these are provided without a cost to families. It is common for one parent to be a fulltime carer for their child, often for many years, leading to loss of financial stability.

6.2.8 Respite

Respite services, particularly for those with a short-life expectancy (less than 6 months), are extremely limited in NZ. Family and friends are often the only option available. This is often what families prefer; however, when families are exhausted, a funded break from care is often beneficial, yet suitable carers are not easily found, nor is funding available. For those with a disability, or long-term health conditions (greater than 6 months), children are assessed for an individual package of care to meet the child's personal care and the family's respite needs. Respite services for those with high and complex health or disability needs are assessed and can include a specific number of bed nights in an appropriate out-of-home service. Or for another family, it may be that close friends, family or suitable carers are able to provide care, either at the child's home or out of home. Out-of-home options are very limited, partly due to parents preferring home-based care, or else such options are for those children with moderately dependent care needs. Out-of-home respite services are not available throughout most of the country for those with very high needs, particularly for younger children.

6.3 Provision of Care for Children

6.3.1 Specialist Care

As previously stated, there is only one specialist PPC service in NZ based at Starship Children's Hospital covering the northern region of the North Island. It currently comprises a medical specialist, nurse practitioner, nurse specialist, social worker, psychotherapist and psychiatrist roles. The aim has been to support children and young people where they wish to be cared for, with a seamless approach across the continuum of settings. The team provides direct care locally and a consultancy service nationally for those with more complex needs throughout NZ as required. There are other services, one in South Island based at Nurse Maude Hospice in Christchurch and two in the same city in the North Island: *True Colours Charitable Trust* and *Rainbow Place*—both of which have dedicated nursing hours, some medical and psychosocial supports to specifically provide palliative care to children and young people. For other places in NZ, care is provided by clinicians in broader paediatric roles, who are well known to these children and families, often having cared for them over many years.

6.3.2 Children's Community Nursing

PPC is holistic in its approach to care, aiming to improve the quality of life for the child or young person and their family/whanau for whatever that time might be. Increasing complexities and uncertainty of prognosis as a result of advancements in care and technology is not only changing the illness trajectory previously expected, but also how care should be delivered [22]. It has been widely agreed [10, 23] that the health and disability care of children should be provided as close to home as possible. There are a number of children's community nursing services in NZ provided by DHBs which include nurse-led care to children and their families. Community nurses are often involved in care for long periods of time, especially with children who have long-term conditions and already have a therapeutic relationship with the child and family. These nurses have knowledge and skills in general paediatric care, high and complex needs and along with support from local paediatricians, developmental services, general practices and the tertiary specialist services are able to provide care in the home. They have the education and skills to manage pain pumps, long intravenous lines and medications required for comfort management. In contrast, many adult-based community or hospice services will only use subcutaneous continuous administration of medications for children at end of life.

Where community children's nurses are not available, adult district or hospice services provide community and out-of-hours end-of-life care for infants, children and young people. Community nurses play a key role in coordination of these children's care and support needs, liaising with clinicians and specialist services depending on the need. Joint visits with specialist PPC services are encouraged and they will attend hospital appointments and discharge planning meetings.

6.3.3 Remote Services and Technology

The smaller and more rural the team caring for a child, the more that is expected of nurses who, in all likeliness, may not have cared for a child with palliative care needs before. In the smallest of communities, it may even be a public health nurse and/or a general practitioner who then link and collaborate with paediatric or PPC services.

The use of home-based video technology is often available (yet not all rural areas have suitable internet speeds) and utilised to support families returning home to local, particularly rural, areas. Depending on the available technology and what the support needs are, this may include a weekly telephone call or videoconference into the home. This may be between a PPC doctor or nurse and the family. In another situation, it may be a video conference directly with a local health centre where the child can be seen and assessed, who then link with medical, or nursing supports at a larger paediatric service. This may be used to continue family support, or for other healthcare professionals, for example, psychosocial supports. Although this is not a replacement for the face-to-face consultation, it enables continued connection with the family and improves equity and access to more specialist care [24]. The overall concept of supporting local services by those with specialist clinical PPC skills and experience to rural areas has been described in Australia as a 'pop-up' model [25]. This acknowledges the need for training and education to build capacity for local healthcare services, often utilising telemedicine and is like the model used to support small local areas in New Zealand.

6.3.4 Hospices

There is no children's hospice in NZ. This is due to a number of reasons but mostly because Auckland is the only city where there is a suitable population to support this service, leaving an inequitable service that cannot be accessed by the greater population. Families also request care in their home and from a financial perspective, there would be a large outlay for services requiring significant travel in order to attend to each child and family. Therefore, it was hoped that by building sufficient clinical expertise in regional areas, supported by the national service, a more equitable and local approach to care could be provided [5, 11].

Children and young people may receive care from adult hospices or their community services to enable care closer to a child's home. A Memorandum of Understanding exists between Hospice New Zealand, some individual adult hospices and the NZ PPC Clinical Network to support collaborative service provision. It is interesting to note that very few children's deaths (1.2%) occur in adult hospices in NZ [6, 7].

6.3.5 Case Example 1

Simon (not his real name) was a 10-year-old boy who had been on the children's oncology ward for several months receiving treatment for a brain tumour. While on treatment, it became obvious that clinically, his symptoms were progressing and scanning revealed the tumours had increased and further treatment would not improve his prognosis. Together with the oncologist, Simon and his parents agreed that returning home and being in their home town with their local friends, family and support networks would be important to them. Reluctantly, they said goodbye to the team that had been caring for them in the ward.

A referral was made to the PPC Clinical Nurse Specialist (CNS) to provide a plan of care for managing Simon's symptoms and assist with discharge planning. Simon was from a rural town which had a small paediatric ward. Contact was made with the paediatric team and the district nursing (adult community) service as the family wanted care at home. The district nursing service provided generalist palliative care in the community but had not looked after a child as young as Simon and were concerned about medication doses and what to expect.

A videoconference session was set up between the local palliative care providers and the PPC CNS to talk through some of the differences they would expect and to answer any questions they might have. They visited Simon weekly to start and when he needed review by a paediatrician in the hospital, the district nursing team joined. Weekly videoconferencing was held for the staff providing the care and the PPC CNS. As Simon's condition deteriorated, it became clearer that home was not going to be the place of care. The team talked with the family and offered options of admission to hospital or possibly the local hospice. Simon's parents went to look at the adult hospice and felt comfortable that the care provided would work for Simon and could provide additional support for them as a family. Simon transferred to the hospice and stayed until he died about 3 weeks later. During this time, weekly videoconferences were held between the hospice and the PPC CNS as part of a regular adult complex case meeting. The hospice was able to give additional support to the family following Simon's death. The CNS consistently reviewed supportive needs and the plan of care with the hospice to see if any concerns or difficulties were raised when caring for Simon and his family. They said, although it was different, all went as well as could be expected, that the family valued the care and support from the staff, so they could spend valuable time as a family and not have to worry about what was going on around them. The hospice continued to provide bereavement support for the family following Simon's death.

6.4 Implications for Nursing Practice

The history and changing cultural context in NZ is considered important in all aspects of healthcare delivery, including palliative care. Utilising the concepts of hope and collaborative communication enables care that is individually focused, culturally supported and family centred.

6.4.1 Hope

Hope, although simply defined as the feeling of expectation and desire for a particular thing to happen [26], in PPC requires a broad and multifaceted understanding about how it can influence the child, parent and healthcare professional. When a child is diagnosed with a condition from which they are likely to die, their parent's hopes and dreams are shattered and they may be left with feelings of hopelessness [27]. One of the myths that is commonly held is that patient and parents must make a choice between 'fighting for a cure' or 'giving up hope' when potentially engaging a palliative care team [28]. PPC healthcare professionals understand that at times, although there is no hope for a cure, they must have open and honest conversations with the child and family; however, they must also foster hope for the child and family [27]. Hope is also used by children and parents to help cope with a serious illness [29], with hope enabling them to get through difficult times [30]. Therefore, the role of the healthcare professional is to foster and support patients and families to maintain their hopes in the midst of a deteriorating condition [27, 29, 30]. Parental hope is likely to change over the course of a child's illness, even on a daily basis; yet, while they still hope for a miracle, it does not mean they are in denial about their child's possible and sometimes imminent death [27].

6.4.2 Communication

Excellent communication between all healthcare professionals and the family, who are partners in care, is fundamental to enabling care that is child and family focused. A collaborative approach to communication in PPC is the expectation. This requires not only the exchange of information but also the development of a collaborative relationship. Collaborative communication enables the establishment of a common goal to guide PPC, with mutual respect and compassion, while developing an understanding of differing perspectives through planned and guided meetings to allow goals to be made in conjunction with the family [30].

A caring nurse relationship is a partnership with the child and family. The way in which a healthcare professional addresses family's needs will understandably impact parents' interpretation of that episode of interaction and care. To explore the family's needs going forward, it is essential that the nurse has a good understanding of what has shaped the narrative of health and wellness in the past [31]. Exploring a family's values and beliefs acknowledges that care is based on what is important for them in the context of serious illness and building a relationship to meet these needs. The ability for staff to demonstrate compassion and have a full understanding of a family's strengths, supports and stressors will certainly help to provide the care a family requires.

PPC clinicians aim to provide open and honest conversations at a level appropriate to the child's developmental level in the context of their family's beliefs and values [31]. Believing that the parents know their child best, it can be important for parents to talk this through with the healthcare professional first, for guidance and help as to how this could be done. Some families have a more pragmatic approach and understanding of life and death and each family will have differing experiences with death which informs the child's understanding. Certainly, in clinical practice, there are parents who do not want to discuss death and dying with their child. This can be very confronting for clinical staff, particularly when the team believe that the child understands his/her own circumstances and is not allowed to talk to his/her parents about it. To share other parents' experiences related to such discussions, healthcare professionals often discuss a well-cited journal article with parents. This article demonstrated that those parents who discussed death and dying with their children did not regret that decision, while the parents who did not, did have regrets as to not speaking with them [32]. Communicating with parents and children around difficult decisions, including advance care planning, requires experience, compassion and knowledge of the family's hopes and goals. Utilising a clear communication process particularly around difficult conversations can be helpful to achieve this [30].

6.4.3 Advance Care Planning/Te Wa Aroha

The PPC service at Starship has led the development of an Advance Care Plan based on the *Allow Natural Death* approach which in fact eliminates the negative terms *Do Not Resuscitate* and *Not for Resuscitation* (Fig. 6.2). This has been endorsed by the NZ PPC Clinical Network and is available for other hospitals to adapt for their organisation [33]. Working in collaboration with Māori and Pacific Island leaders, the term *Te Wa Aroha* (Māori) was gifted by the Chef Advisor Tikanga (senior Maori Advisor the Auckland Hospital Region) to acknowledge the concept of Allow Natural Death. *Te Wa Aroha* means a *time* or a *journey of love*. This term is recognisable and relatable for people in NZ and has changed the approach to communication focusing on the healthcare and support provided for the infant, child or young

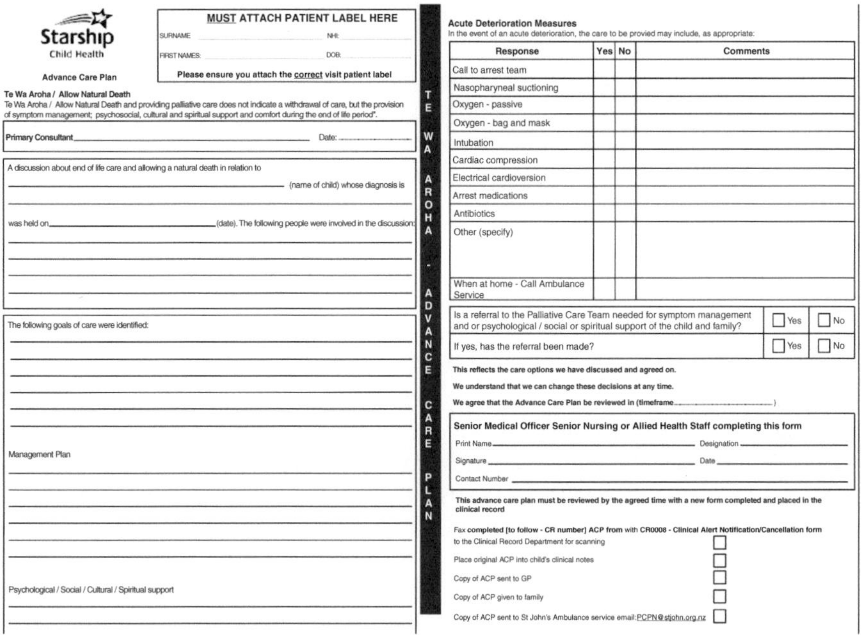

Starship Child Health

Advance Care Plan

MUST ATTACH PATIENT LABEL HERE

SURNAME: NHI:

FIRST NAMES: DOB:

Please ensure you attach the correct visit patient label

TE WA AROHA - ADVANCE CARE PLAN

Te Wa Aroha / Allow Natural Death

Te Wa Aroha / Allow Natural Death and providing palliative care does not indicate a withdrawal of care, but the provision of symptom management; psychosocial, cultural and spiritual support and comfort during the end of life period".

Primary Consultant ________ Date: ________

A discussion about end of life care and allowing a natural death in relation to ________ (name of child) whose diagnosis is ________

was held on ________ (date). The following people were involved in the discussion:

The following goals of care were identified:

Management Plan

Psychological / Social / Cultural / Spiritual support

Acute Deterioration Measures

In the event of an acute deterioration, the care to be provied may include, as appropriate:

Response	Yes	No	Comments
Call to arrest team			
Nasopharyneal suctioning			
Oxygen - passive			
Oxygen - bag and mask			
Intubation			
Cardiac compression			
Electrical cardioversion			
Arrest medications			
Antibiotics			
Other (specify)			
When at home - Call Ambulance Service			

Is a referral to the Palliative Care Team needed for symptom management and or psychological / social or spiritual support of the child and family?	☐ Yes	☐ No
If yes, has the referral been made?	☐ Yes	☐ No

This reflects the care options we have discussed and agreed on.

We understand that we can change these decisions at any time.

We agree that the Advance Care Plan be reviewed in (timeframe________)

Senior Medical Officer Senior Nursing or Allied Health Staff completing this form

Print Name ________ Designation ________

Signature ________ Date ________

Contact Number ________

This advance care plan must be reviewed by the agreed time with a new form completed and placed in the clinical record

Fax **completed [to follow - CR number] ACP from** with **CR0008 - Clinical Alert Notification/Cancellation form** to the Clinical Record Department for scanning ☐

Place original ACP into child's clinical notes ☐

Copy of ACP sent to GP ☐

Copy of ACP given to family ☐

Copy of ACP sent to St John's Ambulance service email:PCPN@stjohn.org.nz ☐

Fig. 6.2 Starship Te Wa Aroha/Advance Care Plan in Te Wa Aroha/Advance Care Plan. Starship Child Health. Auckland 2018

person and family. Starting a conversation with 'if you your child is very unwell, how can we support you to love and care for them?' through to 'if they might not survive this illness, what is most important to you?' Whatever course their illness trajectory might take, the focus will be on how they wish to be loved and cared for, first and foremost [33]. The Advance Care Plan is a tool for collaboration and communication with the child and young person, their family and all key health professionals.

6.4.4 Case Example 2: Te Wa Aroha

Rangi is a 10-year-old Māori boy with a complex medical history including recurrent respiratory infections, intractable seizures, profound intellectual disability and dysphagia with recurrent aspiration episodes. He is cared for by his mother and his parents are separated. The communication between his parents is difficult at times. They do want the best for their son but do not wish to discuss a plan of care, knowing he may not survive additional illness. The family agreed to meet at the hospital Marae (formal Māori meeting house) and each brought with them members of their respective families and an advocate for the child. Kaumātua (Māori elders) led the meeting with clinical staff including a PPC nurse practitioner and social worker. Māori protocol was followed throughout and the discussion included Rangi's situation and concerns about his declining health. Te Wa Aroha (a time or journey of love) was introduced as a way forward to care for him, whatever his future might be. His parents agreed to discuss how he would be loved if he continued to survive, what was important to them if he did not and how much they both wanted to be with him at that time. An advance care plan, Te Wa Aroha, was made for Rangi.

6.4.5 Cultural Support

Cultural support is inherent in individualised care for the child and family. Due to the large Māori and Pacific Island population in NZ, nurses are expected to provide competent cultural care and support, as part of the Treaty of Waitangi agreement. The core principles of partnership, protection and participation including working alongside culturally appropriate services enable improved communication and, subsequently, improved care. This can be useful during times of difficult and challenging health issues for the child, communicating in an appropriate way around death and after a child has died.

There are times where families may choose not to have cultural support for a number of reasons and this needs to be respected and families supported in agreement with their wishes. Respect and sensitivity around cultural needs are as individual as each family, some families adhering strictly to expected cultural norms, while others do not.

6.4.6 Case Example 3: Communication End-of-Life Care for Baby at Home

Tafotila was diagnosed prior to birth with a severe cardiac anomaly and it was thought that she would not likely survive to birth. However, if she did, her family had been given news that she was not expected to survive. Tafotila's parents did not speak English and were new to NZ. PPC worked alongside the support worker from the hospital, to communicate and discuss options for care. The family wanted to be at home and were supported with joint visits from a support worker and PPC nurse specialist. A plan of care was made including options for symptom management which was discussed with the family. When the baby started to have changes in breathing, the mother phoned the support worker for advice on what to do. The support worker communicated with the PPC service and relayed the symptom management advice to the mother who was able to give medication to support her baby's comfort at home; Tafotila died peacefully. The support worker did not just act as an interpreter but also enabled the supportive care for Tafotila and her family by communicating information about medication and comfort. The family may have been more reluctant to give medication without this level of support and care.

6.4.7 Discharge Planning/Symptom Management Plan

The place of death and where end-of-life care is received can be extremely important for NZ families and may require some difficult decision-making, particularly for those families where their usual care team is many miles from their home. They may not have met any of their local care team due to treatment in a specialist centre some distance away from their home. At other times, a child may deteriorate so quickly they cannot make it back to their home. A focus for PPC is certainly to ensure care in the preferred place of care whenever possible.

Providing local care teams with guidance around discharge and managing symptoms at home is often required. Talking through the plans with the child, parents and nursing team is important to know that their care needs can be met in their home environment.

6.4.8 Siblings

Involving and engaging with siblings should also be a focus of communication within the context of caring for the family. Nurses engaging with siblings will enable assessment of possible concerns and need for interdisciplinary referral. For children who have seen their siblings attend countless hospital appointments, investigations and admissions and treatments, it can have a significant effect on their psychological well-being and happiness. This can be expressed by anger, resentment, guilt and loneliness [31]. It is important to ensure that the children's schools are aware of any concerns. NZ has very limited specific PPC local supports for siblings; utilising other service provision through schools and social support systems is required. Acknowledging and discussing issues and identifying means of support for siblings can be helpful in the short term, enabling continuing connections with positive supports such as school, community groups and sports. Some families find encouragement and support by a wider family member taking special care and consideration of the sibling. Other families find it important to have a protected or identified time with a parent, one-on-one if possible.

6.4.9 After a Child Has Died

The care of a child and family after death is equally important. The influence of the Māori culture has normalised not only families choosing to care for their child at home but also for the child's body to stay at home, sometimes up until the day of the funeral, burial or cremation. It is more accepted for families to take their children home so that they are not left alone and to take them to the funeral home/place of funeral in their own personal vehicles and to have close involvement in all stages of the process. Families are supported in their wishes for their child or young person after death, acknowledging they are still the primary carers. To support this involvement and process, the family may choose cooling options as opposed to embalming.

Traditional Māori culture would expect the body to return to the family's ancestral burial ground at their marae (communal sacred place). However, this is becoming more difficult as families can be based significant distances away from the ancestral burial ground, younger generations do not always have cultural connections and financial burden may present challenges. Some families choose cremation for their child, again a move away from the traditional custom of burial [34]. Cultural competency training is mandated in all aspects of healthcare. In PPC, it is essential that clinicians have an understanding of the unique cultural beliefs, traditions and ceremonies for each family. For some families living in NZ, they may be uncertain of their cultural practices or customs due to distance from their family supports and their home country. It is not uncommon for them to ask and seek options and guidance from the health professionals involved in their care.

6.4.10 Grief and Bereavement

Parental grief processes will be somewhat shaped by the differing diagnosis or illness their child has [35]. Parents whose child has a non-malignant diagnosis recognise that their child is going to have a shortened life. Many parents who have a child with a serious illness are likely to experience ongoing grief for many years—from diagnosis, through changes and often decline in their child's overall condition during many hospital admissions. Living with the uncertainly of how long their child is likely to live may mean that they are not 'prepared' for their child's death. Even after years of caring for a child with serious illness and a stepwise deterioration, a child's death can come suddenly. Although not knowing when their child might die, this group of parents are more likely to have had some decision-making around aspects of care, whether it be in the social, physical, emotional or spiritual realms of care their child receives as their child becomes more unwell. This enables parents and families to focus on what is important to their individual family and hopefully minimise some of the regrets they may have around their child's death [35]. Parents who have a child with a malignant condition, where there have been very clear treatment pathways, may find it difficult to move the focus away from treatment and hope for other treatment options even in the child's last weeks of life [35]. Nurses caring for children and their families are often the closest to witness the grief and loss the child and family are experiencing. In NZ, services aimed at supporting families can be limited to what is available locally.

Evidence suggests and acknowledges that everyone will grieve in their own way; there are no right or wrong ways to grieve and grief is as individual as those experiencing it [36]. Following the death of the child, the family may be supported informally by friends and family, their immediate local community and faith and cultural supports. The children's community or adult-based nurses will often provide contact and support to families after the child has died, liaising with specialist services if required for more specialist bereavement support. Healthcare professionals will often attend the funeral or remembrance services as a mark of respect and to offer support for the family. It is after the initial bereavement that follow-up by healthcare teams involved will be required. Clinical experience suggests that some families do not want follow-up visits at all, while others will request ongoing visits provided by a supportive healthcare professional. In many parts of NZ, it may be the family doctor who supports the family and is the link to local services or who may seek advice from specialist services. Even moderate-sized towns in NZ may not be able to provide specialist counselling for the bereaved, particularly for the death of a child; however, adult hospice services in local areas are often utilised to provide ongoing support for families. Specialist paediatric tertiary health services will offer a review of care and contact a family after a child's death, particularly when a child has returned home to their local services for end-of-life care quite quickly, so it can be important for parents to revisit the care the child had and the decisions they made. Additionally, recognition and follow-up around the child's first birthday and anniversary of their death by the healthcare team is a standard practice for most services.

Skylight [36] is a NZ-specific service provider which is utilised to provide specific resources or support for parental and child grief. Skylight has a variety of grief, loss and bereavement information, as well as support materials which can be sent to parents or those supporting a child and family. Other local services such as The National Grief Centre and *Kenzie's Gift* will provide local grief and loss supports.

6.5 Implications for Nursing Education

Education for PPC is provided to generalist nurses through many formal and informal situations. There is, however, limited access to more specialist paediatric palliative care education. A survey of paediatric healthcare professionals identified education in PPC as one of the initial priorities for the NZ PPC Clinical Network. This led to the development of the monthly PPC Education Forum via videoconference which is available throughout the country. This offers a range of speakers from those specialising in palliative care to smaller, more local services. The breadth includes the four levels for all ages: physical, emotional, spiritual and social. Similarly, the University of Auckland provides a bi-yearly paediatric and adolescent palliative care paper as part of their post-graduate palliative care programme.

6.6 Implications for Nursing Research

There are limited research opportunities relating to PPC in NZ. Most research comes through post-graduate training for those involved in PPC, including Masters- and Doctoral-level study, or otherwise through the Ministry of Health for one-off projects. Smaller projects are sometimes undertaken; however, NZ particularly struggles with small numbers of children and their families, due to our small population, the small number of PPC clinical practitioners and the funds available for research projects.

6.7 Conclusion

NZ, while a small country, aims to provide high-quality PPC as close to home as possible. There is only one specialist PPC service, an interdisciplinary team, providing support and consultation to children and their families and healthcare professionals in other regions. There are some regions who have dedicated PPC roles; however, most care is provided by general paediatric or rural services. This chapter presented the cases of Simon, Rangi and baby Tafotila to illustrate the PPC of NZ. The Māori cultural heritage has influenced the approach to care and, in particular, gifted Te Wa Aroha, a time or journey of love, to enable communication and development of advance care planning and care across the paediatric palliative care trajectory.

References

1. https://nzhistory.govt.nz/politics/treaty/the-treaty-in-brief
2. http://archive.stats.govt.nz/Census/2013-census/profile-and-summary-reports/quickstats-culture-identity/ethnic-groups-NZ.aspx
3. https://www.health.govt.nz/new-zealand-health-system/eligibility-publicly-funded-health-services/guide-eligibility-publicly-funded-health-services/new-zealand-residents
4. Fraser LK, Miller M, Hain R, et al. Rising national prevalence of life-limiting conditions in children in England. Pediatrics. 2012;129(4):e923–e29.
5. Bycroft K, Chang E, Drake R. Development of paediatric palliative care services in New Zealand (Aotearoa). In: Silberman M, editor. Palliative care. Perspectives, practices and impact on quality of life: a global view, vol. 1. New York: Nova Science Publication Inc; 2017.
6. Naylor W. National health needs assessment for palliative care, phase 1 report: assessment of palliative care need. Wellington: Cancer Control New Zealand; 2011.
7. Chang E, MacLeod R, Drake R. Characteristics influencing location of death for children with life-limiting illness. Arch Dis Child. 2013;98(6):419–24.
8. McLeod H. Trajectories of paediatric and congenital deaths in New Zealand. Presentation to paediatric palliative care network. Commissioned by Ministry of Health; 2018.
9. Ministry of Health. New Zealand palliative care glossary. Wellington: Ministry of Health; 2015.
10. World Health Organization. 2002. Definition of palliative care for children. https://www.who.int/cancer/palliative/definition/en/. Accessed 26 Jan 2019.
11. Ministry of Health. Guidance for integrated paediatric palliative care services in New Zealand: report to the Ministry of Health. Wellington: Ministry of Health; 2012.
12. Hynson JL. The child's journey: Transition from health to ill health. In: Goldman A, Hain R, Liben S, editors. Oxford textbook of palliative care for children. 2nd ed. Oxford: Oxford University Press; 2012. p. 13–22.
13. Goldman A. ABC of palliative care: special problems of children. BMJ. 1998 Jan 3;316(7124):49–52.
14. Starship. https://www.starship.org.nz/patients-parents-and-visitors/directory-of-services/Palliative-Care/. Accessed 26 Jan 2019.
15. Ministry of Health. Maori health models. Te Whare Tapa Whā: Mason Durie, 2015. Wellington, New Zealand, 2015. https://www.health.govt.nz/our-work/populations/maori-health/maori-health-models. Accessed 26 Jan 2019.
16. Chenery K. Family centered care: understanding our past. Nurs Praxis N Z. 2004;20(3):4–12.

17. Foster M, Whitehead L, Maybee P. Parents and healthcare professional perceptions of family centered care in hospital, in developed and developing countries: a review of the literature. Int J Nurs Stud. 2010;47:1184–93.
18. Paediatric HFAa, Society of New Zealand. Through the eyes of a child: a national review of paediatric speciality services. Wellington: Health Funding Authority and Paediatric Society; 1998.
19. Kuo DZ, Houtrow AJ, Arango P, Kuhlthau KA, Simmons JM, Neff JM. Family-centered care: current applications and future directions in pediatric healthcare. Matern Child Health J. 2012;16:297–305.
20. New Zealand Nurses Organisation. Neonatal palliative care for New Zealand Neonatal units. Comfort as a Model of Care Whakamariertia rite kit e tauria o te tiaki, 2015. Neonatal Nurses College Aotearoa 52p. https://www.nzno.org.nz/Portals/0/Files/Documents/Groups/Neonatal%20Nurses/2016-03%20Final%20Neonatal%20Palliative%20Care%20Nov%202015.pdf. Accessed 25 Jan 2019.
21. https://www.starship.org.nz/for-health-professionals/starship-clinical-guidelines/p/palliative-care-clinical-guidelines/#All
22. Feudtner C. The breath of hopes. N Engl J Med. 2009;361(24):2307.
23. Ministry of Health. Child Health Strategy Wellington 1998.
24. Bradford NK, Young J, Armfield NR, Herbert A, Smith AC. Home telehealth and paediatric palliative care: clinician perceptions of what is stopping us? BMC Palliat Care. 2014;13:29–39.
25. Mherekumombe MF. From inpatient to clinic to home to hospice and back: using the "Pop up" pediatric model of care. Children. 2018;5:55.
26. Oxford Dictionary. 2019. https://www.oxforddictionaries.com/. Accessed 20 Jan 2019.
27. Smith H. Giving hope to families in palliative care and the implications for practice. Nurs Child Young People. 2014;26(5):21–5.
28. Friedrichsdorf SJ, Bruera E. Delivering pediatric palliative care: from Denial, Palliphobia, Pallilalia, to Palliactive. Children. 2018;5:120.
29. Hill DL, Feudtner C. Gallagher MW, Lopez SJ, editors. Hope in the midst of terminal illness, The Oxford handbook of hope (Internet), vol. 2015: Oxford University Press. p. 190–206.
30. Feudtner C. Collaborative communication in pediatric palliative care: a foundation for problem solving and decision making. Pediatr Clin North Am. 54:583–607.
31. Larkin P. Communicating with children and their families during sensitive and challenging times. In: Lambert V, Long T, Kelleher D, editors. Communication skills for children's nurses. 1st ed. England: Open University Press; 2012. p. 90–104.
32. Kreicbergs U, Valdimarsdóttir U, Onelöv E, Henter J, Steineck G. Talking about death with children who have severe malignant disease. N Engl J Med. 2004;351(12):1175–86.
33. Te Wa Aroha/Advance Care Plan. Starship Child Health. Auckland 2018.
34. Muircroft W, McKimm J, William L, MacLeod R. A New Zealand perspective on palliative care for Māori. J Palliat Care. 2010;26(1):54–8.
35. Jaaniste T, Coombs S, Donnelly TJ, Kelk N, Beston D. Risk and resilience factors related to parental bereavement following the death of a child with a life-limiting condition. Children. 2017;4:96.
36. Skylight Trust NZ. https://www.skylight.org.nz/.

Perspectives on Hospice and Palliative Care in the United States

7

Cindy Tofthagen, Ann Guastella, and Jessica Latchman

Contents

7.1	Introduction and Background	105
7.2	Costs of Hospice Services: Policy and Payment	108
7.3	Ethical Issues in Hospice and Palliative Care	109
7.4	Current Trends in Hospice Care in the United States	110
	7.4.1 Integrative Therapies	111
	7.4.2 Telehospice	111
	7.4.3 Regulatory Issues	112
7.5	Current Trends in Palliative Care	114
	7.5.1 Comprehensive Assessment	115
	7.5.2 Community-Based Palliative Care	115
	7.5.3 Telemedicine	116
	7.5.4 Caregiver Support	116
	7.5.5 Advance Care Planning	117
7.6	Conclusions	117
References		118

7.1 Introduction and Background

The hospice movement in the United States (US) began in 1965 when Dame Cicely Saunders, a physician who began the first hospice in the United Kingdom, came to speak at Yale University about care of the dying [1]. Her talk captured the attention

---

C. Tofthagen (✉)
Mayo Clinic, Jacksonville, FL, USA
e-mail: tofthagen.cindy@mayo.edu

A. Guastella · J. Latchman
H. Lee Moffitt Cancer and Research Center, Tampa, FL, USA
e-mail: Ann.guastella@moffitt.org; Jessica.latchman@moffitt.org

© Springer Nature Switzerland AG 2019
L. Holtslander et al. (eds.), *Hospice Palliative Home Care and Bereavement Support*, https://doi.org/10.1007/978-3-030-19535-9_7

of Florence Wald, the Dean of the Yale School of Nursing, who went on to become the founder of the first hospice in the United States in 1974. In between those events, societal views of death and dying were influenced by the views of Dr. Elizabeth Kubler-Ross, who authored the best-selling book entitled *On Death and Dying*, based on over 500 interviews with individuals at the end of life [2]. In the book, she described five stages that terminally ill individuals often experience including denial, anger, bargaining, depression, and acceptance. *On Death and Dying* challenged the status quo of death in America by postulating that death should occur at home, rather than in a hospital and that individuals should have some control over the environment in which they die and the events that take place surrounding their death.

In the US, hospice care is a model for care with people facing a life-limiting illness [3]. Hospice care encompasses expert medical care, pain management, symptom management, and emotional and spiritual support which are personalized to the patient's needs, wishes, and goals. Hospice care is usually provided in the patient's home, but can include freestanding hospice facilities or hospice inpatient units, nursing homes, hospitals, nursing homes, and other long-term care facilities. Care is provided by an interdisciplinary team (Fig. 7.1) [3]. Services address the physical, psychological, and spiritual needs of the patient, as well as their family caregivers (Table 7.1). Hospice patients require different levels of care over the course of their disease and care is based on individual needs, however, ongoing involvement of family caregivers is also necessary.

Our culture was described as "death-denying" by Dr. Kubler-Ross in the 1970s [2]. Almost 50 years later, prolonging life by the use of medical technology has only increased. The majority of people still die in the hospital, often attached to machines to keep them alive. Botox, plastic surgery, and facial fillers promise a more youthful appearance but cannot stop the toll of time on the body. Our oldest and frailest citizens live in nursing homes and assisted living facilities, shielding the rest of the society from witnessing the realities of aging and death. To make the concept of hospice more palatable, some hospices dropped the word hospice from their name, replaced with more non-descript names that are less likely to evoke thoughts of death. Others added palliative care services and their name changed to include the term palliative care, again softening the blow that if you are referred to that agency, you are likely nearing the end of your life. Even some palliative care programs, in an effort to remove the stigma associated with the terminology, have changed their name to supportive care. These are just some of the examples of how as a society, we tend to avoid reminders of our own mortality.

Even with our attempts at denial, 88% of the Americans would prefer to die as comfortably as possible, at home, surrounded by loved ones [4]. Hospice is the primary avenue through which achievement of these goals can be accomplished. Hospice and palliative care has gained acceptance within the medical community and the public; however, misconceptions remain. Hospice may be perceived as a "last resort" after all other treatment options have been exhausted, a place you go to

7 Perspectives on Hospice and Palliative Care in the United States

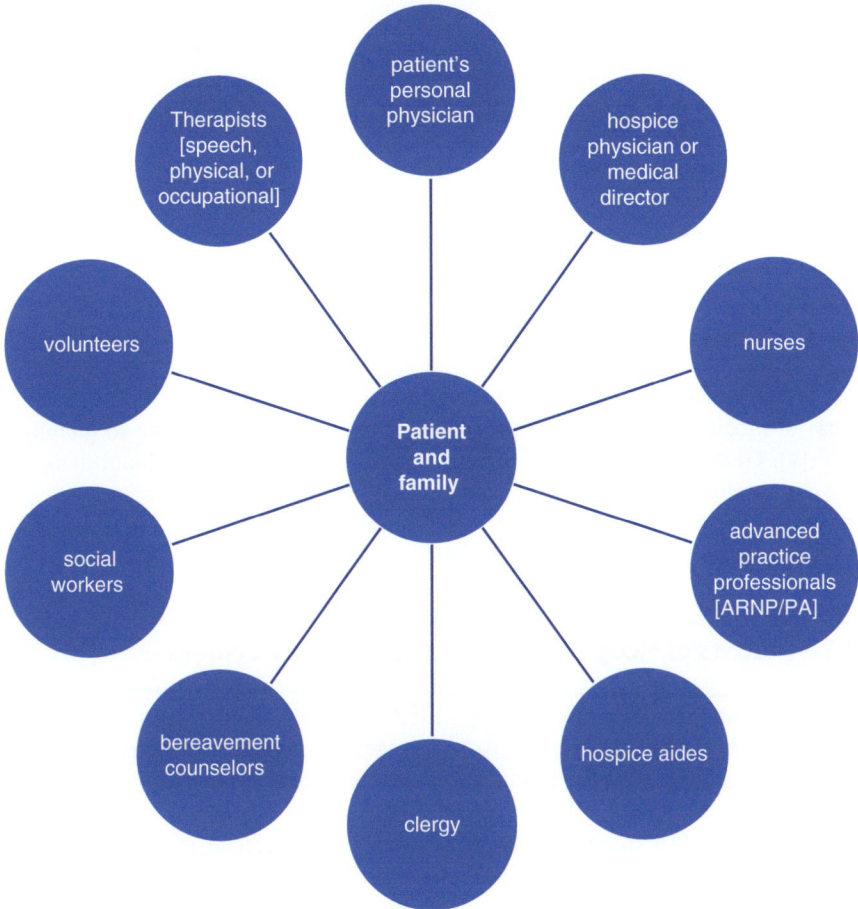

Fig. 7.1 Hospice interdisciplinary team [3]

Table 7.1 Functions of the hospice interdisciplinary team [3]

Manage pain and symptoms
Assist the patient and family members with emotional, psychosocial, and spiritual aspects of dying and provide medications and medical equipment associated with primary life-limiting illness
Instruct the family or significant other on how to care for the patient
Provide grief support and counseling prior to death
Make short-term inpatient care available when pain or symptoms become too difficult to manage at home, or the caregiver needs respite time
Deliver special services such as speech and physical therapy when needed
Provide grief support and counseling to surviving family or friends following death

die, or even a method to hasten death. Individuals may perceive that a referral to hospice is being made as a way to deny access to life-saving treatments or that hospice means "giving up" [4]. The public has even more misconceptions and lack of understanding when it comes to palliative care [5]. Over the last half a century, the hospice movement has shaped societal views, policy, and individual decision-making surrounding death. Yet, how we live is as fundamental to hospice care as how we die. Hospice has an emphasis on supporting quality of life and living each moment to the fullest [4]. Palliative care evolved from the hospice movement, starting in the 1980s. The Institute of Medicine (2015) defines palliative care as "care that provides relief from pain and other symptoms, that supports quality of life, and that is focused on patients with serious advanced illness and their families" ([7], p. 7). There is an emphasis on open communication and supporting autonomy in medical treatment decision-making [6]. Palliative care is one of the fastest-growing areas of medicine; yet, there is a shortage of clinicians with training in palliative care [7]. Given that 75% of Americans over 65 years of age have more than one chronic condition, with an aging population, the need for palliative care is expected to continue to grow [7]. This chapter will discuss the current and emerging practices for hospice and palliative care in the US.

7.2 Costs of Hospice Services: Policy and Payment

Hospice services are covered by Medicare, Medicaid, Veteran's Health Administration, and most private insurance. Medicare is by far the largest payer of hospice services through the Hospice Medicare benefit [7]. The Hospice Medicare benefit was established in 1983 to ensure Medicare patients access to high-quality end-of-life care [8]. To be eligible for hospice, two physicians must attest that an individual has less than 6 months to live. Once enrolled in hospice, Medicare pays a hospice organization a set daily rate to provide services. Daily rates for in-home care range from $150–191 per day based on the length of service. Less than 50% of eligible Medicare recipients ever receive hospice services. The Hospice Medicare benefit affords patient with four levels of care to meet their clinical needs: routine home care, general inpatient care, continuous home care, and inpatient respite care [3]. To ensure quality care and eliminate fraud, numerous regulatory and documentation standards must be met.

Hospice care is provided to the patient and family via a multidisciplinary team of healthcare professionals that typically include physicians, nurses, chaplains, social workers, therapists, home health aides, and bereavement counselors. Hospice care is holistic in nature, providing attention to physical, psychological, and spiritual needs. The vast majority of hospice services are provided in the patient's home. In the home setting, hospice provides care as needed, supporting the family to function as the primary caregivers, with the help and support of the hospice team.

Healthcare at the end of life, as is healthcare across the continuum, is fragmented [7]. A fee-for-service payment system encourages overutilization of care at the end of life by paying for diagnostic tests, expensive (even if futile) treatments, and hospitalizations while not providing payment for even the most essential services that would allow patients to remain at home, have pain and symptoms well managed, and receive assistance with basic human functions that illness and frailty have impaired. Healthcare costs during the last year of life typically exceed the costs for all other years of life combined [7]. Of the two million deaths that occur in the US each year, the majority do not involve hospice. For those who do not choose hospice, final days are often spent in the hospital or intensive care unit, which may not reflect the preferences of the individual or serve his/her needs.

Aggressive medical intervention is the default decision at the end of life. Individuals who wish to forgo aggressive intervention must express their needs for end-of-life care when they are physically and cognitively able [7]. Unfortunately, clinicians, patients, and family members are often hesitant to initiate conversations about end-of-life preferences. Advanced directives, including living wills and healthcare power of attorney, allow individuals to provide information about their preferences, however, two-thirds of Americans do not have an advanced directive [9].

Once enrolled in hospice, patients must typically forgo all treatments with a curative intent [10]. The necessity to stop all potentially curative treatment leads to delays in referral to hospice, especially among people with cancer, who often want to try every available treatment option, even if there is minimal chance for success. The current payment system for hospice has not kept up with rapid advancements in science that make new treatment options, like immunotherapy and targeted therapies for cancer treatment, which may provide palliation of symptoms and allow them to live a little longer with minimal impact on quality of life. In the face of metastatic cancer or heavy disease burden, patients should have the option of enrolling in hospice and receiving cancer treatment. Unfortunately, hospices cannot absorb the high cost of continued cancer treatment and the Hospice Medicare benefit is not enough to pay for these treatments. The current payment system creates an artificial barrier to early referral to hospice, resulting in a variety of unmet patient and caregiver needs at the end of life.

7.3   Ethical Issues in Hospice and Palliative Care

Ideally, palliative care should begin at the same time as diagnosis and treatment of a chronic, life-threatening illness. Patients often live longer when they receive early palliative care [11]. Early referral to hospice allows the patient and family to receive the most benefit, form trusting relationships with the care team, access a wide array of services, and provide maximum input regarding their wishes and preferences for treatment. The median length of service for people enrolled in hospice in 2016 was 24 days and 27.9% of hospice patients were enrolled for 7 days or less [3]. Late referrals mean patients and families may not have time to establish a trusting relationship with the hospice team, symptoms may not be optimally managed, and neither the patient nor their family fully benefit from hospice services.

Studies have consistently shown that patients who have palliative care introduced at onset of diagnosis tend to have better outcomes. Thus, more and more hospital systems have embedded palliative care into their treatment pathways as a way to offer patients more support, decrease cost and improve overall patient outcomes [12]. Many organizations including the American Society of Clinical Oncology (ASCO) have now recommended that palliative care be embedded with standard oncology care for patients with high symptom burden or metastatic disease. However, in many oncology settings, this continues to be a struggle as many oncologists introduce palliative care only when all other treatment options are exhausted [11]. Hence, patients tend to have worse outcomes than those who receive palliative care earlier on in their diagnosis [12].

Hospice and palliative care use varies based on race and ethnicity with Whites enrolling in hospice more often than all other races [13]. African Americans and Asians, although referred to hospice at similar rates, are least likely to enroll in hospice services. Hispanics and African Americans are less likely to have an advanced directive and more likely to prefer aggressive treatments at the end of life [13]. Some of the possible explanations include misperceptions, availability of family support, preferences for aggressive end-of-life treatment, and differences in clinician engagement in the end-of-life discussions. Religious and cultural considerations may also influence hospice utilization. Whether individuals choose to embrace hospice depends on knowledge, perceptions, and availability. End-of-life decision-making should be a focus of community education programs and engagement of racially and ethnically diverse populations in end-of-life decision-making. Further exploration of barriers to hospice and end-of-life care is essential to high-quality end-of-life care for all populations.

Autonomy is a guiding principle in the American healthcare system as well as the hospice movement. Few would dispute the statement that adults have the right to determine which types of available treatment to accept and to refuse. The principle of autonomy also applies to hospice and palliative care in that, given the certainty of a terminal illness, individuals have the right to autonomy regarding certain aspects of their death experience such as where they die and who is present [14]. This becomes controversial when it extends to having control of the timing of death. Three cases involving young women who were put on life support after sustaining life-threatening injuries and the ensuing legal battles to allow each of them to be removed from life support and die peacefully drew national attention. The cases of Karen Ann Quinlan, Nancy Cruzan, and Terri Schiavo influenced legislation and public opinion related to dying and also brought recognition to the importance of advanced directives [15].

7.4 Current Trends in Hospice Care in the United States

Hospice utilization has continued to grow over the last decade, resulting in an overburdened healthcare system. From 2016 to 2017, there was a 2.6% increase in hospice admissions, with a 1.3 million Medicare enrollees receiving hospice services

[16]. 47.5% of enrollees were over the age of 80 while only 13% of enrollees were younger than age 70. As we grow older, our Medicare population grows older which will significantly increase the number of hospice admissions. Our aging population is now seeing our first onslaught of baby boomers which will result in increased hospice utilization.

Hospice utilization may also be influenced by the increase in the number of for-profit hospices. From 2000 to 2017, the proportion of for-profit hospices jumped to 4400 hospices [16] and 67% of hospices that bill Medicare are for-profit hospices, while only 29% are not-for-profit and 3.9% are government owned [3]. The increase in for-profit hospices will lead to increased government spending and cost to Medicare.

7.4.1 Integrative Therapies

As our population ages and our baby boomers get closer to end of life, hospice care will continue to expand. We will likely see a trend toward the use of experiential and alternative therapies in hospice care, in addition to typical hospice services. Alternative and experiential therapies may include physical methods, psychological therapies, and complementary modalities. These modalities are likely to decrease the patient's perception of pain and symptoms, increase tolerance of pain and symptoms, increase adaptive behaviors, and decrease maladaptive behaviors. Physical methods include superficial heat and cold, massage, rehabilitative treatment, and therapeutic exercise. Psychological and behavioral methods include relaxation therapy, meditation, guided imagery, and energy-based healing meditation (therapeutic touch, healing touch, and reiki) [17, 18]. Complementary modalities include traditional Chinese medicine, hypnosis, acupuncture, and Qigong [18, 19].

7.4.2 Telehospice

The emerging trend of telemedicine will extend into hospice care. In hospice, this is referred to as telehospice. Telehospice may be delivered via an I-Pad, smartphone, or home computer with web conferencing software installed, so the physician or advanced practice professional or on-call nurse can communicate remotely with the patient and caregiver [20]. Communication is of the essence when there is a crisis and pain or symptoms are out of control. A family member or caregiver can be talked through simple procedures or administration of additional medications when a patient is in crisis via telehospice. Staff in a nursing home caring for hospice patient can easily use telehospice to reach an on-call physician. The tools for telehospice may include: (1) individual measurement devices—blood pressure cuffs, blood–glucose meters, and other peripheral devices for tracking patients' individual measurements; (2) telehealth workstations—full-scale workstations which can transmit a full work-up of patient physiologic parameters; (3) videophones—telephones that have the capability to allow patients/caregivers and clinicians to see each other and speak directly to each other; and (4) pre-programmed devices—pain medication, hydration, and nutrition can be managed by ambulatory infusion pump, which may not require an in-person professional visit [20]. Telehospice will provide enhanced communication during this time; however, it is unlikely to replace home visits. It will enable hospice staff and physicians to provide care at end of life to those who are out of reach of an actual hospice. This will allow staff to virtually visit seriously ill patients, thereby improving comfort and quality at end of life. It will also be a cost saving measure and benefit to those patients who live in rural and remote areas.

7.4.3 Regulatory Issues

Regulatory scrutiny of hospice compliance will continue with a focus on the following areas: hospice general inpatient care (GIP); live discharges; documentation of terminal illness; and Medicare D prescription claims [3, 21]. In 2012, some hospices billed one-third of GIP stays inappropriately, costing Medicare $268 million [22]. Hospice general inpatient care is used for pain control or symptom management that cannot be managed in other settings such as home or care given in assisted living facilities. Use of the hospice general inpatient care is intended to be short-term and is the second most expensive level of care [22]. General inpatient care can be provided in three settings: (1) Medicare-certified hospice inpatient unit; (2) hospital; or, (3) skilled nursing facility [22]. The Centers for Medicare and Medicaid Services (CMS) staff will review cases for misuse of this level of care, with particular attention paid to care being billed for but not provided, long length of stay, and beneficiaries receiving care unnecessarily [22]. The National Hospice and Palliative Care Organization made the following recommendations to the Centers for Medicare and Medicaid Services: (1) increase its oversight of hospice GIP claims and review Part D payments for drugs for hospice beneficiaries; (2) ensure that the physician is involved in the decision to use GIP; (3) conduct prepayment reviews for lengthy GIP stays; (4) ensure that hospices meet care planning requirements; (5) establish additional remedies for poor hospice performances; and (6) follow up on inappropriate GIP stays [22]. This will allow patients and providers to obtain care that is feasible and more patient-centric and sustainable.

Live discharges are defined as the number of discharges of patients from hospice care over a fiscal year. The Centers for Medicare and Medicaid noted in 2017 that hospices at the 95th percentile discharged 47.6% of their patients alive [22]. The increase in live discharges suggests that patients are being admitted to hospice inappropriately and that they do not have a six-month prognosis for accessing the Hospice Medicare benefit. The use of prognostic indicators remains a challenge for providers in hospice. Therefore, ongoing education by The Academy of Hospice and Palliative Medicine through its annual educational conferences and via other vehicles like an online self-assessment study tool focused on hospice regulatory compliance and publication of the Hospice Medical Director Manual is imperative. These avenues will improve the quality and consistency of the practice of hospice medicine and the care provided by hospices.

Another area of concern seems to be documentation. Documentation of terminal illness will continue to be reviewed by the Centers for Medicare & Medicaid Services [21, 22]. Use of prognostic indicators, the Hospice Medicare physician recertification process, and face-to-face visits to confirm that the patient is appropriate for hospice care remain pivotal. Disease prognostic indicators provide guidelines for hospice physicians, nurse practitioners, and nurses to determine appropriateness for hospice care. Face-to-face visits allow the hospice physician or nurse practitioner to actually visit and assess the patient to make sure that they remain appropriate for hospice care. Documentation by all providers should be comprehensive and show that the patient remains appropriate for hospice care.

Review of Medicare D prescriptions that should have been covered by hospice will also be examined [21, 22]. For patients under Hospice Medicare or Medicaid, hospice programs are required to provide medications and biologicals related to palliation and management of the terminal illness defined in the hospice plan of care. Each hospice is paid by Medicare daily for providing hospice care, regardless of the amount of care given. It was noted in 2012 by the Office of the Inspector General (OIG) that there were situations in which Medicare was paying twice for prescription drugs for hospice beneficiaries. Part D Medicare payments for non-hospice drugs received by hospice beneficiaries during hospice election were $325 million in 2011 compared to $380 million in 2017 [23]. The Office of the Inspector General worked with the National Hospice and Palliative Care Organization to identify four common categories of prescription drugs used to treat symptoms with advanced disease. These categories include anti-nauseants, laxatives, analgesics, and antianxiety drugs and these categories should be covered under the hospice Medicare benefit. In some instances, one or more of these categories may be unrelated to the terminal illness and Part D benefit is responsible. Therefore, any care associated with the primary diagnosis is covered under the Hospice Medicare A benefit.

With the increase in patients requiring palliative care at end of life, there will be an increased need for providers to be trained in palliative care and for new models of providing end-of-life care to be developed. Additional training in palliative care will need to be provided to oncologists and hematologists, general practitioners, geriatric physicians, and nurses [24]. This suggests that palliative care fellowships for physicians and specific educational offerings to physicians and nurses will likely increase to meet the needs of our aging population.

Another trend affecting hospice care is more focus on advance directives [21]. Advance directives will take on increasing importance for patients. Patients will want to dictate how they wish to face the end of life. Legislators and healthcare providers continue to raise awareness of the importance of placing advance directives.

Our changing demographics, in terms of an aging population, will affect how hospices in the United States provide services. Baby boomers, those born between 1946 and 1964 following World War II, represent 29% of the population that began reaching retirement age in 2011. Baby boomers have fewer children and are more mobile than their parents. They will be less likely to have the assistance of family at end of life. This may suggest the need for telehospice, group living at end of life, and palliative care prior to hospice enrollment. For hospices in the United States, this may provide a shift to enrolling patients in a palliative care arm prior to end-of-life care with hospice care.

7.5 Current Trends in Palliative Care

In the US, palliative care is defined as medical care delivered by a healthcare trained specialist that focuses primarily on symptom management, and improving quality of life to patients with any serious, chronic, or life-threatening illnesses [25]. The interdisciplinary team is similar to a hospice multidisciplinary team (Fig. 7.1). The focus is on addressing physical, psychosocial, spiritual, and existential pain [26]. As the population ages, and people experience multiple chronic conditions and frailty, the need for palliative care specialist and creative ways of providing services will increase.

Palliative care differs from hospice in that it does not solely focus on end of life, but can be initiated at any stage of the disease and at any time during the disease trajectory. In fact, it can be used in conjunction with curative treatment. It focuses on a wide spectrum of disease including, cancer, chronic obstructive pulmonary disease (COPD), congestive heart failure, kidney disease, end-stage liver disease, HIV/AIDS, as well as many other diseases [27].

Over the past decade, palliative care has become an emergent field. The need for palliative care specialist and programs throughout the United States has and continues to rise due to a growing need. As the average life expectancy increases and diseases become more chronic in nature, many patients will require palliative care services [11]. The Center to Advance Palliative Care reported in 2018 that palliative care in US hospitals has risen by 178% from 2000 to 2016 [12]. Studies project that the dominant illness for which palliative care will be needed is dementia and cancer [24].

If palliative care needs continue to rise at this alarming rate, healthcare organizations will require more specialty trained palliative care professionals to provide care for these complex patients. This would mean more specialized training programs for nurses and physicians, as well as training for the non-specialist in the community who delivers daily palliative care to patients. Healthcare systems would need more infrastructure and added investment in palliative care programs [24].

According to the National Consensus Project Clinical Practice Guidelines for Quality Palliative care (NCP) fourth edition, two key areas of focus continues to be providing early access to palliative care despite patient's setting, diagnosis, age, or prognosis. The second area of focus is empowering clinicians to introduce palliative care early on in the disease trajectory [26]. In addition to this, the NCP recently added five themes which include; a comprehensive assessment; family/caregiver assessment, support, and education; care coordination during transitions; and culturally inclusive care [26]. The goal is to improve patient outcomes by introducing palliative care early on. Many studies continue to illustrate that palliative care is often introduced too late during the course of the disease, limiting its full benefits to many patients [11].

7.5.1 Comprehensive Assessment

In order to be fully comprehensive, a palliative care assessment should include physical, psychosocial, spiritual, and cultural aspects of care. The team should be interdisciplinary in nature and be delivered by clinicians and palliative care specialist who can provide optimal care in these domains. The team may include physicians, nurses, advanced practice professionals, nurses, chaplains, and social workers, each focusing on their specialized area of care with the intent to care for the patient holistically. The team should also collaborate with patient and caregivers to develop a treatment plan focused on patients' goals, maximizing functionality, and optimizing the quality of life [26]. The palliative care team should also perform continuous assessment and reassessment of the patient's goals and preferences, since they may change over time. Therefore, the care plan must be updated regularly to reflect the current objectives desired by patients and families, in addition to maintaining care focused on optimizing patient outcomes [26].

Providing culturally sensitive care is also a key focus in the current guidelines. The palliative care team must therefore be respectful of all individuals despite race, gender, or ethnicity. By honoring patients' values, beliefs, and traditions, the palliative care team can provide a more comprehensive approach to care. Patients and families can feel more supported and respected, improving the overall quality of life [26].

7.5.2 Community-Based Palliative Care

Community-based palliative care continues to be a challenge and major focus; essentially palliative care services should be delivered to patients wherever they may be receiving care. This can include, but not limited to, the patients home, oncology centers and clinics, nursing homes and skilled nursing facilities, physicians' offices, and outpatient clinics [28]. The goal of palliative care is to meet the needs and challenges of patients despite where their care setting might be. Patients would have optimal symptom, and pain management, as well as psychosocial support which would improve continuity and coordination of care as well as reduce expenditures. Community palliative care specialists can prevent unnecessary hospitalizations, reduce readmission rates, improve 30-day mortality, and decrease overutilization of costly procedures and interventions, thereby, improving overall patient satisfaction and outcomes [28].

However, although community-based palliative care has numerous benefits, the major hurdle continues to be cost. These programs will require a substantial investment, strong infrastructure as well as powerful outreach and marketing if implemented. Programs would need to show their effectiveness by tracking metrics pertaining to the cost of care, mortality rates, and admission and readmission rates if they are to be successful [28].

7.5.3 Telemedicine

Telemedicine in yet another means of delivering quality palliative and supportive care services to patients who critically need it. Although in its infancy, many believe telemedicine can revolutionize the healthcare field. It is defined as the avenue by which patients can receive medical care directly in their home via video communication [29]. The Department of Health and Human Services estimates that more than 60% of all medical facilities and 40–50% of all hospitals in the United States currently use some form of telemedicine, making it a fast-growing field. As the possibilities are limitless, access is easy and its grasp is far-reaching, telemedicine can be an invaluable resource in giving patients improved and increased access to care [29]. This would be especially beneficial to those who have to travel far distances to receive care and for those who are confined to their homes due to illness. For many others, convenience and access are essential since telemedicine eliminates the need to travel or take time out from work to see a specialist. This would improve health promotion and disease prevention, as well as improve comfort, and patient and family satisfaction [29].

Despite its potential benefits to palliative care, there are numerous issues regarding telemedicine which still need to be addressed. For many settings, new infrastructure and equipment would be needed. Staff will have to be trained and new policies and guidelines regarding patient privacy issues and reimbursement policies may be a hindrance [29]. Another issue may be user related, as many elderly and frail patients may not be able to use the technology, although older adults are also embracing technology. However, as more research is done and technology continues to advance, telemedicine may improve access to care. There remain significant opportunities to explore the intersection of palliative care and telemedicine. If actualized, telehealth can enhance clinical care, patient satisfaction and improve quality of life for many suffering from chronic and serious illnesses [29].

7.5.4 Caregiver Support

In addition to patients, palliative care also focuses on the caregiver and family. Since the majority of patient care is done by caregivers, many caregivers can experience caregiver burnout if not supported and educated appropriately [11]. Caregiver burnout encompasses emotional, psychological, and physical stressors such as fatigue, stress, anxiety, and depression. Caregivers who suffer from these tend to have high mortality rates [11]. However, for patients and families who have early onset palliative care, many caregivers tend to be more prepared and less stressed in their role.

They have a better knowledge of symptom management at home and tend to feel more supported in caring for their loved ones [30]. Thus, palliative care can provide for a more comprehensive caregiving experience and patients and loved ones tend to have better outcomes.

7.5.5 Advance Care Planning

Advance care planning continues to be another important aspect of care. It is the process by which patients can delineate their wishes and preferences regarding future medical care while still being able to make medical decisions about treatment choices. Directives are only implemented when a patient loses the ability to make medical decisions on their own. Essentially, they are legal documents directing medical care. The goal of advance care planning is to respect patients' values and beliefs regardless of the disease state [31]. However, patients and families require education and guidance by their healthcare team, which should include the palliative care, in making medically appropriate decisions which are documented in their advance directives. It is the goal of the palliative care team to have advance care directives on all patients in order to provide comprehensive care aligned with patients' goals [26]. The goal is to honor patient's wishes and preferences as well as decisions made by their surrogates and proxies. However, as the overall medical course of the patient changes, advance care planning should be readdressed with the continued focus remaining on honoring patients' preferences. It is also important to note that they can be revoked or changed at any time the patient wishes [31].

7.6 Conclusions

Over the last half-century, hospice and palliative care have been integrated into standard medical practice and palliative care has been delineated as a unique medical specialty with its own science and body of knowledge. In spite of the acceptance within the medical community, public misperceptions, and lack of acceptance of death as a natural phase of life persist. Laws are increasingly in support of the rights of individuals to make their own end-of-life decisions and for those decisions to be honored. Conversations related to end-of-life preferences are more likely to occur between family members than between individuals and their healthcare team.

The need for hospice and palliative care is increasing and will continue to do so as the population ages and chronic health conditions multiply. Palliative care services, which are largely facility based, will need to move into community settings and more professionals will need to develop skills and knowledge to provide palliative care. Telehealth, community palliative care programs, and expanding family caregiver support offer potential to efficiently increase services to meet future needs.

References

1. National Hospice and Palliative Care Organization. History of Hospice Care 2016. https://www.nhpco.org/history-hospice-care.
2. Kubler-Ross E, Wessler S, Avioli LV. On death and dying. JAMA. 1972;221(2):174–9.
3. National Hospice and Palliative Care Organization. Facts and figures: hospice care in America. Alexandria, Virginia: NHPCO; 2018.
4. National Hospice and Palliative Care Organization. Key Hospice Messages n.d. https://www.nhpco.org/press-room/key-hospice-messages.
5. Shalev A, Phongtankuel V, Kozlov E, Shen MJ, Adelman RD, Reid MC. Awareness and misperceptions of hospice and palliative care: a population-based survey study. Am J Hosp Palliat Care. 2018;35(3):431–9.
6. May P, Normand C, Cassel JB, Del Fabbro E, Fine RL, Menz R, et al. Economics of palliative care for hospitalized adults with serious illness: a meta-analysis. JAMA Intern Med. 2018;178(6):820–9.
7. Institute of Medicine. Dying in America: improving quality and honoring individual preferences near the end of life, vol. 638. Washington, DC: The National Academies Press; 2015.
8. National Hospice and Palliative Care Organization. The hospice Medicare benefit. Alexandria, Virginia: NHPCO; 2015. https://www.nhpco.org/sites/default/files/public/communications/Outreach/The_Medicare_Hospice_Benefit.pdf
9. Yadav K, Gabler N, Cooney E, Kent S, Kim J, Herbst N, et al. Approximately one in three US adults completes any type of advance directive for end-of-life care. Health Aff (Millwood). 2017;36(7):1244–51.
10. Cagle JG, Van Dussen DJ, Culler KL, Carrion I, Hong S, Guralnik J, et al. Knowledge about hospice: exploring misconceptions, attitudes, and preferences for care. Am J Hosp Palliat Care. 2016;33(1):27–33.
11. Bakitas MA, Tosteson TD, Li Z, Lyons KD, Hull JG, Li Z, et al. Early versus delayed initiation of concurrent palliative oncology care: patient outcomes in the ENABLE III randomized controlled trial. J Clin Oncol. 2015;33(13):1438–45.
12. Center to Advance Palliative Care. Palliative Care Continues Its Annual Growth Trend, According to Latest Center to Advance Palliative Care Analysis. 2018. https://www.capc.org/about/press-media/press-releases/2018-2-28/palliative-care-continues-its-annual-growth-trend-according-latest-center-advance-palliative-care-analysis/.
13. LoPresti MA, Dement F, Gold HT. End-of-life care for people with Cancer from ethnic minority groups: a systematic review. Am J Hosp Palliat Care. 2016;33(3):291–305.
14. McCormick AJ. Self-determination, the right to die, and culture: a literature review. Soc Work. 2011;56(2):119–28.
15. Fine RL. From Quinlan to Schiavo: medical, ethical, and legal issues in severe brain injury. Proc (Bayl Univ Med Cent). 2005;18(4):303–10.
16. Baxter A (2018) Top payment scrutiny areas in hospice care. https://homehealthcarenews.com/2018/05/top-payment-scrutiny-areas-in-hospice-care/.
17. Burhenn P, Olausson J, Villegas G, Kravits K. Guided imagery for pain control. Clin J Oncol Nurs. 2014;18(5):501–3.
18. Running A, Turnbeaugh E. Oncology pain and complementary therapy. Clin J Oncol Nurs. 2011;15(4):374–9.
19. Hopkins Hollis AS. Acupuncture as a treatment modality for the management of cancer pain: the state of the science. Oncol Nurs Forum. 2010;37(5):E344–8.
20. Castro F (2017) Telemedicine and hospice care, what is telehospice? https://athenetelehealth.com/telemedicine-hospice-care-telehospice/.
21. The Watershed Group (2018) 5 trends to watch in hospice in 2018. http://www.thewatershed-group.com/5-trends-to-watch-in-hospice-in-2018/.
22. National Hospice and Palliative Care Organization. Scrutiny about hospice general inpatient care: information for providers. Alexandria, Virginia: NHPCO; 2017.

23. American Academy of Hospice and Palliative Medicine. Medicare program; FY 2019 hospice wage index and payment rate update and hospice quality reporting requirements. Final rule. Fed Regist. 2018;83(151):38622–55.
24. Etkind SN, Bone AE, Gomes B, Lovell N, Evans CJ, Higginson IJ, et al. How many people will need palliative care in 2040? Past trends, future projections, and implications for services. BMC Med. 2017;15(1):102.
25. Murray SA, Kendall M, Mitchell G, Moine S, Amblas-Novellas J, Boyd K. Palliative care from diagnosis to death. BMJ. 2017;356:j878.
26. Ferrell BR, Twaddle ML, Melnick A, Meier DE. National Consensus Project Clinical Practice Guidelines for quality palliative care guidelines, 4th edition. J Palliat Med. 2018;
27. Kaplan B. Comfort care for cancer patients: exploring distinctions between hospice care and palliative care. Oncol Nur Adv. 2010:42–3.
28. Santa-Emma P, Thomas N, Barclay J, Blackhall L. Current trends in palliative care: a briefing from the palliative care leadership centers. Charlottesville: PCLC at University of Virginia Health System; 2017.
29. Tuckson RV, Edmunds M, Hodgkins ML. Telehealth. N Engl J Med. 2017;377(16):1585–92.
30. Gomes B. Palliative care: if it makes a difference, why wait. J Clin Oncol. 2015;33(13):1420–1.
31. Sudore RL, Lum HD, You JJ, Hanson LC, Meier DE, Pantilat SZ, et al. Defining advance care planning for adults: a consensus definition from a multidisciplinary Delphi panel. J Pain Symptom Manag. 2017;53(5):821–32.

Global Perspectives: Palliative Care Around the World

8

Mary Ellen Walker

Contents

8.1	Palliative Care Defined..	122
8.2	Global Palliative Care Needs and Access...	123
	8.2.1 High-Income Countries..	124
	8.2.2 Low- and Middle-Income Countries...	124
	8.2.3 Children..	124
8.3	Barriers to Palliative Care Implementation..	125
	8.3.1 Opioid Accessibility..	125
	8.3.2 Policy Challenges...	126
	8.3.3 Funding Challenges..	126
8.4	Palliative Care as an Ethical Responsibility...	127
8.5	The Palliative Care Model...	128
	8.5.1 Multidisciplinary Teams...	128
	8.5.2 Palliative Care Services..	129
	8.5.3 Palliative Care Funding..	130
	8.5.4 Palliative Care Policies...	131
	8.5.5 Palliative Care Awareness...	131
8.6	Palliative Care Success Stories..	132
8.7	Nursing Considerations...	132
	8.7.1 Practice Implications...	133
	8.7.2 Education Implications..	134
	8.7.3 Research Implications...	134
8.8	Conclusion...	135
References...		135

M. E. Walker (✉)
College of Nursing, University of Saskatchewan, Saskatoon, SK, Canada
e-mail: mew513@mail.usask.ca

© Springer Nature Switzerland AG 2019
L. Holtslander et al. (eds.), *Hospice Palliative Home Care and Bereavement Support*, https://doi.org/10.1007/978-3-030-19535-9_8

No matter where in the world one lives, death is an experience that touches everyone. Palliative care addresses physical, psychosocial, and spiritual suffering that patients often experience with terminal health conditions [1]. However, around the world, countries vary in the ways in which people would like to be cared for at the end of their lives and the access they have to that care. Although countries all over the world need to improve access to palliative care, the biggest gaps in access to palliative care are to people in low and middle-income countries (LMICs) countries and children [1]. These gaps in palliative care accessibility are a result of challenging sociopolitical systems [2] and a lack of palliative care policy, education, medication availability, funding, and implementation [3]. However, nurses and other health professionals have an ethical responsibility to provide the relief of suffering that palliative care provides [4]. Palliative care can be successfully provided in a variety of contexts with policies and funding that provide multidisciplinary teams, opioid availability, and increased awareness of palliative care's importance. Nurses can specifically address these global palliative care issues through practice, education, and research that show sensitivity to diversity, addresses gaps in care, and increases public awareness. Nurses have a significant role to play in alleviating global suffering through palliative care.

8.1 Palliative Care Defined

All over the world, people suffer from pain and other symptoms of incurable health conditions. Relief from this suffering is a human right, including access to palliative care services that address unnecessary suffering [2, 3, 5, 6]. Palliative care aims to improve quality of life for patients with life-threatening conditions through active, compassionate care that prevents and relieves suffering and promotes living life to its fullest potential [1, 5, 7, 8]. Relief is addressed with early identification; assessment; treatment of physical, psychosocial, and spiritual suffering; and supporting families [1, 5, 7, 9]. Palliative care can be given alongside curative treatments [1, 5] and should be practiced wherever people are dying [10]. The palliative care approach regards death as a normal process, does not hasten or postpone death, supports patients to live actively, and helps families cope during illness and bereavement [1]. These palliative care characteristics make it a holistic and adaptable model of care.

Palliative care is meant to address the care needs of a variety of people at the end of life. However, hospice and palliative care have historically focused on cancer, although most children and adults who need palliative care have noncommunicable, nonmalignant conditions [1, 3, 9]. However, there has been increased awareness that palliative care needs to address chronic diseases [1]. In fact, 93% of palliative care need is generated from noncommunicable disease, yet only 37% of countries have national policies for noncommunicable disease that include palliative care, and palliative care is least likely to have funding compared with other noncommunicable services [4]. It is important to recognize the diversity of palliative care patients in relation to the diseases from which they suffer. To see a list of the common diseases that cause people to require palliative care, *see* Table 8.1.

Table 8.1 Common diseases requiring palliative care for children and adults

Common diseases requiring palliative care	
Children	Adults
Cancer	Alzheimer's and other dementias
Cardiovascular disease	Cancer
Congenital anomalies	Cardiovascular disease
Drug-resistant tuberculosis	Cerebrovascular disease
Endocrine, blood, and immune disorders	Chronic lung disease
HIV/AIDS	Diabetes
Kidney disease	Drug-resistant tuberculosis
Liver cirrhosis	HIV/AIDS
Meningitis	Liver cirrhosis
Neonatal conditions	Multiple sclerosis
Neurologic disorders	Neurodegenerative disorders
Protein energy malnutrition	Parkinson's disease
[1, 3, 13]	Renal failure
	Rheumatoid arthritis
	[1, 9]

8.2 Global Palliative Care Needs and Access

Palliative care is in high demand. Every year, about 20 million people need end-of-life palliative care, of which six percent (1.2 million) are children [1, 2]. Approximately, 37.4% of all deaths require palliative care [1, 4], but less than 10% of adults who need palliative care have access to it [11]. Estimates of the number of people needing palliative care do not include caregivers, the bereaved, orphans, or vulnerable children [1]. It is expected that 12 or more people are emotionally affected with each death, indicating that there is a great need to care for bereaved friends and family [10]. Palliative care is underdeveloped with inadequate access worldwide [1], except a few high-income countries [4, 6]. As of 2014, there were 16,000 hospice or palliative care service units worldwide, and in 2011, only 136 of 234 countries had one or more hospice-palliative care services [1]. Furthermore, only eight countries had integrated palliative care into their health systems [1]. These statistics represent the global shortage of palliative care services.

Although palliative care services are needed throughout the world, palliative care needs and access vary by region and income category [1, 12]. Countries in Europe, Asia-Pacific, and North American regions have high levels of government support for palliative care [11]. However, many central and eastern European countries only have localized palliative care services [6]. Interestingly, palliative care is only beginning to develop in much of the Islamic world [7]. However, even some top-ranked countries struggle to provide palliative care to all [11]. For example, the United Kingdom (UK) has been rated as having the best palliative care services in the world, with comprehensive national palliative care policies, integration of palliative care into the health system, and a strong hospice system [11]. However, the UK is still not providing palliative care to everyone who needs it [11]. The UK example is evidence that even high-income countries have challenges in meeting the demand for palliative care.

8.2.1 High-Income Countries

High-income countries experience challenges in providing palliative care, but they have shown some advantages over LMICs. Rich nations tend to have the best quality palliative care services [11]. Country income level is a strong indicator of palliative care quality and availability [4, 11]. In fact, there is a large country-income gradient for palliative care funding, opioid availability, and integration of palliative services with primary health services [4]. Almost all countries that have integrated palliative care services into their health systems are high-income countries from Western Europe [6]. Most high-income countries have made progress in developing their palliative care systems.

8.2.2 Low- and Middle-Income Countries

LMICs have many challenges in relation to developing and implementing palliative care services. Poor people all over the world have limited access to palliative care, but most of these people live in LMICs [8]. It is estimated that 80% of the need for palliative care is in LMICs [1, 4, 5, 8, 13]. Despite the high need, there is a lack of access to palliative care in LMICs [5, 14, 15], including pain management [8, 11]. The lack of access in LMICs may be due to struggling healthcare systems, a lack of economic and human resources, low educational levels and an inability to provide specialized palliative care education, and lack of access to opioids [3, 7, 14]. People in LMICs experience preventable, premature deaths due to infection and poverty-associated diseases [8]. Furthermore, constrained health systems often have issues of patients presenting late in their disease and under-diagnosis with limited curative therapies, increasing the need for palliative care [3]. In addition, services tend to be based in urban areas [12]. Also, LMICs have high human immunodeficiency virus/acquired immune deficiency syndrome (HIV/AIDS) rates and greater mortality related to malignancies [3]. These issues have made people in LMICs particularly vulnerable to lack of access to palliative care.

8.2.3 Children

Children are another vulnerable group that lacks access to palliative care. Approximately, 98% of all children in need of palliative care are from LMICs [1, 8, 14]. In fact, most young people who need palliative care live in LMICs where curative treatment is less available [3, 14], while most pediatric palliative care is provided in high-income countries [1, 3]. Pediatric palliative care should be available regardless of where a child lives [1], yet 65.6% of countries have no known children's palliative care [3, 14]. In countries with pediatric palliative care, services vary regionally in quality and access [14]. Globally, of the children who need palliative care, 49% live in Africa, 24% live in South East Asia, and 12% live in the East Mediterranean [1]. These regional disparities in pediatric palliative care demand and access indicate a need to improve pediatric palliative care access.

Clearly, there are gaps in access to pediatric palliative care services [13]. These gaps may be due to the important differences between adult and pediatric palliative care. These differences include communication, levels of understanding, assent and consent ethical issues, pharmacokinetics and dynamics in children, transitions into adolescence and adulthood, the people involved with a child's care, and differing conditions requiring palliative care [3]. The conditions that cause pediatric patients to access palliative care are often different from adults, causing the need for pediatric palliative care services to range from hours to years, and into adulthood. Furthermore, the Global Atlas of Palliative Care [1] definition for pediatric palliative care states that palliative care for children should start at the time of diagnosis, but does not make the same recommendation for adults. Pediatric palliative care also has a stronger emphasis on involving the family and gives more attention to life stage development. However, pediatric palliative care is not considered a specialty in some countries, but instead, falls under adult care [14]. In many LMICs, there is a lack of attention children's palliative care education, clinical practice, funding, and research, and palliative care focuses on specific diseases, like HIV and cancer [3]. In fact, children are less likely to receive palliative care than adults [13], and most global efforts directed at children are to reduce mortality [13]. These specific challenges to pediatric palliative care are important to address and are compounded by the barriers to implementing adult palliative care.

8.3 Barriers to Palliative Care Implementation

There are many barriers that are preventing patients from accessing appropriate palliative care. A major barrier to increasing palliative care is the global bias toward treatments that extend life [8]. It is often challenging for sociopolitical systems to allocate money toward health challenges that result in death, especially in LMICs [2]. Furthermore, many people fear death and some medical professionals avoid telling patients about a death prognosis [1, 3]. These factors make the shortage of specialized palliative care professionals important to address [3, 7]. Furthermore, LMICs have additional barriers where palliative care policy, education, medication availability, funding, and implementation are lacking [3].

8.3.1 Opioid Accessibility

There are also many obstacles to treating pain with opioids. Opioids are unavailable to 75% to 80% of the world's population [1, 13]. Australia, New Zealand, Canada, the United States, and European countries account for 90% of opioid consumption [1]. Furthermore, oral morphine is available in less than 20% of pharmacies in the African, East Mediterranean, and South East Asian regions [4]. Restrictive policies in many countries have been implemented to prevent opioid misuse [1, 7, 8, 11]. To address these restrictive policies, human rights organizations have called for the balance of medical use and prevention of illicit use [1]. In addition, there is a lack of supply and distribution systems, especially in rural areas, and the pharmaceutical industry promotes more expensive drugs [1]. Furthermore, misinformation may have turned public attitudes against using opioids for pain control [7, 8]. Adding to the problem, healthcare professionals in many countries are not trained to prescribe, dispense, or provide care to those who need opioids [1, 11]. To provide high-quality palliative care, opioids need to be accessible to patients in hospital and communities [4, 11]. Barriers to opioid access must be addressed to provide optimal palliative care.

8.3.2 Policy Challenges

Lack of palliative care policies in countries all over the world has impacted the ability to provide quality palliative care. More attention needs to be paid to palliative care policy, especially as it related to education and financial support for palliative care [4, 5, 15]. These issues may have hindered countries in increasing access to palliative care and working on legislation that impacts opioid availability [5]. However, lack of research and evidence about palliative care, especially for children, makes policies and guidelines difficult to develop [3]. These challenges are compounded by palliative care not being integrated into many counties' health systems [3, 5]. Policies are an important step in guiding health systems and the health professionals who work in them to address palliative care.

8.3.3 Funding Challenges

Another challenge to optimal palliative care implementation is its funding context. Global palliative care operates in a resource-constrained context where it competes with health technologies, treatment options, complex policy environment, and demand for evidence-based healthcare [16]. Governments and healthcare systems have focused on life-sustaining measures and neglected the suffering of palliative patients [15]. Therefore, resources for palliative care limited worldwide [1, 4]. Even in developed countries like the UK and Canada, half of the palliative funding is from private sources [4]. Funding is often a mix of charity, public, and private sources, which can cause unclear responsibilities, administrative complexity, and unclear sustainability [12]. Furthermore, funding is challenged by corruption [10, 12]. Corruption harms palliative care systems by reducing effectiveness and equity of services, disrupting sustainable growth, degrading ethical practices, and causing donor fatigue [10]. Implementing sustainable funding is a crucial step in providing palliative care.

8.4 Palliative Care as an Ethical Responsibility

Palliative care is an ethical responsibility [4]. Knual et al. [8] believe that this global lack of access to palliative care is a medical, public health, and moral failing. The United Nations Committee on Economic, Social, and Cultural Rights states that it is critical to provide care for chronically ill and terminally ill people, sparing them from avoidable pain and allowing them to die with dignity [1]. The global community has the responsibility to close this gap to relieve pain and suffering, especially for populations that have been largely ignored, such as children, vulnerable populations, or those living through humanitarian crises [8]. To address these shortcomings of palliative care, nurses and other health professionals need to focus on relief of suffering, bringing palliative care to those with the least resources, integrating palliative care into healthcare systems, and increasing quality of life [1].

To make palliative care accessible to those who need it, the system must be culturally, ethically, and socioeconomically appropriate [1]. Healthcare in high-income countries is based on ethical principles that include autonomy, beneficence, non-maleficence, and justice [7]. However, there may be conflict with these Western values in other countries, especially LMICs [7]. Palliative care may not be a priority in many LMICs [10], as some cultures stigmatize death or diseases like cancer, HIV, and tuberculosis [1, 7]. Furthermore, there are different ethical challenges in LMICs. For example, there is an ethical issue related to letting lay-volunteers perform care often otherwise provided by a health professional (wound care, cleaning out maggots, preventing bedsores, promoting good hygiene and nutrition, providing medications, and supporting family members) [7]. However, due to the lack of healthcare personnel in LMICs, many patients would not receive any care without volunteers [7]. In many LMICs, healthcare professionals need to consider family influence, lack of health infrastructure, and poverty when caring for patients [7].

There are often cultural and family values and traditions in developing countries that may be combined with religious or spiritual practices [7]. These values and traditions may influence palliative care in a variety of ways. For example, relatives often influence patients in LMIC in where, how, and by whom they would like to be cared for, especially in joint family systems [7]. A high degree of family decision-making allows the family to advocate for the patient, but it also brings up issues of confidentiality and patient autonomy [7]. Families are often forced to make decisions about how to distribute finite resources for the good of the whole family (children's education, marriages, or healthcare costs) [7]. In fact, living wills and advanced directives are less common to cultural groups with family-centered decision-making, and some cultures believe that talking about death is bad luck [17]. Attitudes and beliefs regarding death and dying vary between countries and between cultural groups within countries [17]. Ethics are an important consideration when addressing the barriers to palliative care and implementing a model that addresses the needs to the people.

8.5 The Palliative Care Model

Palliative care is a relatively new component of healthcare, but palliative care and pain relief are increasingly considered essential to universal healthcare [1, 8]. Studies exploring palliative care have shown that it decreases costs and improves quality of supportive bereavement services and care [1, 2, 15]. Palliative care will become an increasingly important part of the healthcare system as people are living longer with multiple comorbidities, including noncommunicable disease [1, 4, 11, 12]. Palliative care is an essential component of healthcare that can prevent early mortality and suffering from communicable and noncommunicable diseases [1, 4].

The palliative care model emphasizes policy, education, medication availability, and implementation, along with health promotion, early detection, prevention, and timely treatment [1]. Countries that have been successful in providing high-quality palliative care services have several common characteristics. These countries have a strong and effective national palliative care policy framework, high levels of public spending on healthcare services, extensive resources for training generalist and specialist palliative care workers, subsidies to reduce financial burden, access to opioids, and strong public awareness [11, 15]. Palliative care should be a coordinated system where family and patient needs are identified and met, and trained personnel can provide access to symptom relief, including opioids [18]. To achieve this model, palliative care requires multidisciplinary teams; essential medicines including opioids; symptom management; psychological care; patient and family input; bereavement services; institutional support; and ongoing advocacy at the policy level [11, 14, 15]. Palliative care should be delivered based on need, not diagnosis or prognosis [1]. However, each country will choose a different approach based on their health system, the proportion of deaths that need palliative care, and integration of palliative care into healthcare systems [1, 9, 11]. These approaches will need to address the organization of multidisciplinary teams and palliative care services, policies, funding, and public awareness of palliative care services.

8.5.1 Multidisciplinary Teams

Multidisciplinary teams may include a variety of healthcare professionals, such as psychologists/counselors, social workers, spiritual team members, community health workers, volunteers, pharmacists, physicians, and nurses [18, 19]. All generalist or specialist healthcare providers working in primary, secondary, or tertiary health centers should have basic palliative care skills [1, 18]. Health professionals with basic palliative care training should seek consultation from palliative care specialists when needed [9, 18]. At the local level, teams should include at least a primary care nurse and physician with palliative care skills, including assessment, diagnoses, and care delivery [18]. At the regional level, the team should be a physician, nurse, and counselor with advanced training in palliative care, including the ability to prescribe and dispense medication, as well as treat refractory symptoms, emotional crises, and existential distress [18]. At the national level, dedicated palliative beds should be established and staffed with trained professionals [18]. Spiritual care should also be available and provided by appropriately trained professionals to support the care team, patients, and families and sensitive to the religious norms of the family [18].

Training of medical professionals is also an issue that needs to be addressed. In order to meet the demand for palliative care, all physicians and nurses should be trained as specialist or generalist palliative care providers [11]. In fact, Krakauer and Rajagopal [15] recommend that all nursing, medicine, and pharmacy undergraduate programs include basic palliative care training. Therefore, palliative care should be included in all basic health education and continuing education should be provided [11]. Education may also have to be considered for exceptional circumstances. For example, nurses in rural and remote areas may need education to prescribe medications when no doctor is available [14]. There are many important considerations that need to be addressed to prepare health professionals to provide palliative care services.

8.5.2 Palliative Care Services

Palliative care services are where the palliative care system interacts with the patient and whoever the patient considers as family. Services that are necessary to care for palliative patients include home visits, symptom management, end-of-life planning, respite care, and bereavement support [19]. These services should be easy to access and allow patients to receive care and die in their preferred place [19]. Palliative care can be provided in the home, care facility, hospice, hospital, or outpatient facility [1]. Home care may mean having a peaceful death in a familiar place and has been proven to be cost-effective [7]. In addition, palliative care should be provided early in the illness, along with disease-fighting treatments, if appropriate [1, 12, 18]. Well-coordinated services could result in less hospitalization, better satisfaction, symptom management, and quality of life [19]. The results of well-coordinated services benefit the patient and the healthcare system.

To have a healthcare system that can provide services that address palliative patients' requirements, there needs to be adequate resources to provide those services. Knaul et al. [8] recommend that countries should have, at minimum, a package of low cost, essential healthcare (*see* Table 8.2). Knaul et al. [8] recommend an essential package of medicines and equipment that can be used in primary care setting. The essential package is designed to be low cost with off-patent formulations, frugal innovation for equipment, and staffing is based on competencies rather than profession [8]. The essential package should be complemented by social and spiritual staff, social safety nets, and anti-poverty policies [8]. In addition, healthcare systems need to safely provide opioids and ensure that they are readily and continually available to meet patient needs [18]. At minimum, access to immediate and sustained release oral and injectable morphine should be available [8, 18]. If countries provide these basic resources to the palliative care system, they may be able to increase the palliative care accessibility.

Table 8.2 Adapted from Knaul et al. [8] Essential Package of medicines, medical equipment, and human resources for palliative care

Knaul et al. [8] essential package

Medications
- Amitriptyline
- Bisacodyl (Senna)
- Dexamethasone
- Diazepam
- Diphenhydramine (chlorpheniramine, cyclizine, or dimenhydrinate)
- Fluconazole
- Fluoxetine or other selective serotonin-reuptake inhibitors (sertraline and citalopram)
- Furosemide
- Hyoscine butylbromide
- Haloperidol
- Ibuprofen (naproxen, diclofenac, or meloxicam)
- Lactulose (sorbitol or polyethylene glycol)
- Loperamide
- Metoclopramide
- Metronidazole
- Morphine (oral immediate-release and injectable)
- Naloxone parenteral
- Omeprazole
- Ondansetron
- Paracetamol
- Petroleum jelly

Medical equipment
- Adult diapers (or cotton and plastic, if in extreme poverty)
- Flashlight with rechargeable battery (if no access to electricity)
- Nasogastric drainage or feeding tube
- Opioid lock box
- Oxygen
- Pressure-reducing mattress
- Urinary catheters

Human resources (varies by referral, provincial or district hospital, community health center, or home)
- Clinical support staff (diagnostic imaging, laboratory technician, nutritionist)
- Community health workers
- Doctors (specialty and general, depending on level of care)
- Nurses (specialty and general)
- Pharmacist
- Physical therapist
- Psychiatrist, psychologist, or counselor (depending on level of care)
- Social workers and counselors
- Non-clinical support staff (administration, cleaning)

8.5.3 Palliative Care Funding

An important component of any health services is funding. Funding determines the availability, type, content, and quality of services [12]. National policies need to address how palliative care fits with health-care systems and insurance systems [11, 19]. Most sources recommended that palliative care should be integrated with and funded through a universal health system [1, 8], as out-of-pocket payments can limit use and access of services [12]. Some countries have addressed financial barriers to palliative care with policies that provide monetary assistance through subsidies, state-run services, and national pensions [11]. Each country needs to assess their particular context to implement the funding model that will be most successful for their circumstances.

Most high-income countries have mixed funding models, with hospital-based services being provided through the health system and community-based services funded through charities [12]. A complication of charitable funding is that resources vary by location [12]. However, in some countries the only financial support for palliative care is through the charitable sector [11]. Nyatanga [10] suggests that charities should invest in facilities and resources, rather than giving money to governments, and engage with government officials to create transparency in funding. However, cost-effective models can be implemented anywhere [8].

Any method used to fund palliative care should support early, appropriate access; support an appropriate mix of services; be in an appropriate location; be stable and predictable, with clear entitlements that are easy to navigate; and have a long-term perspective to ensure quality, availability, and access to palliative care [12]. Funding mechanisms also need to relate to a country's political, economic, health, cultural, political, and social context, including local in-country variations, economic and policy contexts for effective palliative care delivery [9, 11, 12]. Thoughtful consideration is needed to choose the best funding model for a country.

8.5.4 Palliative Care Policies

Policies that consider a country's context need to be put in place to guide palliative care development. These policies are needed to scale up services and coordinate among agencies at all levels [1]. These policies should include a definition of palliative care, a national strategy, how palliative care fits within the overall health infrastructure, national standards, clinical guidelines and protocols, and recognition of palliative care as a medical specialty [1, 10]. These policies need to be available in a variety of languages and able to adapt to local contexts [5]. Furthermore, policies are needed to support and integrate palliative care training into education programs for professional and nonprofessional workers [1, 15]. Policies are also needed to address important challenges in palliative care, like opioid availability, bereavement support, and reporting outcomes [1, 14, 15]. While evidence to create and implement palliative care policies is lacking for most contexts, it is important to start creating policies to measure need, evaluate policies and programs, and monitor progress [8]. Policies also require careful attention, as they will guide palliative care implementation.

8.5.5 Palliative Care Awareness

A vital component of palliative care is increasing awareness of its value among the public. Work needs to be done to create a context where palliative care is not stigmatized. There needs to be a cultural shift to see death as part of a normal process and value the relief of suffering that palliative care provides [11]. This shift can happen partly through normalizing conversations around death and dying and raising awareness about palliative care and end-of-life decisions [11]. In more and more countries, Death Cafés are opening where people can have open conversations and share ideas about death [11]. Health professionals may be able to raise awareness through conversations with their patients and the public, advocating for better palliative care services, and sharing experiences with people from other countries. Palliative care awareness is an important part of gaining public support for a service from which a large proportion of the public will benefit.

8.6   Palliative Care Success Stories

Despite several challenges in implementing palliative care, some countries have started to make great gains [11]. There are examples of LMICs that have improved the quality of their palliative care systems, such as Panama and Mongolia [11, 14, 15]. Panama has increased its number of patients being served from 1000 to 3000 from 2010 to 2014 due to a primary approach to palliative care services [11]. Panama now has a national palliative care program that provides advice and technical guidance to professional caregivers; introduced palliative care coordinators into the health system; and health staff are trained to provide hospice and home care to patients with advanced disease [11]. In 2000, Mongolia received charitable funding to build awareness in the public, policymakers, and health professionals; develop palliative care training; and increase access to opioids [11]. Mongolia now has 10 palliative care centers, and palliative care services are including in national welfare legislation; all medical and social work schools include palliative education; and affordable morphine is available [11]. Even in the absence of support from the broader health system and lack of macroeconomic gains, some LMICs have had impressive results [14]. These impressive results can be a lesson for health professionals and policymakers on how to improve palliative care with finite resources.

8.7   Nursing Considerations

Nurses are key players in advancing any issue in healthcare, including palliative care. Nurses represent about 70% of the global heath workforce and deliver up to 90% of healthcare services [2]. Therefore, it makes sense that nurses are an important part of the palliative care system. In fact, one study found that most pediatric care contacts with a health professional were with a nurse [19]. Nurses are an important part of the success of palliative care because of their diversity; wide range of expertise; human-centered relationships; holistic and compassionate care; skills to meet individual, family, group, community, and population needs; history of social justice advocacy and leadership; and ability to influence policy [2]. In fact, because palliative care is a human right, nurses are ethically obligated to ensure that all people, especially the most vulnerable, have access to palliative care [2].

Providing healing environments for people with advanced illness is a moral imperative of palliative nursing [2]. Therefore, it is important to review the practice, education, and research considerations for nurses in relation to global palliative care.

8.7.1 Practice Implications

There are special practice considerations that are important for nurses to recognize when providing palliative care. As in all types of nursing care, patients need to be respected for their individual or cultural beliefs and preferences [17]. This consideration is especially relevant in a globalized world. Some nurses may find that accepting decision-making about end-of-life care can be challenging if the patient and his or her family are from a different culture or religion or speak a different language than the nurse [17]. These differences may be especially important considerations when working in organizations that support a different belief system than the patient whom the nurse is caring for. For example, many hospices in India are run by Christian missionaries, but the population is largely made up of people who are Hindu or Muslim [7]. Nurses must be careful about imposing their own beliefs and aware that people at the end of life are vulnerable to suggestion [7]. Patient beliefs and practices may involve customs, ceremonies, or alternative medical treatments that conflict with health professionals' ideas of what is best for the patient [7]. In these situations, nurses need to provide careful attention, active curiosity, and self-reflection and evaluation [17]. Making room for the needs of patients and their families is an important part of the holistic care that palliative nursing provides.

Another large part of the nursing role in palliative care is the physical care that they provide. A critical role is related to pain and symptom management, and nurses may work with patients whose needs change frequently. Nurses will need to make recommendations and communicate pain control needs to prescribing health professionals [18]. Therefore, assessment, planning, intervention, and evaluation need to be done on a continuing basis, while incorporating the needs of the patient and family. Nurses may even need to take on roles with advanced practice requirements, especially in resource-limited areas. For example, nurses may take on the role of prescribing medications if appropriately trained [18]. In circumstances where there are shortages of health professionals, nurses may need to supervise and coordinate nonprofessional health staff and family to provide the care that nurses typically do. Globally, the roles that nurses fulfill in palliative care are diverse, and these roles need to take into account the specific context of a country.

For nurses to have the greatest impact in increasing the quality and access of palliative care, they must become advocates. Nurses must aid policymakers in understanding the economic benefit of palliative care across cultures, including the financial implications of pain and symptom management, and holistic care [2]. Nurses can address the importance of palliative care by creating links between palliative care, national agendas, and transnational agendas [2]. Linking palliative care with the agendas of policymakers may increase that policymakers will see the advantages of palliative care. Increasing awareness of palliative care among the public and discussing its benefits to create demand are ways that nurses can advocate for better access to and quality of palliative care. Palliative care nurses can teach about optimizing quality of life, holistic care, proactive care delivery, and the role of palliative care in addressing the social determinants of health [2]. Advocacy is one of the many ways that practicing nurses can address the needs of current and future palliative care patients.

8.7.2 Education Implications

For practicing nurses to have the knowledge and skills needed to fulfill palliative care needs, nursing education must address palliative care. If generalist nurses are to provide basic palliative care to patients, nursing education programs must include palliative care education and training. Nurse educators and administrators can address the need by making palliative care knowledge part of standard nursing education, training, and licensing [2]. In addition, training and continuing education must also be available for nurses who will work in specialist palliative care roles. This specialist training and education may include varied methods of training and roles in different countries, depending on the needs that specialist palliative care nurses will fulfill. Both specialist and generalist palliative care education must prepare nurses for working in multidisciplinary teams, providing holistic care patients and their families, relief of various kinds of suffering and pain control, and working with patients at a vulnerable stage of life. Special considerations for working with children must also be included. Nurse educators have a significant role to play in preparing nurses across the globe to care for palliative patients.

8.7.3 Research Implications

Nurse researchers have the responsibility of guiding nursing education and practice. However, nursing research has not often made palliative care a research priority [2]. Lack of palliative care research in nursing makes it difficult to implement quality palliative care in nursing education and practice. In fact, the nursing and health research that has addressed palliative care has largely focused on Caucasian patients from high-income countries [18]. Nurses need to address palliative care populations in areas with the greatest need, like LMICs. Therefore, future nursing research regarding palliative care should consider addressing gaps in the palliative care research, such as the impact of location on care, access to medical and nonmedical resources, community attitudes and support, distinct cultures, and local factors [18]. Downing et al. [3] have suggested that research priorities for high-income countries should include service evaluation, decision-making, impact of educational programs, telehealth, preferred place of death, resource utilization and costs, pain management, perinatal palliative care, screening for palliative care, and quality of life measures. They also suggest that research priorities for global children's palliative care should address understanding of death and dying, managing pain in the absence of morphine, funding, training, and assessment for pain management [3]. These research priorities are an important step in addressing palliative care research that will improve nursing practice and increase the quality of care. Nursing research, education, and practice are vital to the relief of suffering that palliative care addresses throughout the globe.

8.8 Conclusion

Nurses are key players in providing access to high-quality palliative care across the world. Nurses work in multidisciplinary teams that care for patients with chronic and terminal health conditions, including physical, psychosocial, and spiritual suffering [1]. However, nurses and other palliative care team members need to recognize and address the global differences in palliative care needs, access, and preferences, with special attention to vulnerable groups. These vulnerable populations include people living in LMICs and children, who often do not receive the palliative care that they need [1]. Nurses have the opportunity to address gaps in palliative care, especially for vulnerable groups, by bringing attention to the global disparities in access to palliative care. These disparities are largely a result of lacking palliative care policy, education, medication availability, funding, and implementation [3]. Nurses can be leaders in guiding palliative care teams to adjust palliative care models to many contexts with attention to policies, funding, multidisciplinary teams, opioid availability, and increased awareness of palliative care's importance. Access to palliative care is a global issue that nurses all over the world can address through their various roles in practice, education, and research. Nurses have the ethical responsibility and opportunity to relieve suffering and improve patients' quality of life wherever they are in the world.

References

1. World Hospice Palliative Care Alliance, World Health Organization. Global Atlas of Palliative Care at the End-of-Life. 2014. https://www.who.int/nmh/Global_Atlas_of_Palliative_Care.pdf.
2. Rosa WE. Integrating palliative care into global health initiatives: opportunities and challenges. J Hosp Palliat Nurs. 2018;20(2):195–200.
3. Downing J, Powell RA, Marston J, Huwa C, Chandra L, Garchakova A, et al. Children's palliative care in low- and middle-income countries. Arch Dis Child. 2016;101(1):85–90.
4. Sharkey L, Loring B, Cowan M, Riley L, Krakauer EL. National palliative care capacities around the world: Results from the World Health Organization Noncommunicable Disease Country Capacity Survey. Palliat Med. 2018;32(1):106–13.
5. Cruz-Oliver DM, Little MO, Woo J, Morley JE. End-of-life care in low- and middle-income countries. Bull World Health Organ. 2017;95(11):731.
6. Wright M, Wood J, Lynch T, Clark D. Mapping levels of palliative care development: a global view. J Pain Symptom Manag. 2008;35(5):469–85.
7. Chaturvedi SK. Ethical dilemmas in palliative care in traditional developing societies, with special reference to the Indian setting. J Med Ethics. 2008;34(8):611–5.

8. Knaul FM, Farmer PE, Krakauer EL, De Lima L, Bhadelia A, Xiaoxiao Jiang K, et al. Alleviating the access abyss in palliative care and pain relief-an imperative of universal health coverage: the Lancet Commission report. Lancet. 2018;391(10128):1391–454.
9. Morin L, Aubry R, Frova L, MacLeod R, Wilson DM, Loucka M, et al. Estimating the need for palliative care at the population level: A cross-national study in 12 countries. Palliat Med. 2017;31(6):526–36.
10. Nyatanga B. Developing palliative care globally: facing the challenge. Int J Palliat Nurs. 2015;21(7):317–8.
11. Economist Intelligence Unit. The 2015 quality of death index: Ranking quality of death across the world. 2015. https://eiuperspectives.economist.com/sites/default/files/2015%20EIU%20Quality%20of%20Death%20Index%20Oct%2029%20FINAL.pdf.
12. Groeneveld EI, Cassel JB, Bausewein C, Csikós Á, Krajnik M, Ryan K, et al. Funding models in palliative care: Lessons from international experience. Palliat Med. 2017;31(4):296–305.
13. Connor SR, Downing J, Marston J. Estimating the global need for palliative care for children: a cross-sectional analysis. J Pain Symptom Manag. 2017;53(2):171–7.
14. Caruso Brown AE, Howard SC, Baker JN, Ribeiro RC, Lam CG. Reported Availability and Gaps of Pediatric Palliative Care in Low- and Middle-Income Countries: A Systematic Review of Published Data. J Palliat Med. 2014;17(12):1369–83.
15. Krakauer EL, Rajagopal MR. End-of-life care across the world: a global moral failing. Lancet. 2016;388(10043):444–6.
16. Harding R, Gwyther L, Mwangi-Powell F, Powell RA, Dinat N. How can we improve palliative care patient outcomes in low- and middle-income countries? Successful outcomes research in sub-Saharan Africa. J Pain Symptom Manag. 2010;40(1):23–6.
17. Thomas R, Wilson DM, Justice C, Birch S, Sheps S. A literature review of preferences for end-of-life care in developed countries by individuals with different cultural affiliations and ethnicity. J Hosp Palliat Nurs. 2008;10(3):142–63.
18. Osman H, Shrestha S, Temin S, Ali ZV, Cleary JF. Palliative care in the global setting: ASCO resource-stratified practice guideline summary. J Oncol Pract. 2018;14(7):431–6.
19. Jagt-Van Kampen C, Kars MC, Colenbrander DA, Bosman DK, Grootenhuis MA, Caron HN, et al. A prospective study on the characteristics and subjects of pediatric palliative care case management provided by a hospital based palliative care team. BMC Palliat Care. 2017;16(1):1–10.

Finding Balance Through a Writing Intervention

Lorraine Holtslander

Contents

9.1 The Finding Balance Intervention Description... 138
9.2 Case Example.. 139
9.3 Conclusions.. 140
References.. 141

Family caregivers provide an immense amount of care and support to patients who are at the end of life yet receive very little attention or support after the death of the patient [1]. Nurses can provide support, information and resources and monitor those at greatest risk of complicated grief and other negative outcomes [2]. Support for family caregivers both during and after the death of the patient is mandated by international guidelines for palliative care and hospice services [3], however, most programs lack sufficient resources and the evidence needed to provide the most effective and efficient bereavement support remains lacking [2].

Many factors contribute to the impact of caregiving on bereavement outcomes including gender and age [4], the caregiving experience [5, 6], formal and informal supports [7], and the unique psychosocial context of each individual [8]. Most family caregivers are older adults caring for a spouse and for them bereavement itself has a significant negative effect on morbidity and mortality [9], including risk of suicide [10], depression [11], loneliness, substance abuse, physical and emotional illnesses [12], pain [13], sleep disturbance [14], and even death [15]. There are very

L. Holtslander (✉)
College of Nursing, University of Saskatchewan, Saskatoon, SK, Canada
e-mail: Lorraine.holtslander@usask.ca

© Springer Nature Switzerland AG 2019
L. Holtslander et al. (eds.), *Hospice Palliative Home Care and Bereavement Support*, https://doi.org/10.1007/978-3-030-19535-9_9

few theory and evidence-based interventions that support the needs of bereaved family caregivers [16]. Writing itself has shown benefit to helping during grief, an excellent example of this can be found in Chap. 3 of this textbook. The Finding Balance Intervention (FBI) was developed based on a grounded theory that revealed the difficulty in finding balance between negative thoughts and emotions and activities of grief [17]. In this grounded theory study, bereaved caregivers defined finding balance as a process of learning to handle the difficult emotions, thoughts, and activities of grief so that they could move forward. One participant described it as "walking a fine line." Another said it was like "being in the middle of two points, one would be the deep grieving; the extreme of it, and the other would be not having any grief at all; looking forward to what you are going to do."

Additional research with older adults who had cared for a spouse showed the FBI was easy to use, acceptable and offered a benefit by increasing restoration-oriented coping and higher oscillation activity between loss and restoration-oriented coping [18]. This oscillation is described in the Dual Process Model (DPM) of coping with bereavement which describes everyday life experiences during grief as an oscillation between both loss and restoration processes [19]. Adaptive, positive coping with grief and bereavement is found in accommodating the loss while also participating in activities that are restoration-oriented. The DPM has shown considerable promise in ongoing research with older adults in bereavement [20]. The DPM was the basis for the development of a scale, the Inventory of Daily Widowed Life (IDWL), through research with 161 older bereaved spouses [21] that demonstrated the importance of having a balance between loss and restoration processes as it predicted more positive outcomes.

The DPM provided a conceptual framework for the FBI as well as the grounded theory of finding balance [17]. The processes of finding balance were identified as three themes and organized into the FBI booklet, including "walking a fine line," "deep grieving," and "moving forward." Activities were chosen through Delphi methods, consultation with local experts and an international expert in bereavement interventions, Dr. Robert Neimeyer; details on the development and testing of the FBI were published in 2016 [18]. The purpose of this chapter is to describe the FBI and provide a case example from research with older adults, bereaved after losing a spouse to cancer. The FBI is an example of an evidence-based writing intervention for bereaved family caregivers. The FBI itself can be found on the author's website at: www.lorraine.holtslander.com

9.1 The Finding Balance Intervention Description

The *FBI* is a booklet that describes the processes of finding balance, with examples from others who have been through this experience and provides writing assignments for each process of finding balance. The writing focuses on identifying emotions and how to deal with these emotions, constructing a support system, and reflecting on the caregiving experience. There are three sections and additional space for creative writing. Instructions are provided such as "find a comfortable place, don't worry about spelling or grammar, and if possible, write for 10–15 min a day." The goal of finding balance during bereavement is described including to feel somewhat in control, to be able to find a new identity, to build self-confidence, to feel comfortable with one's new life, and to be able to look forward to the future. The tool encourages reflection and focused writing, with the overall goal of encouraging a person who is bereaved to find their own unique way of moving ahead in their grief.

Deep grieving is about expressing emotions while also writing about "time out" activities and creating a support system. Writers are encouraged to find a way to express their emotions, be open to them, and then identify someone to call when you need support. Writing about ways to take a "time out" from these difficult emotions includes suggestions such as taking a walk or calling someone. There is space to write a list of supportive people that can be contacted such as family, friends, grief support group members, or counselors to make a supportive directory for when help is needed with specific concerns.

Walking a fine line is about combining two extremes including activities that take one back to grieving and activities that involve looking forward. The writing activity includes a weekly calendar to schedule 3 activities a week that are about grief and three activities that involve taking time for oneself, both keeping a connection to the outside world while honoring the need to rest and relax. This section also encourages the creation of a unique ritual, service, or special event to help remember the person who died such as planting a tree, creating a scholarship, or planning a memorial event.

Moving forward consists of activities that address the process of moving forward such a being thankful, planning the day, reaching out to others, and taking time to care for yourself. Ideas include writing the story of your caregiving, considering how this story might help others, and the lessons learned along the way. Caregivers are asked to write about what makes them feel stronger, such as personal growth through the challenges of caregiving, spiritual beliefs, and how you may now be able to help others in similar circumstances. The case example below illustrates the writing that may be done in the FBI and how reflecting on this was helpful in grief.

9.2 Case Example

Mary is a 75-year-old woman who provided care for her husband John as he journeyed through pancreatic cancer for about a year. Caregiving was very difficult, exhausting and challenging, particularly the management of his extreme pain and nausea. Many nights were disrupted attending to John's needs. Even with the help of family, friends, and a home care nurse, John eventually required admission to a palliative care unit in a local hospital for pain management and sedation. All of these experiences were difficult and traumatic for Mary and left her with strong feelings of sadness, regret, and guilt that she was unable to care for John herself at home where he preferred to be. Mary was also exhausted by the experience and her own health suffered. The home care nurse visited Mary at home approximately

2 months after John's death to offer bereavement support. The nurse could see that Mary was still struggling with difficult memories, sadness, and finding new meaning and purpose for her completely changed life. The nurse offered Mary a small booklet called the Finding Balance Intervention and encouraged her to write in it every day for 2 weeks at which time the nurse would provide a follow-up visit.

In the section entitled "Expressing Your Emotions" Mary wrote: "today I spent time visiting with friends and we reflected on the past good times as couples. I feel lonely for him but also happy to have had him for so many years." Her journaling under "Time Out" included "my faith is most helpful," "games on the computer," "family time," "a good movie," "my art projects" and so on; Mary wrote quite a long list of activities that provided a distraction from difficult emotions. Mary also wrote a long list of supportive people and how they helped her.

Under "Creative Space to Journal" Mary wrote about "feeling torn in half the day John died, one half of me was gone and the other half was alone and had no one to turn to or care for!" As she wrote out her feelings and experiences, Mary came to a realization: "I am now realizing how much John taught me all those years, he never complained and lived today as if there was no tomorrow and so I have come to realize that life is there to enjoy what you can, learn from your mistakes and be grateful for what you had. I pray that God will allow me to help others in coping with life. I cry but mostly when I am alone and it relieves the ache in my heart. I am opening a door in front of me but will always keep the back door ajar! I don't ever want to forget the 50 wonderful years I had with John but I do have to go on and complete my purpose."

Maintaining a balance of daily life involved two long lists of activities coupled with time for yourself and included some creative activities such as writing a book about what she remembers about John, doing more art projects, and continuing to honor John on Father's day, his birthday and in giving a donation in his memory to the hospital where John died. On reflection in the FBI, Mary wrote: "My faith is getting stronger as I look back and see the past 50 years we had together."

Mary's use and feedback on the FBI was similar to others we included in our study [18]. The tool did seem to bring up sadness and difficult emotions, but they also felt they opened up and experienced personal growth. Just thinking and writing about the emotions, thoughts, and their activities was difficult, but the reflection time brought them along in their grief journey. One participant described feeling inadequate and that the suffering of their spouse stayed with them; but reflecting through writing showed how the caregiving experience also gave them time together, to say goodbyes. Telling the story of caregiving was difficult, but after it came out, it felt better. Realizing other bereaved caregivers felt the same way through the examples provided was described as helpful.

9.3 Conclusions

The FBI is a theory-based, evidence-informed self-administered writing tool that offers many possibilities in clinical practice. If the nurse has an opportunity to provide a bereavement support visit to the family caregiver, it could be offered and then follow-up provided as needed. Of course, in cases of complicated grief, the caregiver should be referred for professional support. The FBI could be used in bereavement support groups to have individuals write and then discuss their writing as a group as they feel comfortable to share. Many family caregivers will have adequate coping skills and supports to manage grief on their own, but others certainly would benefit from an intervention that honors their caregiving journey, assists in balancing difficult emotions and activities, gives an opportunity to grieve and offers ways to find a new purpose after caregiving ends.

References

1. Holtslander L, et al. Honoring the voices of bereaved caregivers: a metasummary of qualitative research. BMC Palliat Care. 2017;16(1):48.
2. Holtslander L. Caring for bereaved family caregivers: analyzing the context of care. Clin J Oncol Nurs. 2008;12(3):501–6.
3. World Health Organization. Definition of palliative care [Electronic version], 14 Feb 2002; 2005. http://www.who.int/cancer/palliative/definition/en/
4. Hart CL, et al. Effect of conjugal bereavement on mortality of the bereaved spouse in participants of the Renfrew/Paisley study. J Epidemiol Community Health. 2007;61:455–60.
5. Boerner K, Schulz R. Caregiving, bereavement and complicated grief. Bereave Care. 2009;28(3):10–3.
6. Kim Y, Schulz R. Family caregivers' strains: comparative analysis of cancer caregiving with dementia, diabetes, and frail elderly caregiving. J Aging Health. 2008;20(5):483–503.
7. Buckley T, et al. Cardiovascular risk in early bereavement: a literature review and proposed mechanisms. Int J Nurs Stud. 2010;47:229–38.
8. Holtslander LF, Duggleby WD. The psychosocial context of bereavement for older women who were caregivers fo a spouse with advanced cancer. J Women Aging. 2010;22(2):109–24.
9. Stroebe M, Schut H, Stroebe W. Health outcomes of bereavement. Lancet. 2007;370:1960–73.
10. Erlangsen A, et al. Loss of partner and suicide risk among oldest old: a population-based register study. Age Ageing. 2004;33:378–83.
11. Holtslander LF, McMillan S. Depressive symptoms, grief and complicated grief among bereaved family caregivers of advanced cancer patients. Oncol Nurs Forum. 2011;38(1):60–5.
12. Schulz R, Hebert R, Boerner K. Bereavement after caregiving. Geriatrics. 2008;63(1):20–2.
13. Kowalski SD, Bondmass MD. Physiological and psychological symptoms of grief in widows. Res Nurs Health. 2008;31:23–30.
14. Carter PA. Bereaved caregivers' descriptions of sleep: impact on daily life and the bereavement process. Oncol Nurs Forum. 2005;32(4):E70–5.
15. Christakis NA, Iwashyna TJ. The health impact of health care on families: a matched cohort study of hospice use by decedents and mortality outcomes in surviving, widowed spouses. Soc Sci Med. 2003;57:465–75.
16. Hudson P. Improving support for family carers: key implications for research, policy, and practice. Palliat Med. 2013;27(7):581–2.
17. Holtslander L, Bally J, Steeves M. Walking a fine line: an exploration of the experience of finding balance for older persons bereaved after caregiving for a spouse with advanced cancer. Eur J Oncol Nurs. 2011;15:6.
18. Holtslander L, et al. Developing and pilot-testing a Finding Balance Intervention for older adult bereaved family caregivers: a randomized feasibility trial. Eur J Oncol Nurs. 2016;21:66–74.
19. Stroebe M, Schut H. The dual process model of coping with bereavement: rationale and description. Death Stud. 1999;23:197–224.
20. Chow AY, et al. Dual-Process Bereavement Group Intervention (DPBGI) for widowed older adults. Gerontologist. 2018;2018:gny095.
21. Caserta MS, Lund DA. Towards the development of an inventory of daily widowed life: guided by the dual process model of coping with bereavement. Death Stud. 2007;31:505–35.

Additional Resources

Key messages from a metasummary of qualitative research to honor the voices of bereaved family caregivers can be found at:

https://lorraine.holtslander.com/wp-content/uploads/2019/03/Key-Messages-from-a-Metasummary-of-Qualitative-Research-to-Honor-the-Voices-of-Bereaved-Family-Caregivers-Poster.pdf

Our video series, Honoring the voices of bereaved caregivers, can be found at the following links:

Canadian virtual hospice: information and support on palliative and end-of-life care, loss and grief: www.virtualhospice.ca
Caregiving 101: Dick Strayer – his story. https://lorraine.holtslander.com/media/#Dick-Strayer
Honoring voices after caregiving. https://lorraine.holtslander.com/media/#life-after-caregiving
Honoring voices: walking alongside the caregiver. https://lorraine.holtslander.com/media/#walking-alongside-the-caregiver
Reinventing a life: Sherrill Miller – her story. https://lorraine.holtslander.com/media/#Sherrill-Miller

Keeping Hope Possible

10

Jill M. G. Bally and Meridith Burles

Contents

10.1	Life-Limiting and Life-Threatening Illnesses: Family and Hope.	143
10.2	The Keeping Hope Possible Toolkit: An Intervention for Parents.	144
10.3	Case Vignette.	149
10.4	Conclusions.	151
References.		151

10.1 Life-Limiting and Life-Threatening Illnesses: Family and Hope

Current evidence about families with children who have life-limiting illnesses (LLIs) and life-threatening illnesses (LTIs) described many parents who are adversely affected by their child's diagnosis and the demands of caregiving [1]. The shock of diagnosis, relentless fear of the child's changing health status, possible death of their child, and prolonged and intensive treatment regimens all result in uncertainty [2–4], distress [5–7], feelings of loss of control [8], and burden on the parents of these children. In turn, the health and well-being of parental caregivers are often compromised [2, 9–11], family roles and functioning are altered [9, 12], and overall quality of life may decline [10]. However, many parents have used hope as a supportive personal resource that is sustaining and critical to their caregiving activities and well-being [2, 3, 5].

The importance of hope for parents of children with LLIs and LTIS is evident in existing literature. Hope facilitates optimistic caregiving, and is an influential factor related to parental health, well-being, and coping [13, 14]. Specifically, parents

---

J. M. G. Bally (✉) · M. Burles
College of Nursing, University of Saskatchewan, Saskatoon, SK, Canada
e-mail: jill.bally@usask.ca; meridith.burles@usask.ca

© Springer Nature Switzerland AG 2019
L. Holtslander et al. (eds.), *Hospice Palliative Home Care and Bereavement Support*, https://doi.org/10.1007/978-3-030-19535-9_10

have identified hope as an important survival tool [2, 15], and described it as life-sustaining, positive, and useful [3, 15]. For parental caregivers, hope is rooted in the caregiving experience [16, 17], and is highly individualized and dynamic [16], as well as broad and multidimensional [13]. Many studies showed that hope is strengthened by the positive attitudes and practical help of extended family members [18], improved child health, having faith, and parental resources [13]. Parental hope is threatened by healthcare providers' negative evaluation of the child's health [5], the experience of pain and uncontrolled symptoms by the child, and parental fatigue [2, 5]. Two research studies produced separate grounded theories of hope and the role of hope in the parental journey with an LTI. Both studies identifyied the critical and essential nature of hope, as well as how hope oscillates on a pendulum, being both positive and negative depending on the context [2, 5]. Accordingly, it appears that parents find a balance between maintaining a sense of reality and never letting go of hope which allows them to manage constant uncertainty and feelings of loss of control [5].

Hope has, therefore, been described by parents as an important component of their own well-being, and a critical and essential aspect of their caregiving activities [13, 19]. As such, keeping their hope possible amidst their child's illness and parental caregiving is a crucial part of providing optimal and holistic pediatric hospice palliative care for families. However, there remains a need for improved access to information, strategies, and supportive interventions that can be used by healthcare providers to successfully assess and intervene to promote hope in parental caregivers. In doing so, healthcare providers can assist with maintaining all aspects of parents' health while navigating the difficult experiences and transitions related to their child's illness. Availability of an easy-to-use and accessible toolkit that encourages hope and management of practical and emotional issues can enhance pediatric hospice palliative care and positive health outcomes for families who have children with LLIs and LTIs.

10.2 The Keeping Hope Possible Toolkit: An Intervention for Parents

The Keeping Hope Possible Toolkit was developed from grounded theory research completed with parental caregivers of children who were in treatment for cancer. These parents identified "Keeping Hope Possible" (as depicted in Fig. 10.1) [5] as an important process in their daily work to maintain their own health and well-being during the parental caregiving experience. Keeping Hope Possible for these parents involved managing the challenging internal struggle that encompassed preparing for the worst and hoping for the best. The four related sub-processes that helped parents keep their hope possible emerged from the grounded theory, and included *accepting reality*, *establishing control*, *restructuring hope*, and *purposive positive thinking* [5].

First, parents described the essential initial step in Keeping Hope Possible as *Accepting Reality* in which they experienced feelings of shock and questions about faith and reasons for illness, followed by engagement in reasoning to accept their child's cancer diagnosis and treatment plan [5]. Next, parents discussed having to

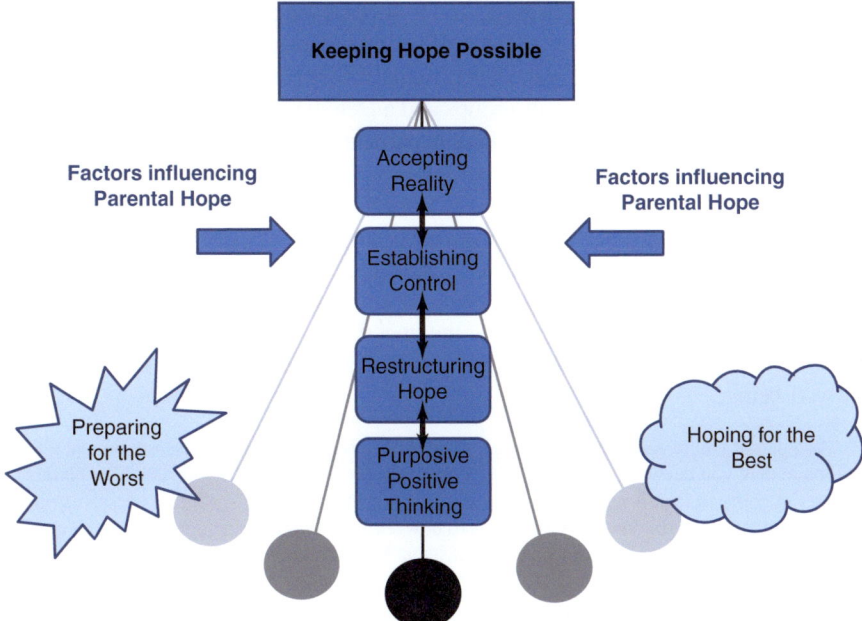

Fig. 10.1 Keeping Hope Possible (Bally, J. M., Duggleby, W., Holtslander, L., Mpofu, C., Spurr, S., Thomas, R., & Wright, K. (2014). Keeping Hope Possible: A grounded theory study of the hope experience of parental caregivers who have children in treatment for cancer. Cancer Nursing, 37(5), 363–372)

Establish Control by identifying their strengths, social supports, relevant knowledge, and their child's needs. In doing so, and focusing on the present moment, parents were able to manage distress and keep their hope possible. These outcomes supported their well-being and caregiving activities. Once parents felt they had achieved some control over their circumstances, they began to *Restructure Hope* which also helped to keep it possible [5]. For parents, this involved adjusting hope as needed in various circumstances such as getting through a medical test, waiting for lab results, or managing their child's acute medical treatment [5]. The last sub-process in Keeping Hope Possible as explained by parents was *Purposive Positive Thinking*. While parents acknowledged the importance of thinking about the negative aspects of their experiences and the worst case scenario, their child's death, they also discussed the importance of finding the positives in all circumstances. Parents stated that this took purposeful work, training, and making the choice to think positively so as not to get perpetually immersed in the difficult and negative aspects of illness and caregiving [5].

These four sub-processes of Keeping Hope Possible were used as a creative and helpful theoretical framework for guiding the development of a psychosocial support intervention for parents who are caring for their children with LLIs and LTIs. However, subsequent research was undertaken to verify the relevance and importance of the four sub-processes, and to support the development of the theory-based hope intervention prior to refinement and implementation with parents of children with a variety of LLIs and LTIs. Namely, the next steps in research involved significant consultation via focus groups and a Delphi approach with a national and international group of experts including parental caregivers, nurses, physicians, social workers, play therapists, and community members involved in pediatric care for families of children with LLIs and LTIs [20]. The focus groups were conducted with 18 participants, and data analysis highlighted the relationship between children's physical and psychological care needs and parents' overall health and well-being. For example, one parent openly discussed the difficulties and sadness associated with her child's illness and the uncertainty about his health from day to day. She found that enhancing her own knowledge base helped with her own sense of well-being:

> As a parent you're given this diagnosis that your child has this whatever disease. For us, we found that, you know, knowledge is power and the more you can teach yourselves the better you're going to feel. It was almost a calming mechanism if we could educate ourselves on everything, like right down to blood cells to how – whatever chemotherapy did to each cell and, you know, all the – you know, the knowledge behind it kind of almost soothed our soul a little bit.

It was also revealed that families experience many unmet support needs, and therefore, opportunities exist for enhancing palliative and hospice care provided to parents of children with serious illness. For example, focusing on communication, one parent noted an opportunity for improvement in meeting her needs as demonstrated in the following quote:

> For us something that we wished we could have had – we wished we could have had more one on one candid conversations or an opportunity to have one on one candid conversations with our doctors that excluded our child so we can ask questions because he was seven at the time. He was fully aware of what we were saying and what we were talking about. We just wish we could have asked more questions without him there. Not to keep him out of it, but just so we could ask maybe more blunt questions or more questions that we really wondered about.

Another parent discussed the opportunity for providing holistic care using novel therapies such as mindfulness and meditation. She said:

> I love the idea of the meditation, and we talk about it but I think it rarely is implemented. And mindfulness, it's about retraining, it is about retraining our brain. And those who might be negative might need more work, or it might be an impossibility, but to retrain our brain to think about a situation that's positive, or at the very least focus on the present rather than the what if. It really takes it on a daily basis.
>
> The question is who is going to do it? Is it the child's caregiver? Is it the nurses? Is it the team? And then eventually, once the parents learn then they can do that on their own. But I think it's a really, it's a new philosophy which I think is really proving itself to be effective.

Similarly, the Delphi research involved 68 members who participated in three rounds of surveys aimed at better understanding how to support parents in keeping their hope possible [20]. Additionally, the Delphi was conducted to support the identification of helpful resources used by formal and informal caregivers including healthcare providers, community members, and parents. The findings included eight themes that were interrelated with the basic social process of Keeping Hope Possible, including: (1) *Organize Basic Needs*; (2) *Connect with Others*; (3) *Prioritize Self-Care*; (4) *Obtain Meaningful Information*; (v) *Take Things Day by Day*; (6) *Advocate for Parental Participation*; (7) *Manifest Positivity*; and, (8) *Celebrate Milestones* [20]. Figure 10.2 is a model depicting the relationships amongst the Keeping Hope Possible sub-processes and the thematic findings of the Delphi study.

In addition to the focus groups and the Delphi, a metasynthesis was completed to review the qualitative literature related to parents' experiences in caring for a child with an LLI or LTI [21]. Through a systematic and exhaustive search of existing literature, a total of 23 articles were selected for inclusion. Findings from the data analysis demonstrated that parents undergo significant and persistent distress related to their complex experiences and uncertainty, in which they particularly struggle with their own compromised health and negative thoughts of their child's possible death [21]. Three important processes emerged including: the devastation of living with uncertainty; the emergence of hope; and, moving forward with life [21]. The findings from this qualitative metasynthesis added to our knowledge of parental

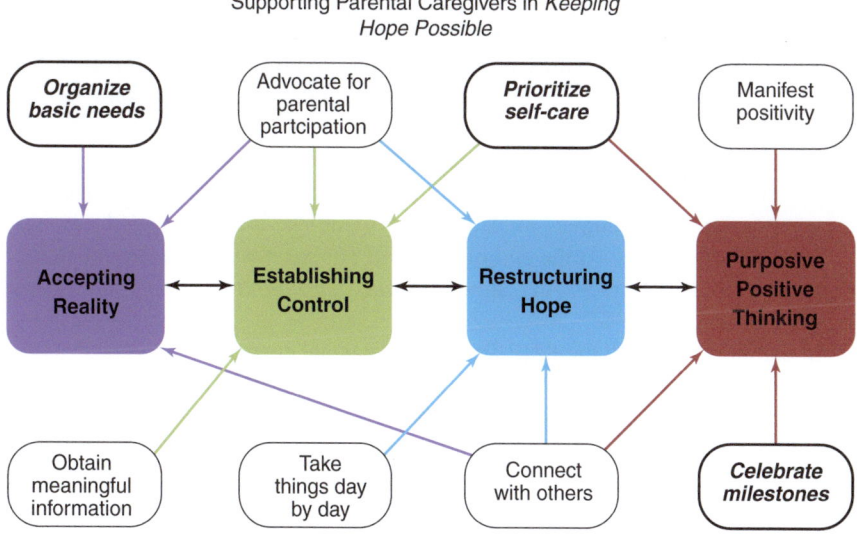

*Bold & Italicized = unique findings

Fig. 10.2 Supporting parental caregivers in Keeping Hope Possible (Smith NR, Bally JM, Holtslander L, Peacock S, Spurr S, Hodgson-Viden H, Mpofu C, Zimmer M. Supporting parental caregivers of children living with life-threatening or life-limiting illnesses: A Delphi study. Journal for Specialists in Pediatric Nursing. 2018 Oct; 23(4):e12226)

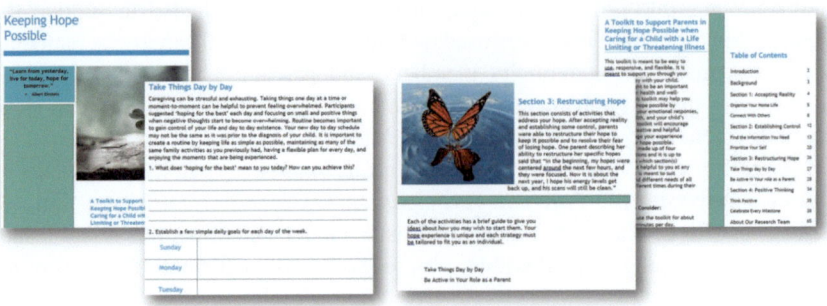

Fig. 10.3 The KHP Toolkit (Author)

experiences, as well as care and support needs, and therefore, informed the refinement of the KHP Toolkit.

Once refined, the KHP Toolkit (Fig. 10.3) is made up of four sections pertaining to the grounded theory sub-processes including *Accepting Reality, Establishing Control, Restructuring Hope,* and *Positive Thinking.* Each section is comprised of activities related to two of the eight themes identified through the Delphi research which aim to support parents in keeping their hope possible by reflecting on emotional responses, their own health, and their child's experiences. The activities are collected within a colourful, wire-bound booklet that is easily transported and accessible. Each section is colour coded for easy identification, and pictures and supportive quotes are used throughout, along with inclusion of space for creative writing. The specific activities vary by section, and address both practical and psychosocial issues. For example, one section includes a table to compile lab and test results, whereas another relates to self-care and generating ideas to prioritize one's own well-being. Mindfulness activities are also included, including those that facilitate distraction and a focus on the present such as colouring pages and labyrinths. Space to document milestones and memories is also provided, amongst various other activities. At the end of the KHP Toolkit, there is a calendar so that parents can keep track of appointments, special moments, and other commitments.

In the introduction to the KHP Toolkit, parents are encouraged to choose a section or multiple sections that might be most relevant and helpful at the given time. Specifically, the Toolkit is meant to be flexible, and suit the unique and diverse needs of all parental caregivers at different times during their experience. It is suggested that parents could aim to use the Toolkit for approximately 15 min per day, or as they prefer, and time allows. By ensuring that it is portable and flexible, parents control how and when they use the Toolkit such as while waiting for appointments, or in the evening once their child is asleep. In addition, parents are reassured when given the Toolkit that there are no right or wrong answers, there is no need to worry about spelling and grammar, that it will remain their own, and that the contents do not have to be shared with anyone. The images included in Fig. 10.3 depict a few pages of the KHP Toolkit that highlight its contents and organization.

The Toolkit is currently undergoing evaluation in an ongoing study that aims to assess its effectiveness based on participant outcomes following its use over several weeks. Specifically, parents are being randomly assigned to one of two groups that either start using the KHP Toolkit at that time, or two weeks later (as such, both groups receive the toolkit but at different times). Participants complete four quantitative measures to assess their hope, feelings of control, distress, and uncertainty prior to use of the Toolkit, and after having used it for 2 weeks, 4 weeks, and 3 months which enables comparison across the two groups and at different time points. In addition, brief qualitative evaluation interviews are being conducted to learn more about parents' experiences with, and the acceptability and feasibility of the intervention, as well as to close the research process with each parent. To date, we have obtained supportive feedback from participants about the KHP Toolkit, and specifically, the sections that resonate most strongly. While the Toolkit holds potential as an accessible support intervention for use with this population, the research and data analysis are ongoing. The following case vignette reflects a composite case that captures aspects of multiple participants' experiences as a means for demonstrating how a registered nurse, nursing students, and other healthcare providers in acute care and community settings can integrate the KHP Toolkit to support parents during uncertain and often traumatic experiences.

10.3 Case Vignette

While waiting to see their child's physician, Mariella and her partner, Ryan, talk quietly to avoid disturbing the child while he naps. Meanwhile, a nurse, Lisa, prepares equipment for the appointment in the corner of the room. Lisa notices that Mariella appears tired and pale, raising concern. She asks the couple if they have any questions or concerns that could be discussed while they wait for the physician. The couple exchange pensive glances, and nod to indicate they do have some concerns. Additional discussion reveals that Mariella is struggling to manage her son's care while Ryan is at work and that she is not sleeping much at night due to immense worrying, despite being exhausted. Ryan wants to play a greater role in the caregiving process, but he needs to maintain his long work hours since his work provides the family's main income. Along with fatigue, the couple are very worried about their child's symptoms and question whether treatment is having a beneficial impact. Lisa remembers that the family has been given several information sheets about the child's condition at previous appointments but does not know if they have been suitable in explaining what the family could expect in terms of the treatment process and outcomes.

Lisa asks Mariella and Ryan about whether they have met with the clinical social worker and suggests arranging a meeting to coincide with the child's next appointment. After confirming their interest and that she would set up the appointment, Lisa does not wish to let their concerns and struggles go unaddressed in the meantime. She obtains a copy of the KHP Toolkit for each of the parents and asks them if they would be interested in learning more about how its use could be beneficial to their coping. Mariella appears very interested and notes "I am willing to try anything that might help." Ryan indicates that he is not really interested but will listen to the explanation regardless. As Lisa goes through the introduction and a few of the activities included in the Toolkit, Mariella nods approvingly, stating "I'm not big on writing, but I like the idea of the colouring." Ryan warms to the idea of giving the Toolkit a try, but mainly as a way to support Mariella. Pleased that they are willing to consider using it, Lisa explains the flexible nature and that they can start at the beginning or another section, noting "there is no wrong way to use the Toolkit." As Lisa leaves the room, she can hear the couple flipping the pages and talking about the sections as their son continues to doze.

Two weeks later, Mariella and Ryan are back with their child for another treatment appointment and to see the clinical social worker. While waiting, Mariella mentions to Lisa that she has used the Toolkit a few times in the evening in the past weeks and is coming up with ideas to try to cope better. Specifically, she indicates an interest in finding out more about respite care from the social worker, noting that "someone mentioned it once, but I didn't think I needed help. I mean, my mom lives nearby, but I don't like to bug her since she works a lot too." Mariella also mentions wanting to find out if there is a support group for parents of children with similar conditions so she can ask questions about what to expect. She recalls: "It would be nice to hear from someone who has been through it from the parent's side." Lisa confirms that the clinical social worker can help her with both of those things and suggests writing what she finds out in the Toolkit so that it is easy to find after.

A few weeks later, Lisa is again on shift at the clinic when Mariella and Ryan come in with their child. The Toolkit is sticking out of Mariella's bag, so Lisa inquires about whether she is continuing to use it. Mariella reports that she forgets about it sometimes, but that she has been enjoying the colouring pages on days in which she is particularly nervous and jittery. "Trying to take things one day at a time, or even one hour at a time, has been helpful too," she notes. Ryan nods in agreement, saying "there's so much we don't know and can't control. I just wish I could be home more so Mariella didn't have to do everything with our son." Lisa takes Ryan's comment as a sign he might have looked at the Toolkit as well, and asks what he thought in general. "You know, I actually found it useful. Like, no one has ever asked me how I feel, and I don't want to talk about my feelings really, but it was good to write some down," Ryan replies. Mariella expresses her agreement, stating "I still want to talk to the social worker and other parents, but this book has given me some ideas about what questions to ask and a place to write them down." As the physician enters the room, the conversation shifts focus to their son and how he has been since the last visit.

Later that afternoon, Lisa is chatting with the social worker who mentions that she was going to help Mariella and Ryan organize respite care and apply for financial support so that Ryan would not have to work as much. "Please don't hesitate to let me know if other families ask about this, Lisa. Sometimes people are embarrassed, but it's the least we can do to tell them what programs are out there," says the social worker. Lisa confirms that she will do this, and adds that she is glad that the situation might improve a bit for Mariella and Ryan while they continue to care for their son.

10.4 Conclusions

As the case vignette illustrates, the KHP Toolkit has potential to be adapted into the acute care or community setting because it is accessible, flexible, and easy to use. In this case, the parents were able to look at it while waiting for an appointment, and then take it home to use as preferred. Its flexibility and portability have been particularly valued by parents who have used it, with indications that it has broad appeal because it combines some practical activities and some aimed at fostering coping, such as positive thinking and mindfulness. While the Toolkit does not contain illness-specific information or that for specific supports, it aims to facilitate identification of questions to ask about at appointments, as well as other sources of information and support including other parents and the Internet. Furthermore, some sections of the Toolkit offer prompts for reflection and writing which participants tended to value more than a blank notebook, despite that some kept a separate journal. Another valued feature of the Toolkit was the potential to facilitate conversations between family members, such as discussing positive events that had occurred or coming up with an inspirational quote. Participants valued different aspects of the KHP Toolkit, but commonly expressed that the focus on hope was their favourite part.

Accordingly, this theory-based support intervention demonstrates promise as a tool that can be easily integrated into existing pediatric hospice palliative care, and used alongside existing support services. The availability of such tools can assist nurses and other healthcare providers in understanding and addressing the holistic health needs of families who are navigating care of an ill child. The need to do so is imperative given the significance that Keeping Hope Possible can have for the well-being of parental caregivers, and in turn their child and other family members. As such, additional evaluation and possible refinement of this support intervention is needed, along with wider implementation in diverse pediatric healthcare and community settings.

References

1. Steele R, Davies B. Impact on parents when a child has a progressive, life-threatening illness. Int J Palliat Nurs. 2006;12(12):576–85.
2. Barrera M, Granek L, Shaheed J, Nicholas D, Beaune L, D'Agostino NM, et al. The tenacity and tenuousness of hope: parental experiences of hope when their child has a poor cancer prognosis. Cancer Nurs. 2013;36(5):408–16.
3. De Graves S, Aranda S. When a child cannot be cured-reflections of health professionals. Eur J Cancer Care. 2005;14(2):132–40.
4. Sallfors C, Hallberg LRM. A parental perspective on living with a chronically ill child: a qualitative study. Fam Syst Health. 2003;21(2):193.
5. Bally JM, Duggleby W, Holtslander L, Mpofu C, Spurr S, Thomas R, Wright K. Keeping hope possible: a grounded theory study of the hope experience of parental caregivers who have children in treatment for cancer. Cancer Nurs. 2014;37(5):363–72.
6. Patel SK, Fernandez N, Wong AL, Mullins W, Turk A, Dekel N, et al. Changes in self-reported distress in end-of-life pediatric cancer patients and their parents using the pediatric distress thermometer. Psychooncology. 2014;23(5):592–6.

7. Rosenberg AR, Dussel V, Kang T, Geyer JR, Gerhardt CA, Feudtner C, Wolfe J. Psychological distress in parents of children with advanced cancer. JAMA Pediatr. 2013;167(6):537–43.
8. Bjork M, Wiebe T, Hallstrom I. Striving to survive: families' lived experiences when a child is diagnosed with cancer. J Pediatr Oncol Nurs. 2005;22(5):265–75.
9. Cadell S, Kennedy K, Hemsworth D. Informing social work practice through research with parent caregivers of a child with a life-limiting illness. J Soc Work End Life Palliat Care. 2012;8:356–81.
10. Eiser C, Eiser JR, Stride CB. Quality of life in children newly diagnosed with cancer and their mothers. Health Qual Life Outcomes. 2005;3(1):29.
11. Monterosso L, Kristjanson LJ, Phillips MB. The supportive and palliative care needs of Australian families of children who die from cancer. Palliat Med. 2009;22(1):59–69.
12. Angstrom-Brannstrom C, Norberg A, Strandberg G, Soderberg A, Dalqvist V. Parents' experiences of what comforts them when their child is suffering from cancer. J Pediatr Oncol Nurs. 2010;27(5):266–75.
13. Kylma J, Juvakka T. Hope in parents of adolescents with cancer: factors endangering and engendering parental hope. Eur J Oncol Nurs. 2007;11(3):262–71.
14. Reder EA, Serwint JR. Until the last breath. Exploring the concept of hope for parents and health care professionals during a child's serious illness. Arch Pediatr Adolesc Med. 2009;163(7):653–7.
15. Horton TV, Wallander JL. Hope and social support as resilience factors against psychological distress of mothers who care for children with chronic physical conditions. Rehabil Psychol. 2001;46(4):382–99.
16. Samson A, Tomiak E, Dimillo J, et al. The lived experience of hope among parents of a child with Duchenne muscular dystrophy: perceiving the human being beyond the illness. Chronic Illn. 2009;5(2):103–14.
17. Thampanichawat W. Maintaining love and hope: caregiving for Thai children with HIV infection. J Assoc Nurses AIDS Care. 2008;19(3):200–10.
18. Amendolia B. Hope and parents of the critically ill newborn. Adv Newborn Care. 2010;10(3):140–4.
19. James K, Keegan-Wells D, Hinds PS, Kelly KP, Bond D, Hall B, Mahan R, Moore IM, Roll L, Speckhart B. The care of my child with cancer: parents' perceptions of caregiving demands. J Pediatr Oncol Nurs. 2002;19(6):218–28.
20. Smith NR, Bally JM, Holtslander L, Peacock S, Spurr S, Hodgson-Viden H, Mpofu C, Zimmer M. Supporting parental caregivers of children living with life-threatening or life-limiting illnesses: a Delphi study. J Spec Pediatr Nurs. 2018;23(4):e12226.
21. Bally JM, Smith NR, Holtslander L, Duncan V, Hodgson-Viden H, Mpofu C, Zimmer M. A metasynthesis: uncovering what is known about the experiences of families with children who have life-limiting and life-threatening illnesses. J Pediatr Nurs. 2018;38:88–98.

Reclaiming Yourself

11

Shelley Peacock and Melanie Bayly

> *Grieving is a natural process. It is through our losses that we can transform ourselves and find new meaning in life.*
> —James Van Praagh

Contents

11.1	For Whom the Intervention is Appropriate	153
11.2	The Intervention	154
11.3	Case Example	156
11.4	Conclusions	158
References		159

11.1 For Whom the Intervention is Appropriate

The *Reclaiming Yourself* tool was developed with and for bereaved older adult spouses to persons with dementia. Dementia is a terminal condition that includes a wide range of chronic cognitive disorders whose symptoms include impaired memory, poor judgement and thinking, difficulty communicating, and mood and behavioural changes (such as aggression), along with increased mobility concerns for the person living with dementia [1]. The number of people living with dementia is growing at an alarming rate worldwide, given ageing of the population, and because there is currently no cure for dementia [2]. In 2015, 46.8 million people were living with dementia, a number which is projected to almost double by 2035 [3]. Persons living with dementia require essential support from others, particularly family members, over the course of their illness. Almost all persons with dementia living in the community or residential care settings receive some sort of assistance from

---

S. Peacock (✉)
College of Nursing, University of Saskatchewan, Saskatoon, SK, Canada
e-mail: shelley.peacock@usask.ca

M. Bayly
Reproductive Psychology Lab, University of Saskatchewan, Saskatoon, SK, Canada
e-mail: melanie.bayly@usask.ca

© Springer Nature Switzerland AG 2019
L. Holtslander et al. (eds.), *Hospice Palliative Home Care and Bereavement Support*, https://doi.org/10.1007/978-3-030-19535-9_11

informal carers such as unpaid family or friends, whether for self-care, household activities, or activities outside the home [4]. The caregiving journey with dementia is lengthy and complicated owing to the relentless, progressive nature of dementia which results in most persons with dementia eventually requiring 24-hour care in a long-term care setting.

The complexity of the journey with dementia makes for unique and differing caregiving experiences compared to other types of family carers including those who care for someone living with cancer, cardiovascular disease, or chronic obstructive pulmonary disease, for example [5]. Caring for someone with dementia is associated with negative consequences such as caregiver burden, social isolation, depression, and anxiety [6–8]. There may also be positive outcomes of caring for a relative with dementia, including (but not limited to) gaining a sense of meaning, accomplishment, and increased self-efficacy, as well as improved relationship quality [9, 10]. These experiences, both positive and negative, can influence how a family carer manages their role and can carry over into their bereavement.

Grieving is also a pervasive experience over the journey with dementia. Family carers to persons with dementia not only anticipate loss that has yet to occur, but also grieve for the losses that have already occurred or are occurring [11]. The losses that family carers may grieve include changes in lifestyle, relationships, hopes for the future, and feelings of security; these are often coupled with a sense of losing and grieving their relative with dementia as their illness worsens [12]. It is important to note that the journey with dementia does not end with the death of a relative with dementia, and family members desire support after the death [13]. Indeed, spousal carers to persons with dementia are more likely to experience higher levels of grief and complicated post-death grief compared to other carers [14, 15]. Research demonstrates that older adult spouses are among those in greatest need of support during bereavement [14]. Despite these needs, research suggests that the support provided to bereaved carers to persons with dementia is exceedingly limited, particularly when the family member died in long-term care [16]. As such, we developed the *Reclaiming Yourself* tool for older adult spouses to persons with dementia, in order to support them to positively navigate their bereavement.

11.2 The Intervention

The *Reclaiming Yourself* tool was developed from the *Finding Balance* tool, which was created to support older adult spouses to persons who died of cancer [17]. The *Reclaiming Yourself* tool is a self-administered psychosocial writing tool, intended to support bereaved carers to their spouse with dementia as they navigate bereavement and reclaim their selves after their experiences with caregiving, grief, and loss. The content of the *Reclaiming Yourself* tool was informed by rich interviews with bereaved spousal dementia carers, who described their experiences navigating bereavement including the important factors which facilitated the process [18]. For these carers, a key element of navigating bereavement was in *reclaiming self*; that is, bereavement involved not only maintaining a connection to the deceased spouse while re-fashioning a self without them, but also reconnecting to significant pre-caregiving activities and relationships.

After an initial draft of the *Reclaiming Yourself* tool was created, it was circulated among experts in the field including current professionals, academics, and bereaved carers to persons with dementia who provided feedback via a *Delphi* process. Three rounds of expert feedback were incorporated to assist with refining the tool to benefit and support the bereavement experience of older adult spouses. The resulting psychosocial writing tool consisted of three sections: (a) *Deep Grieving*; (b) *Embracing Self*; and (c) *Moving Forward*. Each of these sections includes quotations from bereaved spousal carers to persons with dementia that encapsulate aspects of bereavement and reclaiming self, as well as creative space for journaling.

Deep Grieving consists of activities which are intended to address the feelings of grief that bereaved spousal carers to persons with dementia may be navigating. These include acknowledging and expressing emotions, plans for how to achieve a 'time out' from difficult emotions, and the creation of a support system directory consisting of key people who can be contacted and their contact information, and how they can be helpful. These activities are meant to facilitate grief and give the work of grief purpose.

Embracing Self consists of activities focused on reclaiming elements of self that may have been diminished or lost through the long caregiving journey. The first activity involves reflection on activities and relationships engaged in prior to substantial caregiving, and then helps carers view how they align with current interests and relationships. This is followed by a scheduling activity wherein spousal carers are asked to schedule three activities a week to perform, and document three different ways they will take time for themselves that week. Taking time for self is essential to navigating bereavement. Finally, bereaved carers are asked in this section how they would like to keep remembering their partner and to find a way to sustain their connection through memory.

Moving Forward is focused on activities that address the process of moving forward in one's life *post*-caregiving. This includes an activity on voicing any regrets related to the caregiving journey; while this can be challenging for some carers, it has been found that this activity is enormously helpful in letting go of guilt. Additionally, carers are asked to identify and acknowledge the positive aspects of the long caregiving journey such that it may balance out those expressed regrets. Bereaved carers are encouraged to accept past events and let go of their regrets. The final activities are focused on resilience and strength: carer reflection on personal growth as a result of their rich experiences, things that foster inner strength, and how their story of caregiving might help others.

Initial evaluation of the *Reclaiming Yourself* tool was completed with 16 bereaved spousal carers to persons with dementia (primarily female, $n = 12$) living in the Canadian provinces of either Saskatchewan ($n = 8$) or Manitoba ($n = 8$). A research assistant met with each participant to explain the tool and provide them with a copy, which they were asked to use during the course of 1 month. Participants completed quantitative measures of grief, depressive symptoms, and balance between restoration and loss prior to using the *Reclaiming Yourself* tool and after 1 month of use; they also completed an interview about their experiences with the tool. While no significant differences in grief, depressive symptoms, or loss/restoration balance were found pre–post intervention, participant interviews provided useful and insightful feedback regarding the tool and its potential benefits. Significant feedback from those interviews informed the tool refinement and a final online version has been developed to make the tool widely available.

11.3 Case Example

May lost her 78-year-old husband David to Alzheimer's disease, 9 months before she began using the *Reclaiming Yourself* tool. David had been diagnosed 6 years before his death; May was his primary carer for five of those years until she could no longer manage his complex needs. During this period, May experienced numerous losses as David's cognition and health declined. Shortly after his diagnosis, David and May continued to enjoy travelling to many of the places they loved to visit; eventually, they could no longer travel, even to visit their children in other cities. May and David's social circle withered as he had difficulty participating in the activities they used to enjoy with their friends, such as going to the movies, brunch at a neighbourhood diner, and playing cards. May also felt that some of their friends were uncomfortable with the changes in David and did not always know how to act or behave around him. May maintained her weekly tennis game for as long as possible, but when David could no longer be left alone at home, she had to give up that activity as well.

As David's dementia progressed, he had difficulty sleeping, would occasionally become agitated, and sometimes unexpectedly tried to leave their home. This was a very difficult time for May and it took a toll on her physical, emotional, and mental health. She explained that she loved David very much and felt proud that she was able to fulfil her marriage vows in taking care of him 'in sickness', but began to feel exhausted and isolated as David's care needs increased. Moreover, she grieved the losses they were experiencing as David's capabilities and subsequently the nature of their relationship changed.

The most intense period of grief for May was when David made the necessary transition to a local long-term care home. Although his needs (most importantly to keep him safe) were best met in this environment, May wished that she could have continued taking care of him in the home they shared for almost 50 years. In fact, May would often describe the day David moved to his long-term care home as the hardest or worst day of her life. However, her health started to improve after this transition to long-term care and she visited David every day, usually around mealtimes to ensure he ate well and was not alone. David soon did not walk independently, needed increasing help with basic care, and eventually did not always recognize his wife of 53 years. May continued to visit and felt that even when David could not carry on a conversation with her, he became calm and serene when she described memories from their past or told stories about her day. When David died,

May and their two sons were by his side, and she felt that he was at peace. While it was a relief that David had died so his suffering was over, May couldn't help but wish for even one more day with him.

Although May in many ways felt prepared for David's death and had begun to grieve many losses during her caregiving journey, she missed him terribly and found it difficult to structure her days without seeing him. May continued to visit the long-term care home where David had lived and died; however, this time she was visiting as a volunteer. As May worked through her grief, the social worker from the long-term care home suggested that May might benefit from writing about her feelings and experiences and she was provided with a copy of the *Reclaiming Yourself* tool. May kept the tool on the end table beside her favourite chair and would pick it up every few days to work through the activities or journal about something she was experiencing or thinking during that time.

As she worked through the tool (sometimes going back to read over and over again what she had already written), May realized that she still had a lot of complex feelings around David's move to the long-term care home, including relief from the 24-hour care but also guilt and regret over not being able to continue to care for him on her own, in their own home. She found it helpful to fully acknowledge these feelings even when they were painful and felt that writing about them lifted their weight on her; being able to read them on paper was far different from working through them in her mind.

May thought that the greatest benefit of the tool was in how the various activities in each of the sections fostered reflection in a structured way. This was enormously helpful for her to acknowledge and express her feelings, and ultimately facilitated her ability to reframe some of her complicated caregiving experiences. The quotations in the tool from other bereaved carers helped May to feel less alone, as she had not attended a support group and did not feel as though many of her friends truly understood what it was like to care for a partner with dementia. May also appreciated the writing format of the tool because it allowed her to document memories and reflect on how she was doing over time. She wrote down her emotions each time she picked up the tool (sometimes at three in the morning, when she couldn't sleep) and dated/timed each writing entry so that she could look back on it later. May appreciated that she was able to reflect on how she was making progress through her bereavement and see how much had changed and grown already since David's death. She realized that she was doing much better than previously, including while she was caregiving, and this helped her to keep reconnecting to activities (like her weekly tennis game) and friends who had been a large part of her pre-caregiving life.

May shared her experiences with caregiving and bereavement that she had written in the tool with her two sons. It was through this sharing that her sons told her that they now better understood her caring for their dad and realized how incredibly strong she was in caring for him. In that sharing, May's sons had questions and reflections of their own to explore with their mom. Although May always felt that she could ask her sons for support, practical assistance was difficult since they did not live in the same city and their experiences with caregiving and grieving were very different from her own, but no less important. Following one of the activities in the tool, they together reflected on how they could keep a connection to David and decided to participate in May's local *Walk for Alzheimer Disease*. Additionally, May decided to continue volunteering once a week at the long-term care home where David lived and died.

May used the tool for a month and continued journaling even after she had completed all of the activities. The act of writing became important to May, as she perceived it to be therapeutic and cathartic. Having the words of her experiences on paper helped her to understand and also confirm her own feelings and thoughts about her journey with David and his dementia. She felt that using the tool had allowed her to express and reflect on things that she hadn't previously considered, which supported her through her bereavement journey. May was eventually able to let go of her feelings of regret over David's transition and subsequent move to the long-term care home and focused instead on all of the ways she had cared for him and continued to do so when he was no longer living in their own home. She realized how strong she really had been through caregiving and David's death, and this spurred her motivation to keep reconnecting with valued people and activities. May told her social worker that the *Reclaiming Yourself* tool would be helpful for other bereaved spouses to persons with dementia. She suggested that the tool be provided as early after the death of a spouse as possible, since it offered a structured way to work through bereavement and could provide other bereaved carers with the knowledge that they are not alone.

11.4 Conclusions

The case example of May and David illustrates how bereaved spousal carers to persons with dementia can use the *Reclaiming Yourself* tool, and how it may be of benefit. The three sections (*Deep Grieving*, *Embracing Self*, and *Moving Forward*) prompt spouses to reflect and work through their bereavement in a healthy and structured way. The case example reflects qualitative feedback received from pilot-testing of the tool, in which participants reported the tool offered a structured approach to navigating bereavement, operated as a catalyst for emotional expression, and facilitated reflection. While a writing intervention may not resonate with all bereaved carers, for many, this format offers unique benefits for reflection and giving voice to thoughts, emotions, and memories, as well as ways to move forward in one's grieving. This tool helps to fill a need for bereavement support for the population [16] who have experienced an intensive period of caregiving and may struggle with grieving prior to and following the death of their spouse.

The *Reclaiming Yourself* tool therefore has the potential to support older adult spouses to positively navigate their bereavement. Moreover, the tool is convenient, cost-effective, and responsive to the experiences of bereaved spouses. It can be used by individual spouses, or the various sections can augment activities and discussions that may be found in a bereavement support group. The tool is widely available via a webpage (http://research-groups.usask.ca/reclaimingyourself), which includes information about the tool and access to both an online and printable version. It is also part of other family carer interventions for persons with dementia (e.g., *My Tools4 Care—in Care*; https://www.mytools4careincare.ca/). Future considerations for the tool include testing it with a larger group of bereaved spouses and developing a version of the tool to support adult daughters who had their mother die with dementia. Currently, the *Reclaiming Yourself* tool represents a step forward in supporting older adult spouses of persons with dementia in their bereavement.

References

1. Alzheimer Society of Canada. What is dementia? 2018. https://alzheimer.ca/en/Home/About-dementia/What-is-dementia. Accessed 12 Nov 2018.
2. World Health Organization. Dementia. Geneva: WHO; 2017. https://www.who.int/news-room/fact-sheets/detail/dementia. Accessed 18 Jan 2019.
3. Prince M, Wimo A, Guerchat M, Ali GC, Wu TT, Prina M. World Alzheimer report 2015: the global impact of dementia. London: Alzheimer's Disease International; 2015. https://www.alz.co.uk/research/WorldAlzheimerReport2015.pdf. Accessed 18 January 2019.
4. Kasper JD, Freedman VA, Spillman BC, Wolff JL. The disproportionate impact of dementia on family and unpaid caregiving to older adults. Health Aff. 2015;10:1642–9. https://doi.org/10.1377/hlthaff.2015.0536.
5. Gill T, Gahbauer E, Han L, et al. Trajectories of disability in the last year of life. New Eng J Med. 2010;362:1173–80.
6. Brodaty H, Woodward M, Boundy K, Ames D, Balshaw R. Prevalence and predictors of burden in caregivers of people with dementia. Am J Geriatr Psychiatry. 2014;22:756–65. https://doi.org/10.1016/j.jagp.2013.05.004.
7. Cooper C, Balamurali TBS, Livingston G. A systematic review of the prevalence and covariates of anxiety in caregivers of people with dementia. Int Psychogeriatr. 2007;19:175–95. https://doi.org/10.1017/S1041610206004297.
8. Pinquart M, Sörensen S. Spouses, adult children, and children-in-law as caregivers of older adults: a meta-analytic comparison. Psychol Aging. 2011;26:1–14. https://doi.org/10.1037/a0021863.
9. Lloyd J, Patterson T, Muers J. The positive aspects of caregiving in dementia: a critical review of the qualitative literature. Dementia. 2016;15:1534–61. https://doi.org/10.1177/1471301214564792.
10. Peacock S, Forbes D, Markle-Reid M, Hawranik P, Morgan D, Jansen L, Leipert B, Henderson S. The positive aspects of the caregiving journey with dementia: using a strengths-based perspective to reveal opportunities. J Appl Gerontol. 2010;29:640–59. https://doi.org/10.1177/0733464809341471.
11. Hovland C. Welcoming death: exploring pre-death grief experiences of caregivers of older adults with dementia. J Soc Work End Life Palliat Care. 2018; https://doi.org/10.1080/15524256.2018.1508538.
12. Thompson G, Roger K. Understanding the needs of family caregivers of older adults dying with dementia. Palliat Support Care. 2014;12:223–331. https://doi.org/10.1017/S147895153000461.
13. Shanley C, Russell C, Middleton H, Simpson-Young V. Living through end-stage dementia: the experiences and expressed needs of family carers. Dementia. 2011;10:325–40.
14. Chan D, Livingston G, Jones L, Sampson EL. Grief reactions in dementia carers: a systematic review. Int J Geriatr Psychiatry. 2013;28:1–17.
15. Crespo M, Piccini AT, Bernaldo-de-Quirós M. When the care ends: emotional state of Spanish bereaved caregivers of persons with dementia. Span J Psychol. 2013;16:1–8. https://doi.org/10.1017/sjp.2013.97.

16. Arruda EH, Paun O. Dementia caregiver grief and bereavement: an integrative review. West J Nurs Res. 2017;39:825–51. https://doi.org/10.1177/0193945916658881.
17. Holtslander L. A finding balance writing intervention. In: Neimeyer RA, editor. Techniques of grief therapy. New York, NY: Routledge; 2012. p. 120–2.
18. Peacock S, Bayly M, Gibson K, Holtslander L, Thompson G, O'Connell M. The bereavement experience of spousal caregivers to persons with dementia: reclaiming self. Dementia. 2018;17:78–95. https://doi.org/10.1177/1471301216633325.

Living with Hope Program

12

Wendy Duggleby

Contents

12.1 Older Persons Receiving Palliative Homecare... 161
12.2 Living with Hope Program... 162
12.3 Case Example... 165
12.4 Conclusions.. 166
References.. 166

12.1 Older Persons Receiving Palliative Homecare

Palliative and end-of-life care is becoming more essential with the increasing number of persons aging worldwide [1]. A large portion of older persons in the last year of their life have a high prevalence of symptoms and a need for services to assist with essential activities of daily living [2]. These symptoms include psychological distress, as people receiving palliative care deal with issues of grief, uncertainty about the future, and physical symptoms [3]. Hope is an important psychosocial resource for persons receiving palliative care [4] and has been described as essential to attaining both a meaningful life [5] and a dignified death in peace and comfort [4]. Hope has also been linked to quality of life in persons who are receiving palliative care [6] with hopelessness associated with feelings of despair and wishes for hastened death [7, 8]. Hope has been defined by persons with terminal illness as the possibility of a desirable future within uncertainty [9]. It is situational and future-focused (with future redefined as minutes, hours, or days). Multiple types of hope coexist and what older persons are hoping for is desirable [9]. In order to maintain

---

W. Duggleby (✉)
Faculty of Nursing Level 3, Edmonton Clinic Health Academy, University of Alberta, Edmonton, AB, Canada
e-mail: wendy.duggleby@ualberta.ca

© Springer Nature Switzerland AG 2019
L. Holtslander et al. (eds.), *Hospice Palliative Home Care and Bereavement Support*, https://doi.org/10.1007/978-3-030-19535-9_12

hope, older persons receiving palliative homecare described how they reached inwardly and outwardly to find meaning and purpose, as well as a re-evaluated their hope in the light of terminal illness and finding positive possibilities [9].

An important aspect of holistic palliative care is to work with people to maintain and enhance their level of hope [10]. Several hope interventions for people receiving palliative are have been developed and found to have potential to increase hope [6, 11–14]. These interventions included: (a) forgiveness therapy [14]; (b) dignity therapy [13]; (c) short-term life review activities [11]; (d) art therapy [3]; (e) resilience therapy [15]; (f) the opening of a new palliative day care program [12]; (g) Hope Communication Tool [10]; and, (h) the Living with Hope Program [16]. However, only the Living with Hope Program was specifically developed for older persons (60 years of age and older) receiving palliative homecare. Older persons experience psychological distress as younger adults do, but have been found to use different methods of maintaining hope [4, 17]. For example, older persons utilize strategies for finding meaning and purpose, such as life review, to maintain hope in the context of suffering [4]. As well, because persons with terminal illness receiving palliative homecare also experience fatigue, interventions that are short, easy to use, and acceptable to this population are important for nurses to use [18]. Thus, this chapter will highlight the Living with Hope Program that was developed for and found to increase hope in older persons receiving palliative homecare.

12.2 Living with Hope Program

The Living with Hope Program (LWHP) was developed from research exploring the experience of hope of older persons receiving palliative homecare [4]. Older persons described wanting to "live with hope." They described their hope for "not suffering any more", "living life to the fullest" in the little time they have left, a peaceful death, life after death and hope for a better life in the future for their family [19]. They lived with hope by (a) acknowledging "life the way it is"; (b) searching for meaning; and, (c) positive reappraisal. This meant that they first had to acknowledge that their life had changed. Within their changed life, they had to find meaning. Only then could they find possibilities for hope. Symptoms and spirituality influence all of these processes. An example of these processes is from the description of an older man who had been a farmer. When he retired, he and his wife moved into a neighboring town. After retirement, he spent a great deal of time in his garden and was very proud of the beautiful flowers and plants he was able to grow. When he was diagnosed with advanced cancer, he started to have symptoms that interfered with his mobility. It became increasingly difficult to tend his garden, so he began losing hope that he would be able to continue to have a beautiful garden. However, he explained that one day in thinking about his garden, he decided that because of the decline in his health, he needed to really think about what was important to him. He decided that his hope had changed and now he hoped that tomorrow he would be able to sit outside with his grandchildren. No longer was it important to have a garden that was beautifully cultivated, but his hope was to share his joy of nature with his grandchildren.

Based on the findings from the study and using a Delphi approach with an expert panel, hope activities were selected that would assist older persons receiving palliative care to "live with hope" [15]. The LWHP has two components. The first involves viewing a short film (12 min), which is based on the research team's grounded theory study, and showcases terminally ill persons and their family members talking about how they maintain their hope. Its purpose was to achieve video modeling which occurs when viewers identify with the individuals on the film and perceive themselves as capable of performing a specific task [20, 21]. Viewers of the film are able to identify with the persons in the film and feel confident that they are able to maintain their hope, as well, at the end of life. The film is available online at www.nurs.ualberta.ca.

After viewing the film, participants then choose to begin one of three hope activities: (a) begin to write or ask someone to help you write one or more letters to someone; (b) begin a hope collection; or, (c) begin an "About Me" collection. The important instruction is to *begin* one of the activities, as finishing is not important. It does not matter which activity is chosen. The first activity of writing or asking someone to help them write a letter involved choosing someone the participants wanted to write a letter to and give them the letter if they want, but do not have to. For example, older persons receiving palliative homecare have sent letters to family, hid letters in their home so their family could find them after their death, and published a letter to their community in a community newsletter.

Instructions for the second activity of beginning a hope collection were to collect anything the participants wanted that gave them hope. These included poems, writings, pictures, photographs, and music.

The third activity of beginning an "About Me" collection was to begin to tell a story about the older person's life. This story could be written, audiotaped, or a collection of pictures. Older persons receiving palliative homecare have made collages of pictures that are important to them, written in journals about what they want to be remembered by, planted a tree with a journal of their life story. Figure 12.1 shows instructions on how to complete each of the three hope activities [6].

A mixed-method evaluation of the LWHP was completed with 60 palliative homecare clients randomized into treatment or control group [6]. Baseline measures of hope [Herth Hope Index (HHI)] and quality of life [McGill Quality of Life Questionnaire (MQOLQ)] were repeated 1 week later. A qualitative evaluation of the LWHP was then completed with those in the treatment group. Subjects receiving the LWHP had significantly higher hope (Factor 1: temporality and future) ($U = 255$, $p = 0.005$) and quality of life scores (MQOLQ physical and existential well-being subscales) at day 7 ($U = 294.5, p = 0.027$) than those in the control group. Qualitative data confirmed this finding with the majority (61.5%) of subjects in the treatment group reporting that the LWHP increased their hope. For example, some participants suggested that the LWHP gave them a purpose:

> "It gave me a purpose, something I had to do and accomplish. It was something I knew I could do when there is so many things I can no longer do". Another participant said it increased their hope because it gave them something positive to focus on: "It very much increased my hope and that of my families. It gave us all something to focus on and not my cancer".

Choose One of These

1. Write or ask someone to help you write one or more letters to someone:

- Choose people you want to write a letter to.
- Ask someone to help you write the letter or letters.
- You can give the letter to the person if you wish, but you don't have to.

2. Begin a Hope Collection:

- You can collect anything you want that gives you hope.
- These may include poems, writings, pictures, drawings, photographs, music, stories etc.
- Place your collection in a special binder or box.

3. Begin an "About Me" Collection:

- Tell your life as a story.
- In your story tell about your ups and downs beginning as young as you can remember.
- You can tell your story however you would like to do this. Some examples may be collecting cards, pictures or writing a journal.
- You can put your story in a scrapbook or you can audio or videotape your story so others can learn about you.

©LWH 2004

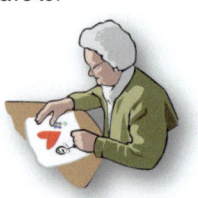

Fig. 12.1 Instructions for hope-focused activities. Reprinted with permission from Duggleby et al. [6]

Forty-six percent of the participants worked on their activities without assistance. The participants spent on average 260 min per week on their hope activity. No significant relationships were found among hope and quality of life and the amount of time spent on the activity, which activity was chosen, or the amount of help received.

A follow-up study was conducted to understand how the LWHP increased hope [22]. Thirteen older persons receiving palliative homecare and a family member were interviewed about their experience using the LWHP at 1 week and 2 weeks. Fifty-two transcripts were analyzed using thematic qualitative analysis. The findings suggested that the participants experienced the following while participating in the LWHP: (a) reminiscing; (b) leaving a legacy; (c) positive reappraisal; and, (d) motivational process. Participants described that reminiscing (personal life review) about their past experiences helped them to evaluate their life and recall happy memories. Reminiscence, recall of memories of one's life, has been found to stimulate bonding with others and promote positive feelings [23]. Reminiscing has also been found to help older persons finding meaning in their lives [11].

Leaving a legacy was described as leaving something behind for family members and future generations. At the same time, leaving a legacy was something that helped them to find value in their life. Positive re-appraisal occurred while using the LWHP as the activity encouraged them to think about hope and other positive thoughts. While using the LWHP, participants described how it motivated them to undertake activities they had been putting off in their personal lives. Hope as a motivational process has been found to increase participation in life and life satisfaction [24]. The LWHP provided the framework to encourage them to start activities they wished they had started a long time ago.

12.3 Case Example

M. was a 62-year-old Caucasian woman with advanced cancer and had been receiving palliative homecare for 3 months. She had a high school education, lived alone (divorced), but had two children close by who helped her when they could.

After watching the Living with Hope film, M. decided that she wanted to begin the 'About Me' activity. She said she chose this activity as she felt that it was important—"good for her kids to know more about her." She felt that people, like herself "don't talk about themselves," so even her family would not know about her life's experiences. She wanted to share some of her experiences with them. For her 'About Me' activity, she decided to start a scrapbook with pictures and memorabilia that were important to her. She described her experience doing the 'about me' activity:

> Well, when I first got started and picked the book that I was going to use, and then realized I'd have to, uh, find some pictures and some memory things like ribbons and certificates and things, it, uh, it actually made me get excited, because, uh, I thought, well, I'd never done something like this for *me*, I've always worked on albums and things for others, so I was actually kind of excited about this, and, um, thinking about all the other different things I could put into this scrapbook. So that's what I was thinking about.

Her daughter also commented that doing the hope 'About Me' activity would be fun for her and her mother. "I think this is a good idea, especially because this should have been done years ago, and, and this is, this'll be fun to do, and I'm looking forward to seeing how it's going to turn out!" She was looking forward to seeing her mother's hope activity.

For M., this hope activity was something that she had not taken time to do before. She started out thinking she was doing this for her family, but also discovered she was doing this for herself. In working on the hope activity, she was reminiscing about her life. The outcome was positive feelings.

M. also described how working on this hope activity had been a motivational process: "the fact that it made me get busy on this, uh, project, my story of my life *[chuckles]*, which I think is funny…" M. felt that the LWHP increased her hope by having her focus on positive experiences. When asked if the LWHP changed her feelings of hope, she said:

> Added—added to it [hope]—enhanced it—enhanced it a little bit. It kind of gave me, uh, more "This is going to be a positive thing"; like, it just added to my already positive thinking. But this is going to be a fun activity, and going through these pictures has been, has been, um—well, just going down memory lane for even just the, the old, old pictures, they're fun to look at, they're funny, and it brings back a lot of memories. Yeah.

She also talked about how she felt the LWHP would help others:

> I think it'll help other people as far as the doctors and the nurses to help people who are in these positions, maybe in the sense that if they've been diagnosed with a serious illness, rather than become negative about it, they can do things that can change their outlook and become more positive.

Her daughter also felt that the LWHP helped her mother to focus on positive memories and gave her something else to think about rather than focusing on her terminal illness. She said:

> "So if they're doing something like this, it might take their mind off of where they're at for a little while, and just give their mind something else to think about—and hopefully, it's a positive thing."

Focusing on positive experiences, not just the negative experiences, has been found to help people who are receiving palliative care deal with and transcend their suffering [9]. Based on M.'s experience, the LWHP "added" to her hope, enhanced it which was the purpose for developing the LWHP.

12.4 Conclusions

Healthcare professionals, in particular nurses, have recognized that hope is important for their people with advanced disease and their families [25]. The LWHP is an evidence-based, easy-to-use, self-administered intervention that can potentially increase hope and improved quality of life of persons receiving palliative homecare. A significant positive association has been found between the hope of persons receiving palliative care and the hope of their family caregivers [26] and healthcare providers [25]. This suggests that if nurses work with their patients to foster hope, the hope of family caregivers and nurses' own hope maybe enhanced as well. These additional benefits underscore the importance of fostering hope in persons receiving palliative homecare.

References

1. Parliamentary Committee on Palliative and Compassionate Care. Not to be forgotten: care of vulnerable Canadians. Ottawa, ON: Parliamentary Committee on Palliative and Compassionate Care; 2011.
2. Gill TM, Han L, Leo-Summers L, Ghahbauer EA, Allore HG. Distressing symptoms, disability and hospice services at the end of life: prospective cohort study. J Am Geriatr Soc. 2017;66(1):41–7.
3. Collins A, Bhathal D, Field T, Larlee R, Paje R, Young D. Hope Tree: an interactive art installation to facilitate the expression of hope in a hospice setting. Am J Hosp Palliat Med. 2018;35(10):1273–9.
4. Duggleby W, Wright K. Transforming hope: how elderly palliative patients live with hope. [Reprint in Can J Nurs Res. 2009;41(1):204–17; PMID: 19485053]. Can J Nurs Res. 2005;37(2):70–84.

5. Eliott JA, Olver IN. Hope, life, and death: a qualitative analysis of dying cancer patients' talk about hope. Death Stud. 2009;33(7):609–38.
6. Duggleby WD, Degner L, Williams A, Wright K, Cooper D, Popkin D, Holtslander L. Living with hope: initial evaluation of a psychosocial hope intervention for older palliative home care patients. J Pain Symptom Manage. 2007a;33(3):247–57.
7. Mystakidou K, Tsilika E, Parpa E, Pathiaki M, Galanos A, Vlahos L. The relationship between quality of life and levels of hopelessness and depression in palliative care. Depress Anxiety. 2008;25(9):730–6.
8. Rodin G, Lo C, Mikulincer M, Donner A, Gagliese L, Zimmermann C. Pathways to distress: the multiple determinants of depression, hopelessness and the desire for hastened death in metastatic cancer patients. Soc Sci Med. 2009;68(3):562–9.
9. Duggleby W, Hicks D, Nekolaichuk C, Holtslander L, Williams A, Chambers T, Eby J. Hope, older adults and chronic illness: a metasynthesis of qualitative research. J Adv Nurs. 2012;68(6):1211–23.
10. Olsman E, Leget C, Willems D. Palliative care professionals' evaluations of the feasibility of a hope communication tool: a pilot study. Prog Palliat Care. 2015;23(6):321–5.
11. Ando M, Morita T, Akechi T, Okamoto T. Japanese Task Force for Spiritual Care. Efficacy of short-term life-review interviews on the spiritual well-being of terminally ill cancer patients. J Pain Symptom Manage. 2010;39(6):993–1002.
12. Guy MP, Higginson IJ, Amesbury BD. The effect of palliative daycare on hope: a comparison of daycare patients with two control groups. J Palliat Care. 2011;27(3):216–23.
13. Hall S, Goddard C, Opio D, Speck PW, Martin P, Higginson IJ. A novel approach to enhancing hope in patients with advanced cancer: a randomised phase II trial of dignity therapy. BMJ Support Palliat Care. 2011;1(3):315–21.
14. Hansen MJ, Enright RD, Klatt J, Baskin TW. A palliative care intervention in forgiveness therapy for elderly terminally ill cancer patients. J Palliat Care. 2009;25(1):51–60.
15. Rosenberg AR, Bradford MC, Barton KS, Etsekson N, McCauley E, Curtis JR Wolfe J, Baker KS, Yi-Frazier JP. Hope and benefit finding: results from the PRISM randomized controlled trial. Pediatr Blood Cancer. 2018;66(1):e27485.
16. Duggleby W, Wright K, Williams A, Degner L, Cammer A, Holtslander L. Developing a living with hope program for caregivers of family members with advanced cancer. J Palliat Care. 2007b;23(1):24–31.
17. Herth K. Hope in older adults in community and institutional settings. Issues Ment Health Nurs. 1993;14(2):139–56.
18. Duggleby W, Williams A. Methodological and epistemological considerations in utilizing qualitative inquiry to develop interventions. Qual Health Res. 2016;26(2):147–53.
19. Duggleby W, Wright K. Elderly palliative care cancer patients' descriptions of hope-fostering strategies. Int J Palliat Nurs. 2004;10(7):352–9.
20. Gagliano ME. A literature review on the efficacy of video in patient education. J Med Educ. 1988;63:785–92.
21. Krouse HJ. Video modelling to educate patients. J Adv Nurs. 2001;33(6):748–57.
22. Duggleby W, Cooper D, Nekolaichuk C, Cottrell L, Swindle J, Barkway K. The psychosocial experiences of older palliative patients while participating in a living with hope program. Palliat Support Care. 2016;14(6):672–9.
23. Westerhof GJ, Bohlmeijer E, Webster JD. Reminiscence and mental health: a review of recent progress in theory, research and interventions. Ageing Soc. 2010;30(4):697–721.
24. Smedema SM, Chan JY, Phillips BN. Core self-evaluations and Snyder's hope theory in persons with spinal cord injuries. Rehabil Psychol. 2014;59(4):339–406.
25. Olsman E, Duggleby W, Nekolaichuk C, Willems D, Gagnon J, Kruizinga R, Leget C. Improving communication on hope in palliative care. A qualitative study of palliative care professionals' metaphors of hope: grip, source, tune, and vision. J Pain Symptom Manage. 2014;48(5):831–8.
26. Duggleby WD, Williams AM. Living with hope: developing a psychosocial supportive program for rural women caregivers of persons with advanced cancer. BMC Palliat Care. 2010;9(1):3.

Creativity, Optimism, Planning, and Expert Advise (COPE): A Problem-Solving Intervention for Supporting Cancer Patients and Their Family Caregivers

13

Cindy Tofthagen and Sherry S. Chesak

Contents

13.1	Introduction	170
	13.1.1 Creativity	170
	13.1.2 Optimism	171
	13.1.3 Planning	171
	13.1.4 Expert Information	171
	13.1.5 Symptom Management	171
	13.1.6 Applying COPE to a Problem	171
13.2	Summarizing COPE Research	174
	13.2.1 COPE for Cancer Caregivers	175
	13.2.2 COPE in Nonmalignant Conditions	175
	13.2.3 COPE for Patients	176
13.3	COPE and the Educate, Nurture, Advise, Before Life Ends (ENABLE) Intervention	176
13.4	Discussion	177
13.5	Conclusions	178
References		178

Sara is a 59-year-old wife and mother of one adult son. She has been receiving treatment for metastatic breast cancer for 3 years. Due to progressive fatigue and difficulty with concentration, she had to quit her job as an accountant 3 months ago. She is undergoing her 4th type of chemotherapy which makes her nauseated. She does not sleep well, waking up several times during the night and having trouble getting

---

C. Tofthagen (✉)
Mayo Clinic, Jacksonville, FL, USA
e-mail: tofthagen.cindy@mayo.edu

S. S. Chesak
Mayo Clinic, Rochester, MN, USA
e-mail: chesak.sherry@mayo.edu

© Springer Nature Switzerland AG 2019
L. Holtslander et al. (eds.), *Hospice Palliative Home Care and Bereavement Support*, https://doi.org/10.1007/978-3-030-19535-9_13

back to sleep. Her feet are numb from earlier chemotherapy and she has almost fallen once or twice.

Jim is Sara's husband of 24 years, who is the owner of an auto repair shop. He works long hours but fortunately, his schedule is flexible so he can take off to go with Sara to her appointments and take care of her on the days she needs help. Their 22-year-old son, Adam, comes by a few times a week and brings groceries and helps with housework and small home repairs. Adam will be graduating from college in 2 months and the whole family is concerned about whether Sara will be able to attend the graduation.

While Sara is receiving her chemotherapy, her nurse Marci, mentions that there is a new program to help people with cancer and their family caregivers. The program is called COPE. She recommends that Sara and Jim attend.

13.1 Introduction

COPE is an acronym for *c*reativity, *o*ptimism, *p*lanning, and *e*xpert information. COPE is a psycho-educational intervention that teaches problem-solving skills to help manage symptoms and other problems that persons with cancer may encounter at home. COPE can be adapted for use with either family caregivers or patients. It is based on the Prepared Family Caregiver Problem-Solving Model, a problem-solving technique that can be used to address any number of concerns [1]. In addition to problem-solving skills, COPE provided information to support caregivers in their role and teaches techniques to better manage symptoms at home, including knowing when to seek professional help [2].

The COPE intervention was developed from a book entitled the *American Cancer Society Complete Guide to Family Caregiving* [2]. With the authors' permission, the content was adapted for in-person delivery by registered nurses and tested in clinical trials [3]. The goals of the COPE intervention are to improve caregiver effectiveness, satisfaction, and self-efficacy. Outcomes may also include improved symptom management and quality of life (QOL) [3, 4]. The elements of COPE can be taught and applied in a variety of situations. In this chapter, we will discuss the four elements of COPE and provide an example of how creativity, optimism, planning, and expert information could be applied to Sara's situation. We will also discuss previous research related to COPE and opportunities for future adaptation and implementation into clinical settings.

13.1.1 Creativity

Individuals are encouraged to use creativity to overcome challenges, with the understanding that creativity must remain within the boundaries of safe and recommended clinical care. Viewing the problem as a challenge that can be overcome is important, as is identifying possible obstacles that could prevent the person from reaching their goal. Ways to think creatively about the problem might include talking to someone else about the problem and getting their viewpoint, thinking about something that has worked in a similar situation in the past and revising that to fit the new problem, evaluating whether the goal is realistic, and brainstorming.

13.1.2 Optimism

Optimism as it pertains to COPE means focusing on good things that are happening, expecting to succeed, practicing positive self-thoughts, self-talk, and self-care. At the same time, being realistic about the seriousness of the problem and attentive to the situation is also stressed. Reflecting on prior problem-solving successes and what worked in those situations helps build confidence in the ability to manage current problems.

13.1.3 Planning

Devising a plan is an important aspect of problem-solving. In order to develop a plan, it is important to gather all the information first. Avoiding making assumptions but instead looking at the problem objectively helps in developing a sound plan. Working together to develop the plan and thinking about what resources will be needed to carry out the plan are important, as well as seeking professional help when needed. After a plan is solidified, carrying out the plan and making adjustments when things do not work out are important aspects of the problem-solving approach.

13.1.4 Expert Information

Finding sources of trustworthy information and learning how to access information in a timely fashion are important. Information should come from reliable sources such as healthcare professionals and reliable websites should be stressed. Identifying when to seek professional help is important to both self-care and caregiving. Having a point of contact with each healthcare provider and getting to know them can help facilitate access to expert information. Teaching patients and caregivers when to seek professional help is a critical part of the COPE intervention.

13.1.5 Symptom Management

In addition to teaching the COPE framework, the COPE intervention provides information on how to manage physical, emotional, and long-term side effects of cancer and cancer treatment (Table 13.1). This includes information to help with understanding the specific symptom, when to get professional help, what can be done to prevent and manage that symptom, possible challenges, how to monitor progress, and what to do when the plan doesn't work.

13.1.6 Applying COPE to a Problem

This section will provide examples of how the COPE problem-solving framework can be applied to a patient problem, using the previous scenario.

Table 13.1 Symptoms addressed in the ACS guide for caregivers

Emotional responses	Physical side effects	Long-term side effects
Anxiety	Nausea/vomiting	Lymphedema
Depression	Constipation	Sexual issues
	Diarrhea	
	Fever and infections	
	Pain	
	Mouth sores	
	Skin problems	
	Loss of appetite	
	Bleeding	
	Tiredness/fatigue	
	Sleep problems	
	Hair loss	
	Confusion	

Sara and Jim decide to attend the classes that Marci suggested. The classes taught them how to use the COPE program to help manage Sara's symptoms. Together, they decided to use the COPE problem-solving model to figure out how to get Sara to Adam's graduation. Sara immediately implemented techniques they learned in the COPE program to help promote sleep and rest, as well as to conserve energy.

Using *creativity*, Sara and Jim started thinking realistically about the potential obstacles that might interfere with her getting to the graduation. They identified the main potential barriers as fatigue and weakness. Neuropathy makes her legs weak and they sometimes tremble or give out. The graduation is from 6 to 8 pm and she is normally exhausted by that time of day. In brainstorming possible options, they realize that they need to arrive early to allow plenty of time to walk from the car and find a seat. To avoid a fall, Sara will need to use some type of assistive device, which she has not done before. Also, they are not sure of available options.

Thinking *optimistically*, Sara realizes that attending the event will be a logistical challenge and she is worried that she may lose her balance or become too exhausted to make it through the whole event. She is also determined to see her only child graduate from college and knows that once she sets her mind to something, she will find a way to make it happen. She remembers similar times in her life where she was faced with a challenge and succeeded in achieving her goal.

Jim and Sara devise a *plan*. They decide to ask Sara's oncologist about getting a wheelchair and a handicapped parking permit. If not, Adam might be able to ride with them and Jim can drop them off at the front door and help Sara find a place to sit until Jim parks and joins them. They have three prong canes for sale at the local drug store, and Sara is relatively confident that she can walk from the door to her seat with the cane without losing her balance. Jim decides to visit the venue where the graduation is taking place in advance to see the layout, how far they will have to walk, and whether there are special accommodations for people in wheelchairs. In order to have enough energy, Sara decides that she will take a nap in the early afternoon and Jim will help her by making sure everything she needs to get ready for the graduation is laid out in advance.

When Sara sees nurse Marci again, she talks with her about their plans, and Marci provides her *expert opinion*. She expresses concern about Sara being out in a large crowd during chemotherapy due to increased risk of infection, yet she understands that being there to see her son graduate from college is important to Sara. She calculates where Sara will be in her chemo cycle on the day of the ceremony and determines that if chemo proceeds as planned, Sara will be hitting her nadir, the point when her risk of infection is highest. Marci confers with the oncologist and the decision is made to delay that chemotherapy by a week to allow for Sara's blood counts to recover. She also completes the disabled parking permit form, gets it signed by the doctor, and tells Sara where she can purchase a lightweight wheelchair if needed. Sara and Jim's plan is successful and they bask in pride as their son receives his degree.

The steps in the COPE problem-solving model may seem intuitive to nurses, as we use similar problem-solving skills when caring for patients; however, patients and caregivers often lack confidence in their ability to successfully manage symptoms and other problems that arise as a result of cancer or its treatment. Even when patients and caregivers possess strong problem-solving skills, implementing the COPE problem-solving techniques can teach them how to approach a problem systematically, and help them see problems from a different perspective. The information about managing symptoms is likely new to them or has been buried in the onslaught of information they have received in the course of treatment. A methodical approach such as COPE helps people develop confidence in their problem-solving ability and can lead to improved symptom management and coping ability; yet, there are still gaps in the research and practice that we will explore. These gaps represent important areas for future research and implementation into practice. Table 13.2 summarizes published studies evaluating the COPE intervention.

Table 13.2 Randomized, controlled trials of the COPE intervention

References	Population receiving COPE	Sample size	Design	No. of sessions	Components of COPE	Outcomes
McMillan and Small [3]; McMillan et al. [4]	Caregivers of hospice patients with cancer	329	RCT	Three face-to-face visits and five phone calls	COPE problem-solving techniques Assessment and management of pain, constipation, and dyspnea emphasized; caregivers provided the textbook containing information on more symptoms	*Patient*: lower symptom distress after caregiver participation in COPE *Caregiver*: QOL, the burden of patient symptoms, and caregiving task burden all decreased in COPE group, compared to usual care and attention control

(continued)

Table 13.2 (continued)

References	Population receiving COPE	Sample size	Design	No. of sessions	Components of COPE	Outcomes
McMillan et al. [6]	Caregivers of hospice patients with heart failure	40 (19 received COPE)	RCT	Three face-to-face visits and five phone calls	COPE problem-solving techniques; targeted common symptoms in heart failure (dyspnea, edema, angina, constipation); recommendations for caregiver self-care	COPE had no significant effect on caregiver or patient outcomes
McMillan and colleagues, [8]	Outpatients undergoing cancer treatment	534	RCT	Three face-to-face visits and two phone calls over 9 weeks	COPE problem-solving techniques: assessment and management of most distressing symptoms, as selected by the participant	COPE improved symptom intensity. COPE did not affect QOL, anxiety, or depression
Meyers et al. [5]	Patients enrolled in phase I, II, or III cancer clinical trials, and their family caregivers	476	RCT	Three face-to-face visits over first 30 days in trial	COPE problem-solving techniques: assessment and management of symptoms, as selected by the participant	*Patient*: no difference in QOL compared to usual care *Caregiver*: QOL remained relatively stable over a 6-month period, while QOL steadily declined in usual care group

13.2 Summarizing COPE Research

The following sections will provide an overview of studies that have included COPE as an intervention. Opportunities for additional research will also be presented.

13.2.1 COPE for Cancer Caregivers

When COPE has been implemented with family caregivers of persons with cancer at the end of life, it has positive effects for both the caregiver and the care recipient (patient) [3–5]. When caregiver-related outcomes were studied, participation in the COPE intervention has demonstrated efficacy in improving quality of life and decreasing caregiver burden when compared to usual care or attention alone [4, 5]. In the first study of the COPE intervention, caregivers received COPE in a face-to-face format, in three sessions over a 9-day period. The intervention focused on the management of three of the most common symptoms at the end of life: pain, dyspnea, and constipation. When patient outcomes were evaluated within the same study, symptom distress improved, although there were no changes in symptom intensity, compared to the other groups [3]. At no time in this study did the patient (care recipient) participate in the COPE intervention. This highlights the importance of the caregiver in relation to better management of patient symptoms. When taught in conjunction with enrollment in a clinical trial, caregiver QOL remained relatively stable over a 6-month period, while caregivers who did not engage in COPE demonstrated progressively declining QOL over the same period, suggesting a sustained benefit of the COPE intervention [5].

13.2.2 COPE in Nonmalignant Conditions

Few studies have evaluated COPE in disease processes other than cancer. Thinking that COPE might be useful outside of oncology, researchers revised the intervention to address the symptoms experienced by hospice patients with heart failure (COPE-HF). They pilot-tested in a group of 40 caregiver/patient dyads, with unexpected results [6]. COPE-HF was adapted to address the needs of family caregivers in managing symptoms such as dyspnea, edema, angina, and constipation and also provided recommendations for self-care such as exercise, social interaction, and spiritual practices. Caregivers received three face to face visits and five phone calls with a nurse trained to deliver the COPE-HF. There were no improvements in any caregiver or patient outcomes when compared to usual care. When caregivers in the study were interviewed by the researchers, caregivers who were new to the caregiving role found the information more useful, while those who had been in a caregiver role for a year or more did not perceive COPE-HF as adding to the skills or knowledge they had already developed [7]. Recommendations made as a result of this study include introducing COPE earlier in the disease trajectory, as soon after diagnosis as possible, and tailoring the information based on the needs of the caregiver. It should also be noted that at least one caregiver found the symptom management content useful in managing their own symptoms; therefore, integrating more information to support self-care and focus on caregiver health and well-being may be useful for future iterations of COPE.

13.2.3 COPE for Patients

Unfortunately, large studies delivering COPE to cancer patients have not demonstrated the same improvements in QOL that occur in caregivers receiving COPE, although data indicate that COPE may lead to improved symptom management. In a clinical trial funded by the Patient-Centered Outcomes Research Institute (PCORI), outpatients undergoing cancer treatment were randomized to receive the COPE intervention in three sessions, usual care, or three supportive care nursing visits where active listening and emotional support without COPE is provided [8]. The research team hypothesized that those receiving COPE would show improved quality of life, anxiety, and depression. Unfortunately, no differences in any of these primary outcomes were seen. However, patients receiving COPE experienced less symptom intensity than those in other groups.

The first study to deliver COPE via use of technology rather than face to face was a web-based version of COPE, designed for patients with chemotherapy-induced peripheral neuropathy [9]. Participants found it easy to use and said the information was helpful. Neuropathy symptoms worsened over the course of the study, which was expected with increasing exposure to the drugs that were causing their neuropathy. However, interference with usual activities decreased, suggesting that participants may have implemented embedded suggestions for home safety, use of assistive devices, and improving function. These findings provide preliminary evidence that the delivery of COPE interventions via technology is acceptable to patients and can be useful in supporting symptom self-management.

13.3 COPE and the Educate, Nurture, Advise, Before Life Ends (ENABLE) Intervention

The COPE framework was a key component in the development of the Educate, Nurture, Advise, Before Life Ends (ENABLE) intervention, an early palliative care educational intervention developed for cancer patients and their caregivers [10, 11]. ENABLE utilizes a manualized, in-person and telephonic format, administered by nurses, advanced practice nurses, and social workers to encourage patient activation, self-management, and empowerment. The intervention includes teaching of skills and coaching in problem-solving, symptom and self-care management, addressing emotional and spiritual needs, communication, and decision support. The ultimate goal is to empower patients and their caregivers to be actively involved in their healthcare from the time of diagnosis [12]. The COPE framework provides the basis for the problem-solving component of the ENABLE intervention, as it affords methods for problem-focused coping versus avoidant- and emotion-focused coping [10]. While ENABLE was originally designed for use with cancer patients, it has since been adapted for use with patients with other serious chronic illnesses and their caregivers [12, 13].

The ENABLE intervention has been developed and tested through a number of trials with cancer patients and caregivers, with development and testing occurring in four phases. Phase I included stakeholder development processes and tested in-person delivery of the intervention [14]. Phases II and III entailed effectiveness research with randomized controlled trials (RCTs) and tested efficacy of the intervention with modified versions, including addition of telehealth elements and a life review component [11, 15]. Finally, phase IV trials studied rural implementation [15]. Outcomes from a phase II study, in which investigators assessed patients' reaction to the ENABLE intervention with a qualitative descriptive design, included themes of enhanced problem-solving skills, better coping, feeling empowered, and feeling supported or reassured [16]. Caregiver-related outcomes from an RCT conducted in phase III demonstrated improvements in depression and stress burden relative to usual cancer care [17]. In another phase III RCT, there was some evidence to suggest that the intervention may positively impact caregiver grief scores after patients die [18]. Patient-related outcomes from phases II and III RCTs indicated improvements in QOL, mood, survival rates, and symptom intensity compared to those receiving usual care [11, 15]. Finally, two RCTs in phase III indicated maximized benefits for both patients and caregivers with early versus delayed palliative care and ENABLE initiation [11, 19]. Further research has also been conducted with ENABLE and COPE among patients with other chronic illnesses and their caregivers [19].

13.4 Discussion

Interventions based on the COPE problem-solving framework [1] and *ACS Complete Guide to Family Caregiving* can improve QOL and reduce caregiver burden [3, 5, 10]. Once COPE problem-solving techniques are learned, they can be applied in virtually any situation, potentially increasing capacity to deal with caregiver-related stress more effectively. The positive effects have only been demonstrated among caregivers of cancer patients and may or may not hold true for caregivers of people with other chronic illnesses [7]. Interviews with caregivers suggest that COPE would be more beneficial to them, had they received the information earlier in the disease trajectory. There is a need for future research evaluating whether COPE is indeed more effective when delivered early in the disease trajectory or can benefit caregivers of those with different or multiple chronic conditions.

Knowledge in oncology is evolving at a rapid pace. Pharmacogenetics, individualized medicine, and immunotherapies are not only changing the cancer treatment landscape but are also changing symptom science. Therefore, all symptom-related content should be continually updated to reflect current standards of care. As scientific knowledge has evolved, patient care has become more hurried and fragmented, making it more challenging for patients and caregivers to get information and have their needs and concerns adequately addressed. In order for a psycho-educational intervention such as COPE to be most effective, the content should be tailored to the individual needs of each participant and adapted to fit the current healthcare environment.

The majority of studies to date have implemented COPE using face-to-face individual meetings, with nurses who have received special training. This is time-consuming, expensive, and impractical in most settings. Future studies should continue to evaluate whether distance interventions, delivered via electronic platforms, are also effective. Delivery of COPE in a group setting should also be explored. This would offer a less costly and more time-efficient delivery method that could provide an additional benefit of increased social support.

When COPE has been implemented with oncology patients, rather than caregivers, it did not have the same effects on QOL that it had with caregivers; however, it did improve aspects of patient symptoms [8]. The authors speculated that the three visits provided were insufficient in the setting of ongoing cancer treatment and that information overload, difficulty concentrating due to feeling poorly, or other patient-related factors may have interfered with them being able to absorb and apply the content. Future iterations of COPE may be able to address these issues through the use of technology. Other electronic interventions have successfully incorporated electronic symptom assessment combined with self-care support and communication coaching to improve symptom distress [20]. The dose of intervention needed varies and providing a COPE intervention to patients when it is most convenient, and when they have the time and motivation to focus on mastering the content, is likely to be more beneficial than a one-size-fits-all approach. Electronic delivery would also allow individuals to select content that is most relevant to any symptoms or problems they are experiencing, as well as having the ability to access COPE information at the time of need.

13.5 Conclusions

COPE is a psycho-educational intervention that combines problem-solving techniques with symptom management information. Clinical trials have demonstrated that COPE improves QOL and alleviates cancer caregiver burden and distress. It also may be helpful in managing patient symptoms during cancer treatment. There are barriers to widespread implementation of COPE in clinical settings that might be addressed through the use of technology. Future opportunities include electronic delivery and adaptation for use in non-malignant chronic conditions.

References

1. Houts PS, Nezu AM, Nezu CM, Bucher JA. The prepared family caregiver: a problem-solving approach to family caregiver education. Patient Educ Couns. 1996;27(1):63–73.
2. Bucher J, Houts P. The American Cancer Society complete guide to family caregiving. Atlanta, GA: American Cancer Society; 2011.
3. McMillan SC, Small BJ. Using the COPE intervention for family caregivers to improve symptoms of hospice homecare patients: a clinical trial. Oncol Nurs Forum. 2007;34(2):313–21.

4. McMillan SC, Small BJ, Weitzner M, Schonwetter R, Tittle M, Moody L, et al. Impact of coping skills intervention with family caregivers of hospice patients with cancer: a randomized clinical trial. Cancer. 2006;106(1):214–22.
5. Meyers FJ, Carducci M, Loscalzo MJ, Linder J, Greasby T, Beckett LA. Effects of a problem-solving intervention (COPE) on quality of life for patients with advanced cancer on clinical trials and their caregivers: simultaneous care educational intervention (SCEI): linking palliation and clinical trials. J Palliat Med. 2011;14(4):465–73.
6. McMillan SC, Small BJ, Haley WE, Zambroski C, Buck HG. The COPE intervention for caregivers of patients with heart failure: an adapted intervention. J Hosp Palliat Nurs. 2013;15(4):PMID:24288455.
7. Buck HG, Zambroski CH, Garrison C, McMillan SC. "Everything they were discussing, we were already doing": hospice heart failure caregivers reflect on a palliative caregiving intervention. J Hosp Palliat Nurs. 2013;15(4):218–24.
8. McMillan S, Small B, Tofthagen C, Haley W, Meng D, Rodriguez R, et al. Patient outcomes of a self-care management approach to cancer symptoms: a randomized clinical trial. Washington, DC: Patient-Centered Outcomes Research Institute; 2019.
9. Tofthagen C, Kip KE, Passmore D, Loy I, Berry DL. Usability and acceptability of a web-based program for chemotherapy-induced peripheral neuropathy. Comput Inform Nurs. 2016;34(7):322–9.
10. Dionne-Odom JN, Lyons KD, Akyar I, Bakitas MA. Coaching family caregivers to become better problem solvers when caring for persons with advanced cancer. J Soc Work End Life Palliat Care. 2016;12(1–2):63–81.
11. Bakitas MA, Tosteson TD, Li Z, Lyons KD, Hull JG, Li Z, et al. Early versus delayed initiation of concurrent palliative oncology care: patient outcomes in the ENABLE III randomized controlled trial. J Clin Oncol. 2015;33(13):1438–45.
12. Bakitas M, Dionne-Odom JN, Pamboukian SV, Tallaj J, Kvale E, Swetz KM, et al. Engaging patients and families to create a feasible clinical trial integrating palliative and heart failure care: results of the ENABLE CHF-PC pilot clinical trial. BMC Palliat Care. 2017;16(1):45.
13. Wells R, Stockdill ML, Dionne-Odom JN, Ejem D, Burgio KL, Durant RW, et al. Educate, nurture, advise, before life ends comprehensive heartcare for patients and caregivers (ENABLE CHF-PC): study protocol for a randomized controlled trial. Trials. 2018;19(1):422.
14. Bakitas M, Stevens M, Ahles T, Kirn M, Skalla K, Kane N, et al. Project ENABLE: a palliative care demonstration project for advanced cancer patients in three settings. J Palliat Med. 2004;7(2):363–72.
15. Bakitas M, Lyons KD, Hegel MT, Balan S, Brokaw FC, Seville J, et al. Effects of a palliative care intervention on clinical outcomes in patients with advanced cancer: the project ENABLE II randomized controlled trial. JAMA. 2009;302(7):741–9.
16. Maloney C, Lyons KD, Li Z, Hegel M, Ahles TA, Bakitas M. Patient perspectives on participation in the ENABLE II randomized controlled trial of a concurrent oncology palliative care intervention: benefits and burdens. Palliat Med. 2013;27(4):375–83.
17. Dionne-Odom JN, Azuero A, Lyons KD, Hull JG, Tosteson T, Li Z, et al. Benefits of early versus delayed palliative care to informal family caregivers of patients with advanced cancer: outcomes from the ENABLE III randomized controlled trial. J Clin Oncol. 2015;33(13):1446–52.
18. Dionne-Odom JN, Azuero A, Lyons KD, Hull JG, Prescott AT, Tosteson T, et al. Family caregiver depressive symptom and grief outcomes from the ENABLE III randomized controlled trial. J Pain Symptom Manag. 2016;52(3):378–85.
19. Zubkoff L, Dionne-Odom JN, Pisu M, Babu D, Akyar I, Smith T, et al. Developing a "toolkit" to measure implementation of concurrent palliative care in rural community cancer centers. Palliat Support Care. 2018;16(1):60–72.
20. Berry DL, Hong F, Halpenny B, Partridge AH, Fann JR, Wolpin S, et al. Electronic self-report assessment for cancer and self-care support: results of a multicenter randomized trial. J Clin Oncol. 2014;32(3):199–205.

Dementia

14

Rhoda MacRae, Margaret Brown, and Debbie Tolson

Contents

14.1	Global Prevalence	182
14.2	Risk Factors and Causes	182
14.3	Alzheimer's Disease	183
14.4	Vascular Dementia	183
14.5	Dementia with Lewy Bodies	184
14.6	Early/Young Onset Dementia	184
14.7	Frontotemporal Degeneration/Dementia (FTD)	185
14.8	Comorbidities and Dementia	185
14.9	Dementia as a Dynamic Concept	186
14.10	As Dementia Progresses	187
14.11	Terminology and Definitions	187
14.12	Defining Advanced Dementia	188
14.13	Features of Advanced Dementia	188
14.14	Palliative Care	189
14.15	Palliare	190
	14.15.1 Dementia Palliare: Best Practice Principles	191
14.16	Care Empathia	192
	14.16.1 Dementia-Specific Issues to Consider When Meeting Care Needs	192
	14.16.2 Working with the Embodied Memory, Senses and Emotions	193
14.17	Fundamentals of Advanced Dementia Care	194
14.18	Preventing and Minimising Stress and Distress	195
14.19	Discussion	196
14.20	Conclusions	196
References		197

R. MacRae (✉) · M. Brown · D. Tolson
Alzheimer Scotland Centre for Policy and Practice, School of Health and Life Sciences,
University of the West of Scotland, Lanarkshire, UK
e-mail: Rhoda.macrae@uws.ac.uk; margaret.brown@uws.ac.uk; Debbie.tolson@uws.ac.uk

© Springer Nature Switzerland AG 2019
L. Holtslander et al. (eds.), *Hospice Palliative Home Care and Bereavement Support*, https://doi.org/10.1007/978-3-030-19535-9_14

Dementia is an umbrella term describing a progressive neurodegenerative syndrome caused by illnesses such Alzheimer's disease that cause structural and chemical changes to the brain. The cognitive impairments most notably affect memory, orientation, comprehension, calculation, learning capacity, language and judgement. Consciousness is not affected. The impairment in cognitive function is commonly accompanied and occasionally preceded, by deterioration in emotional control, social behaviour or motivation [1].

14.1 Global Prevalence

Over 50 million people live with dementia worldwide and this is predicted to increase to 152 million by 2050 [2]. Almost 9.9 million people develop dementia each year, the majority (63%) of whom reside in low- and middle-income countries [3]. A recent systematic review of global trends in prevalence suggests that the incidence of dementia may be declining in high-income countries, but rising in low-income countries [2].

14.2 Risk Factors and Causes

Age remains the strongest risk factor for dementia, but dementia is not an inevitable consequence of growing old [1]. Modifiable risk factors include: (a) mid-life hypertension, (b) low educational attainment, (c) diabetes mellitus, (d) tobacco use, (e) physical inactivity, (f) obesity, (g) alcohol use, (h) mid-life depression, (i) social isolation and (j) cognitive inactivity [4]. There is evidence that a healthy lifestyle that includes regular physical exercise, maintaining a healthy weight, not smoking or drinking alcohol, having a healthy balanced diet low in fat, salt and sugar may reduce the risk of dementia as well as other conditions such as stroke, heart disease and cancer [5].

There is broad agreement that two proteins in the brain are heavily involved in causing changes in the brain. Beta-amyloid, which reaches abnormal levels in the brain of someone with Alzheimer's and forms plaques (Tau protein) that collect between neurons and disrupt cell function [3]. Scientists do not fully understand how these proteins relate to each other or what causes them to build to damaging levels. Resilience and vulnerability factors may play a part, metabolic factors, our ability to metabolise cholesterol and glucose, reduce inflammation and oxidative stress are also implicated [3].

An example of the complex ways these neurodegenerative conditions present or not, is highlighted by the 'Nun Study', an ongoing epidemiological study of a population of 678 Catholic sisters before and after death (https://www.psychiatry.umn.edu/research/research-labs-and-programs/nun-study). Detailed information about the lifestyles of the nuns and post mortem analysis of their brain tissue suggests that dementia-related disabilities are not simply a reflection of resultant brain damage, but involve a more complex picture of brain plasticity (flexibility) to compensate for damage. The theory of cognitive reserve suggests that those who benefit from greater education engage in more cognitive and physical activity and experience good social networks may build up a protective cognitive reserve so that more extensive pathology is required for impairments to become evident [6].

Tentatively, there is consensus that amyloid and its relationship to tau is central, understanding the brain function and the way various components interact with each other within the whole body at an earlier stage is the focus of current research. For an example of accessible multimedia talks that explain the science of brain health, see https://www.ted.com/talks/lisa_genova_what_you_can_do_to_prevent_alzheimer_s.

Although the boundaries between the different types of dementia are not necessarily distinct, it is thought that Alzheimer's disease and vascular dementia account for more than 80% of cases. These all have different pathologies, sometimes mixed pathologies and the types have sub-types, highlighting the complexity within dementia and its many causes.

14.3 Alzheimer's Disease

Alzheimer's disease (AD) is the most common type of dementia. It accounts for 60–75% of all cases. In AD, there is a build-up of amyloid which is deposited in large numbers on the surface of the nerve cells in the brains of people with the disease; over time, chemical connections between the brain are lost, cells die and the brain shrinks as gaps develop in the temporal lobe and hippocampus which are responsible for storing and retrieving new information [7]. This in turn affects people's ability to remember, speak, think and make decisions. Often, the first symptom people notice is problems with day-to day memory, other early symptoms include difficulties finding the right words, solving problems, making decision or perceiving things in three dimensions [7]. These symptoms tend to progress at a steady rate over time. Acetylcholinesterase (AChE) inhibitors can be used in the early stages to slow progression or alleviate symptoms temporarily; these should always be used in conjunction with non-pharmacological interventions to promote cognition, independence and well-being [8].

14.4 Vascular Dementia

It is estimated that vascular dementia accounts for around 15% of cases. Vascular dementia is caused by reduced oxygen supply to the brain, associated with hypertension, high cholesterol, diabetes and stroke. Damage to the brain may happen suddenly when there is an interruption to the blood supply through a blockage, bleed or clot, causing a stroke. A series of smaller strokes over time may cause symptoms to progress in a stepwise fashion. Primary impairments include poor concentration, problem solving, thinking quickly, language and functional difficulties. Secondary prevention treatment to address the underlying causes is the focus with vascular dementia. Mixed presentations involving vascular and Alzheimer's disease are common.

14.5 Dementia with Lewy Bodies

The minimum incidence of dementia with Lewy bodies (DLB) is around 6%; however, there is evidence to suggest that DLB is not always diagnosed and may account for 10–15% of all dementias [9]. Reasons for under diagnosing are complex, but it is thought that DLB is overlooked in people with Parkinson's as Lewy bodies are also found in the brains of people with Parkinson's disease. Diagnostic criteria for DLB were only established in 1996, so some DLB symptoms such as fluctuating cognition and disrupted REM sleep patterns may not have been routinely screened for when making a differential diagnosis until the 2000s. The risk factors for DLB are unknown; it tends to affect more men than women [9].

Lewy bodies are tiny, spherical protein deposits that develop inside the nerve cells. Their presence in the brain interrupts normal communication between nerve cells by disrupting the action of important chemical messengers. Memory is less affected in the early stages and the primary impairments are: visual hallucinations, REM sleep disturbance, parkinsonian features, fluctuations in cognition, attention and arousal [10]. Antipsychotics can worsen the motor features of the condition and in some cases cause severe antipsychotic sensitivity reactions [8].

14.6 Early/Young Onset Dementia

People with dementia whose symptoms begin before 65 years are often described as having early or young onset dementia. It is estimated that they account for around 5–10% of all those with dementia [5, 11]. However, this figure could be higher because of the difficulties diagnosing early-onset dementias which have a more varied differential diagnosis than late onset; often, memory impairment is not the most prominent symptom. Alzheimer's disease accounts for around one-third of early-onset dementia opposed to two-thirds with later onset. Vascular dementia accounts for around 20% of younger people with dementia. Frontotemporal dementia (FTD) is also common in people under 65 years and in about 40% of FTD cases, there is a family history of the condition [12]. Alcohol-related dementia and dementia with Lewy bodies together account for another 20% of people with young onset. The rarer forms of the condition such as dementia with Parkinson's, Posterior Cortical Atrophy, Huntington's disease and Creutzfeld Jakob disease account for another 20%. People with learning disability, particularly Down's syndrome are at greater risk of developing dementia at a younger age and one in three people with Down's syndrome will have Alzheimer's in their 50s [13].

The support needs of younger people with dementia maybe be different from those who are older; they maybe in employment when symptoms begin or they are diagnosed; they may have dependent children and still have financial commitments such as mortgages. Support organisations also report that younger people, who are perhaps more likely to be otherwise fit and well, may struggle to accept they have a cognitive impairment. Family caregivers of people with young-onset dementias are reported to experience greater caregiver burden, distress, depression and sleep disturbance [14]. The troubling experiences related to the changes in behaviour and personality of their loved one often result in high levels of emotional and psychological difficulties that healthcare providers need to be able to respond to effectively [14].

14.7 Frontotemporal Degeneration/Dementia (FTD)

Frontotemporal dementia (FTD) is a leading cause of young-onset dementia. The term frontotemporal dementia or degeneration covers a range of conditions, the most common subtype being frontal or behavioural variant FTD, also known as Pick's disease. Others include Primary Progressive Aphasia (PPA), Semantic Variant PPA (svPPA) or Semantic dementia. About 10–20% of people with FTD will also develop a motor disorder and the most common are Amyotrophic Lateral Sclerosis (ALS), which is the most common form of Motor Neurone Disease (MND), Corticobasal Syndrome (CBS) and progressive supranuclear palsy [12].

FTD usually affects people between the ages of 45 and 64 years and in 30–50% of cases; there is a strong family history [11]. Familial FTD has been linked to specific genes, C9orf72, GRN Progranulin and Microtubule-associated protein tau. These genes mutate and affect the proteins essential to the normal function of brain cells. Pharmacological interventions such as AChE inhibitors or memantine are not suitable for FTD [8]. As with other young-onset dementias, the atypical presentation of FTD may make it difficult to diagnose, as it may resemble a midlife crisis, depression or mental illness [11]. Life expectancy from the initial onset of symptoms averages 6–9 years.

Behavioural variant FTD accounts for around 60% of all FTD cases. Changes in personality and behaviour may be the most obvious signs coupled with difficulty planning, organising and making decisions. Unlike Alzheimer's, people with behavioural variant FTD tend not to have problems with day-to-day memory. The presentation of socially inappropriate, disinhibited, impulsive, apathetic and even aggressive behaviours early in the FTD disease process and often at younger age can be especially difficult for family caregivers. Language-variant FTD accounts for around 40% of FTD. People with FTD and motor disorders will experience difficulties with movement that include twitching, stiffness, loss of balance and co-ordination. If someone has FTD and MND/ALS, they can deteriorate more quickly than someone with FTD alone [12].

14.8 Comorbidities and Dementia

People living with dementia who are over 65 years have on average four comorbidities while people without dementia have on average two [15]. The most common other health conditions include hypertension (53%), painful conditions (34%) and depression (24%); diabetes, stroke and visual impairments are also common [16]. People with dementia are most likely to be admitted to hospital in the UK with preventable conditions: a fall, fractured hip or hip replacement, urinary tract infection and chest infection [17]. They are over three times more likely to die during their first admission to hospital for an acute medical condition than those without dementia [17].

Depression is particularly common among people with advanced dementia and negatively affects their cognition and self-concept. Dementia is an important risk factor in the development of delirium which can worsen dementia symptoms, enhance mortality risk and precipitate admission to hospital.

Pain is often under recognised, yet commonly experienced by people with dementia and advanced dementia across care settings. Identifying and treating pain can be complex; people with dementia may be unable to communicate that they are in pain and become agitated or withdrawn. Validated pain assessment tools are available, but often not implemented and there is a need to evaluate pain management strategies [18]. Yet, given that we know the prevalence of comorbidities amongst people living with dementia, the often painful conditions such as osteoarthritis that come with older age mean that we need to take proactive steps to identify and manage pain.

Knowing the person, picking up on changes in mood, facial expressions, body language and verbal expressions are all important with identifying pain. Not attributing agitation and distressed behaviour to the dementia is important; if the person has unexplained changes in behaviour or shows signs of distress, assessment of pain should be undertaken. The *Abbey Pain Scale* remains in popular use in the UK despite the UK Guidelines for the assessment of pain in older people stating that a valid Numerical Rating Scale or verbal descriptors can be used with people who have mild-to-moderate cognitive impairment or dementia. For those with more severe impairment, the Pain in Advanced Dementia (PAINAD) and Doloplus-2 are recommended [19].

There does appear to be a discrepancy in health outcomes for people with dementia and comorbidities. Atypical symptoms lead to diagnostic overshadowing, or in other words the problems are seen as worsening dementia rather than a comorbidity. Communication difficulties, lack of person-centred care, poor medication management and a gap in knowledge in caring for people with dementia and comorbidities all contribute to overshadowing. This failure to prevent, diagnose and treat comorbidities in people with dementia is leading to people with dementia having a reduced quality of life and an earlier death than people who have the same medical conditions, but do not have dementia [19].

14.9 Dementia as a Dynamic Concept

The experience of dementia is shaped by: the person you are; physical health and psychological well-being; brain changes; life experiences; relationships; environment; in other words, it will be influenced by a wide range of biological, social and psychological aspects [20]. Studies have shown that functional improvement can be achieved by people with dementia in association with environmental changes; conversely people can deteriorate rapidly in response to negative social experiences

[21]. For example, environments with no visual cues, low or glaring light sources, that are noisy, unfamiliar and disorientating are inevitably disabling. The concept of malignant social psychology [22] is also important; this is when people make generalisations or assumptions about how dementia affects people and then treat them based on those. For example, 'dementia will cause incontinence' or 'people with dementia will be incontinent', can lead people and healthcare professionals to treat people in a way that does not recognise the individual abilities of the person. If we recognise this, we can make environments *enabling*, work with people in a person-centred way, one that recognises their abilities and retained functions, thus enabling people with dementia to live well for longer. It is important that we continue to work in this way as the condition progresses, as people can live with advanced dementia for many months or years. Whilst living well with dementia is an important message, especially following diagnosis, planning for advanced dementia and dying well is equally important [23]. Not everyone living with dementia will go on to live with advanced dementia. Some will die while their dementia is in the early or moderate phase. We now focus on approaches to palliative care for those who progress to living with advanced dementia.

14.10 As Dementia Progresses

As the underlying illnesses run their course, symptom severity and healthcare needs increase in terms of both complexity and intensity. Views are changing as to how the progression of dementia is described, although many refer to three stages, namely: mild or early stage, moderate or mid stage and advanced, severe or late stage. The uniqueness of the dementia experience makes it difficult to recognise when the different stages begin. This uncertainty brings with it both practical and ethical dilemmas associated with truth telling and knowing when and what information to share with individuals and family. Sometimes, it can seem obvious to relatives that a person's condition is advancing, but there are many unknowns with dementia prognostication creating dilemmas in practice in terms of answering questions about what will happen next including how quickly an individual might decline and what to expect [24]. The estimates of those who have severe (or advanced) dementia vary from 17% [25] to 21% [26]. Prince et al. [5] reported 12.5% in the UK; however, this also varies with residence. For instance, in Scotland, 90% of care home residents are estimated to have dementia and of those, 35% had advanced dementia [27]. This compares to estimates in the Scottish community dwelling population of 18.6% [28].

14.11 Terminology and Definitions

Dementia symptoms in the later stages are complex and although the term 'advanced dementia' is widely used, it is poorly defined [29]. The tendency to equate later stages of dementia with death and dying fails to recognise that people can and do live for months and years with dementia-specific palliative care needs. This has prompted international calls for a new narrative to capture the continuum of healthcare needs associated with advanced dementia that includes both living with and dying with advanced dementia [29].

14.12 Defining Advanced Dementia

Notwithstanding that, some question the use of dementia staging, yet there are known consequences of not defining when a person has progressed to a more advanced stage of their illness. These consequences include the impact on planning care, on access to specialist services and on the wider support available to individuals and their families. In Scotland, failure to define and recognise advanced dementia has been associated with the perpetuation of inequalities and unfair cost regimes which inappropriately respond to advanced dementia as a social problem [28]. This means that people with advanced dementia are often charged for care, whereas people with other terminal conditions receive care that is free at the point of delivery. Moreover, they may not have access to the expert nursing and specialist palliative care services they need (and deserve). It is reasonable to speculate more generally that the observed low uptake of generic palliative care services by people with dementia might be attributed to the common failure to recognise when a person with dementia requires palliation [30].

Although defining when a person has reached advanced dementia is complex due to the fluctuations in a person's health and the unpredictable pattern of decline in cognitive and physical function, it is important for the reasons outlined above. Informed by the research cited herein [31], the definition below was developed for the Scottish Fair Dementia Care Commission through a managed democratic process involving expert healthcare practitioners and family caregivers:

> Advanced dementia is associated with the later stages of illness when the complexity and severity of dementia-related changes in the brain lead to recognisable symptoms associated with dependency and an escalation of health care needs and risks. Addressing advanced dementia-related health needs requires expert health care, nursing and palliative care assessments together with insights provided by family caregivers and others, particularly when the person has difficulty communicating their own needs and emotions. Advanced dementia involves living, sometimes for years, with advanced illness and the advanced dementia continuum includes the terminal stages of death and dying. The experience of advanced dementia is unique to the individual and dependent on the aetiology of the underlying illness, comorbidities and other factors relating to health, personality, biography and socio-economics ([31], p. 14–15).

14.13 Features of Advanced Dementia

Although there are no typical symptoms and the experience of these will be unique, there is a pattern of physical decline with loss of communication skills in many people and some can experience severe cognitive impairment ahead of physical decline. The different illnesses causing dementia give rise to both shared and unique problems and an illness-specific understanding of the anticipated advanced dementia experience is important. Some of the most important aspects of the advanced dementia experience include neuropsychiatric symptoms, disorientation, communication problems, multiple functional impairments, immobility, incontinence and weight loss. The cumulative impacts of these complex health needs are profound and impact on all care needs.

As the collective impacts of these progressive health problems increase, the illness experience is shaped by the aetiology of the underlying type, comorbidities, personality, biography and socio-economics. It is also significantly influenced by the person's premorbid personality, life experience, coping strategies, interpersonal relationships and their personal close and extended social environment. There are few direct accounts that convey the lived experience of advanced dementia; one is from Clare et al. who vividly describe the lives of people with advanced dementia living in care homes [32]. Their lived experience was shaped by losses resulting from their dementia and their situation; despite feelings of fear, lack of control, loss, frustration and boredom, people displayed many constructive ways of coping. Their situation and emotional response to it were grounded in a strong retained sense of self and identity [32]. The subjective experience, the fundamentals of care and the management of dementia-related symptoms including sensory changes, sleep disturbance, pain management and situations that trigger stress and distress all require attention.

As van der Steen [33] explains, the cognitive decline which is inevitable in advanced dementia impacts on how individuals can contribute to care-related decision-making and if possible, future planning should begin while the person has the cognitive ability to express their own preferences. Accordingly, practitioners should be mindful that family caregivers occupy a central position in decision-making about the person with advanced dementia and that the sustainability of family caring will be a critical determinant within decision-making processes.

As understanding of the complex needs arising from advanced dementia deepens, it is clear that evidence to inform practice is urgently needed alongside stage-specific residential and non-residential dementia care services. Alzheimer's Disease International [34] argues that care systems must be responsive to the needs of people with advanced dementia, proposing that specialist services should provide care, supervision and training to specialists, non-specialists and all involved in advanced dementia care provision including family members.

14.14 Palliative Care

The interest in a palliative care approach to dementia has been motivated by concerns that some healthcare professionals fail to recognise dementia as a terminal neurodegenerative illness. A recent literature review concluded that people with dementia are less likely to receive palliative care than others with different terminal illnesses and that family members were often ill informed about what to expect in advanced dementia [35]. Jones et al. [36] report that fragmented services and poor assessment of needs undermine the quality of palliative care available to people with dementia. Although there have been policy formations with respect to the palliative care approach in dementia care, 'we are someway from a general or even widespread acceptance, let alone adoption of a broadly defined palliative care approach to dementia care' ([34], p.71).

An important contribution to this debate is offered by van der Steen et al. [24] who present a view of optimal palliative care for older people with dementia. They debate how services could be shaped to deliver dementia-specific palliative care, whether they should be in discrete new services which can act as a beacon of best practice, or should existing services including hospices be extended [33]. The European White Paper on Dementia and Palliative Care (EAPC) proposes that the goals of care at the mild stage of dementia should prioritise maintenance of function and as dementia progresses to the moderate and severe stage, maximisation of comfort is the priority. The White Paper also proposes bereavement support for family caregivers [24]. The objectives of palliative care set out in the EAPC guidelines are articulated in a slightly different way in the Canadian Comfort Care booklet [37]. Designed for use in care homes, it focuses on the avoidance of burdensome or futile treatment and the prevention and treatment of pain, pressure sores and shortness of breath, eating and swallowing difficulties, infections and agitation.

We concur with Kidd and Sharpe and suggest viewing advanced dementia as a continuum which includes living the best life possible as well as experiencing the best end of life [23]. This perspective responds to a call for a new positive practice narrative for advanced dementia. One such approach is Dementia Palliare and it is to this we now turn our attention.

14.15 Palliare

The term Palliare, meaning to cloak in support was chosen to make a distinction between palliative care with its roots in non-dementia-specific palliation and end-of-life care to a new advanced dementia-specific approach focused on living the best life possible. People with dementia have a right to high-quality care throughout their illness. It follows that this creates an obligation for anyone involved in the provision of care to a person with advanced dementia to have the necessary knowledge, skills and resources to achieve best practice. The Palliare Project (2014–2017) was a partnership of seven European countries (Czech Republic, Finland, Portugal, Scotland, Slovenia, Spain and Sweden) funded by the EU Erasmus + Higher Education programme. It created an educational framework and practice approach to help support people with advanced dementia who are not yet requiring end-of-life care who are nonetheless reliant on the support of family caregivers and/or professionals for their health and well-being [29]. It offers an approach to providing advanced dementia-specific extended palliative care that flows through the continuum of the progressive advanced dementia experience, focused on living the best life possible.

The *Dementia Palliare Best Practice Statement* details the knowledge and skills that practitioners require to deliver good-quality Palliare [31]. To our knowledge, this is the first interprofessional practice education framework to focus specifically on integrated and prudent advanced dementia care [38]. Palliare practitioners require not only the knowledge and skills to provide direct care, but a commitment to sustain family caring, which will often need to be coupled with a determination to lead and champion practice and service-level changes [24, 38].

14.15.1 Dementia Palliare: Best Practice Principles

The Dementia Palliare Best Practice Statement [31] is an interprofessional learning framework intended to guide practice learning and promote an integrated approach in response to six areas:

1. Protecting rights, promoting dignity and inclusion
2. Future planning for advanced dementia
3. Managing symptoms and keeping well
4. Living the best life possible
5. Support for family and friends
6. Advancing Dementia Palliare practice

The value base underpinning Palliare is founded upon a human rights approach, in which person-centred care that is relationship-aware involves empathy, compassion and dignity. As well as managing the full range of dementia, later life and comorbid symptoms, it recognises the central role of family caring and the needs that family members have during and after their caregiving responsibilities have ended. A partnership approach which, as far as possible, includes the person with advanced dementia, family and friends is essential for future planning and the well-being of family caregivers. Where possible, future planning should begin when the person has the capacity to be central to decision-making. It advocates creative and person-centred approaches that acknowledge an individual's preferences and choices to support living, rather than simply existing with advanced dementia. It is an approach that supports the avoidance of interventions that are unhelpful or unwanted by the individual that is informed by the subjective experience of living with advanced dementia, the high levels of psychological distress family caregivers experience and the need for better dementia palliative care.

The Palliare Framework sets out a new vision that requires a nuanced understanding of advanced dementia and a practice approach that recognises the complexity of healthcare needs and is empathetic to the progressive experience of living with advanced dementia. It promotes a positive approach that asks healthcare providers to lead and promote reform and be willing to develop new services and new practice models that take palliative care in new directions. In the next section, we explore selected aspects of this experience and a new approach called *Care Empathia* that we believe can support high-quality dementia palliative care.

14.16 Care Empathia

To assess and meet the care needs of the person living with advanced dementia requires knowledge, empathy and skill. In-depth specialist knowledge is essential for understanding the advanced neuropathological changes in dementia and their impact on the person. Empathy and understanding about how the person might feel and the skills to address fundamental care needs are critical to quality of life. Informed by the Palliare study outcomes, the Care Empathia approach frames practice-based learning about dementia around three domains focusing education though a head (knowledge), heart (empathy) and hands (psychomotor skills) framework [39]. This approach begins to address the concern that dementia education has been limited in all professional groups until relatively recently, resulting in a serious deficit in skilled dementia care practice.

14.16.1 Dementia-Specific Issues to Consider When Meeting Care Needs

The healthcare issues that require attention as dementia progresses include the impact of reduced self-awareness, altered perceptions and changes in sensory experiences resulting from brain pathology. Consideration is needed about the presence of pain, constipation, dehydration and malnutrition. Skin integrity, oral health and medication reconciliation are key areas of assessment as the person nears the end of life. This complex picture can result in the person living with dementia experiencing excessive stress. Unrelieved stress can have serious consequences in distressed behaviour; this can include agitation, aggression, screaming and refusal of care. This can result in this period being a difficult one for the person, their family, nurses and care practitioners.

The damage to brain function at this stage has little to do with the person's primary diagnosis or type of dementia since early focal damage is now likely to be global. The result is changes in all aspects of the person's function, responses, cognition and communication. Meeting care needs requires a constant consideration of all of these changes while carrying out assessments and providing care.

The lack of self-awareness of limitations (anosagnosia) can lead to the person acting in ways that appear strange and at odds with their advanced illness; for example, they may refuse to rest or stay in bed. Actions such as refusing medication and trying to leave the environment may also result. Part of the progression may include a deterioration in visual perception of objects and the environment (agnosia). This creates a world that can be increasingly difficult to comprehend, the environment becomes difficult to interpret and daily objects become unfamiliar. Trying to eat and drink, dress or go to the toilet can be impossible if the person cannot recognise a spoon, shoes or toilet seat. Wayfinding in a now unfamiliar environment creates anxiety and fear. Additionally, some people can develop an inability to recognise faces (prosopagnosia), even familiar ones. This can be distressing and almost beyond understanding for family and friends. Memory and understanding may be deeply damaged and the dual loss of not knowing what is happening around them and the lack of ability to remember what is happening is devastating. Communication abilities also begin to narrow as language diminishes and reception of information is limited. This dark picture is one that, while sad and difficult to understand, can be improved by excellent knowledge and skilled care.

14.16.2 Working with the Embodied Memory, Senses and Emotions

Crucially, emotions are preserved throughout the illness and remain a strength of the person, giving a much-needed window into their world. It is possible to identify anxiety, fear, pain, anger and contentment with sensitive and empathetic attention [40]. By remaining aware of this emotional aspect of the person, care can also be enhanced. Reacting to the person's distress response by assessing pain, discomfort, fear and potential misperceptions can improve their quality of life and quality of end of life. Communication is enhanced through using the remaining senses with an emphasis on gaining attention through vision, improving what the person can hear by reducing complex language, speaking clearly and using positive nonverbal actions to reinforce information. Another asset at this period of the illness is the preservation of embodied memory. The memory of experiences and people may have been affected, but the tacit knowledge of the body in action can be supported to improve daily activity. By knowing the person's previous pattern of movement, caregivers can ensure that this is applied to personal care, dressing and eating and drinking. A multi-sensory approach is needed to overcome the cognitive loss by using a range of visual and auditory prompts together with aids and adaptations to allow care to progress. This focus on remaining strengths of emotion and embodied memory can improve and enhance the care experience for the person and all other partners in care.

An emotionally focused, embodied approach can also underpin ways of addressing more specific concerns for care during this period. This includes the crucial and common symptom of pain, frequently missed in the person with advanced dementia [41]. The limited ability to report pain results in changes in the person's behaviour, responses and actions. These are frequently misunderstood and related to the changes caused by dementia rather than pain responses. A cluster randomised trial of 60 clusters in 18 care homes using active and systematic pain management showed a reduction of a range of agitated behaviours [42]. The recommended assessment tools that do not require the person to answer questions, but use observation and discussion with family and caregivers to support decisions about pain management, are the Pain in Advanced Dementia (PAINAD) and Doloplus-2 [19]. It remains a key approach to consider pain first, assess, treat and reassess, as sudden changes in behaviour in advanced dementia are most always the result of a physical change, often pain-related, affecting the person rather than directly related to the dementia.

14.17 Fundamentals of Advanced Dementia Care

Personal care including washing and dressing also creates difficulties as the person no longer recognises objects or their purpose and can become resistive to washing, dressing, toilet visits or oral care. Reactions can be severe and providing support and assistance can become a considerable source of distress for family and caregivers. Being able to provide care that is welcome to the person can be achieved by understanding the fear that can be generated by care activities. The neurobiological principles of fear response and threat perception are exacerbated in advanced dementia when understanding the actions of others is severely diminished. Personalised care using threat-reducing responses and relationship-focused approaches can improve care experiences in care homes [43]. In addition, specific and detailed knowledge about the impact of specific care activities can smooth the experience considerably. For example, water in baths and showers is invisible to the person and when the purpose is no longer recognised, the sensation on the body can be sudden and unexpected, causing negative reactions. Dressing is an activity we strive to do independently from early childhood and the experience of 'being dressed' can create anxiety, particularly when individual items of clothing are no longer recognised. Going to the toilet when the objects housed there no longer have meaning is likely to result in refusal to sit on the toilet. Oral care is vital to maintain general health and avoid dental pain. Accessing the person's mouth may result in biting and pulling away. Interventions for personal care of the body must recognise the previous embodied habits and attempt to reflect these in carrying out activities; these can include mirroring, chaining and bridging [44].

- Mirroring is where the caregiver carries out the task in a mirror image of the person's actions; this can be used for tooth brushing, for example. Standing next to the person facing the mirror, both the caregiver and the person perform the same actions.
- Bridging can include having the person hold an object while the care activity is carried out, such as a hairbrush while having their hair brushed or an electric razor while the caregiver shaves the person. This approach to carrying out an action can remind the body about the activity and increase cooperation.
- Chaining is used when the person has sufficient movement to carry out a task and requires only physical prompting to begin the activity.

Appetite reduces in old age and a lack of interest in eating and drinking is exacerbated in advanced dementia by lack of recognition of food and a diminishing ability to manage the mechanical aspects of chewing and swallowing. Approximately 90% of people who reach the stage of advanced dementia will have issues related to eating [45]. An assessment by a speech and language therapist and dietician can be helpful. However, careful and skilled supported eating and drinking is possible until swallowing is compromised. In a study of six people with severe dementia living in a care home, a multisensory approach linked to an integrated teaching programme and reporting system with families and staff was piloted. The findings included a successful eating and drinking experience together with maintenance of body weight over the period of the study [46]. The alternative to this intensive support is a range of invasive procedures including intravenous fluids and percutaneous endoscopic gastronomy (PEG). Neither option can replace the pleasure nor the experience of eating and drinking and external tubing likely to be pulled and dislodged by the person who will not understand the discomfort experienced. PEG feeding studies have not shown any prevention of aspiration pneumonia and the process does not improve survival or reduce the incidence of pressure ulcers [45].

14.18 Preventing and Minimising Stress and Distress

Minimising stress and preventing distress is the thread that should be present in all aspects of care for the person with dementia. Experiencing dementia is stressful; trying to maintain personhood in the face of this irreversible condition is exhausting and anxiety-provoking. The aim of care should be to provide a biopsychosocial environment designed to manage and minimise stress. All aspects of the environment should compensate for cognitive changes, from the built environment to the people who support the person. Design of environments for dementia can be accessed from a range of design guides (e.g., https://www.kingsfund.org.uk/projects/enhancing-healing-environment/ehe-design-dementia). Some of the most important features include managing noise levels and improving lighting. Making use of colour, contrast and signage can enable the person to *wayfind*, access toilets and personal possessions. Relational stress is equally important and working with family and caregivers to understand the environmental impact and support communication strategies is key. Communicating in an emotionally engaged way, sharing knowledge about the person and being in a partnership is central to improving quality of life for the person with advanced dementia. Distress can occur where the optimal care and environment are not available or where there is unrelieved pain, illness or emotional upset. Distress should be assessed and interventions developed urgently to intervene. There is a concern that anti-psychotic medication may be a primary intervention rather than a last resort and considerable effort has been made to publicise the dangers of inappropriate use of this medication in dementia [8].

Non-pharmacological interventions and caring approaches should favour the emotional and embodied strengths of the person with advanced dementia; these can include music, sensory stimulation and Namaste care approaches. Personalised music can stimulate preserved brain areas and create emotional connections. Initiatives such as Alive Inside in the USA (http://www.aliveinside.us/) and Playlist for Life in Scotland (https://www.playlistforlife.org.uk/) have promoted the value of personalised music to enhance quality of life. However, a recent Cochrane review of music-based therapeutic interventions found only limited evidence for impact on emotional well-being, quality of life and symptoms of depression [47].

Sensory stimulation in dementia has been explored through interventions such as multisensory environments; these include stimulation using fibre optics, bubble tubes and colour changing lights; some studies showed a positive impact on distressed behaviour and low mood [48]. A sensory focused day provision for people with severe dementia used mixed methods to support staff and family members to use a range of sensory stimulating activities, including soft toy animals, music and fabrics; it produced outcomes including improvements in quality of life [49]. Namaste care is shown to reduce pain and behavioural disturbances, improving quality of life for people with advanced dementia living in care homes [50]. *Namaste Care* is a structured intervention using sensory, embodied and emotional interventions to give comfort and pleasure to people with advanced dementia, intended to enhance quality of life [50].

14.19 Discussion

Healthcare professionals providing care for those with advanced dementia are required to understand the neuropathology and have insight into the subjective experience of the condition in order to provide a biopsychosocial and spiritual approach to care that meets not only the complex fundamental care needs but, also minimises the stress and distress that often comes with living with a neurodegenerative condition. Many of the healthcare workforce are not educated in dementia care, yet are often expected to provide quality care. Those experienced and expert in providing palliative care equally will have had little or no education in dementia care or dementia palliative care. The impact that this lack of education may have on their confidence and motivation to work with people with dementia is likely to be a negative one. The impact this may have on the recipient of care is just as likely to be a negative one. One could argue that this negative spiral further stigmatises not only people with dementia but also devalues the complexity of dementia care, advanced dementia care and dementia specialist palliative care. We would argue that there is pressing need for healthcare practitioners to be educated in advanced dementia palliative care and for approaches such as Care Empathia and Palliare to be adopted more widely. Palliative care principles are applicable to advanced dementia care, but there is an urgent need for more research specific to the dementia field [34]. As Kydd and Sharp point out 'If dementia is not seen as a chronic illness then services will not be geared to providing enabling strategies to live well, if dementia is not seen as a disability then services will not be geared to develop inclusive buildings and communities and if dementia is not seen as a terminal illness then services may fail to address good end of life care' ([23], p.6).

14.20 Conclusions

This chapter offers extensive information regarding the various forms of dementia and their impact on the health and well-being of the person and their loved ones. Those who go on to live with advanced dementia with all the complex healthcare needs this entails require a palliative approach to help avoid the many distressing and inappropriate interventions. A palliative approach that includes aspects of specialist advanced dementia care can help address the complex ethical care dilemmas, provide comfort and fully involve families and loved ones during life and after death. Frameworks such as the Best Practice Statement for advanced dementia care and the White Paper defining optimal palliative care in older people with dementia offer nurses and other healthcare professionals approaches to provide dementia-specific palliative care [24, 31]. Care Empathia presents how we can provide the fundamentals of advanced dementia care in an empathetic and embodied way so that we are maximising quality of life and support people to die well.

References

1. World Health Organisation. Dementia. Geneva: WHO; 2017. https://www.who.int/news-room/fact-sheets/detail/dementia0. Accessed 6 Mar 2019.
2. Prince M, Ali GC, Guerchet M, Prina AM, Albanese E, Wu YT. Recent global trends in the prevalence and incidence of dementia, and survival with dementia. Alzheimers Res Ther. 2016;8(1):23.
3. World Alzheimer Report. The state of the art dementia research: new frontiers. London: Alzheimer's Disease International (ADI); 2018.
4. Norton S, Matthews FE, Barnes DE, Yaffe K, Brayne C. Potential for primary prevention of Alzheimer's disease: an analysis of population-based data. Lancet Neurol. 2014;13(8):788–94.
5. Prince M, Knapp M, Guerchet M, McCrone P, Prin M, Comas-Herrera A, Wittenberg R, Adelaja B, Hu B, King D, Rehill A, Salimkumar D. Dementia UK. 2nd ed. London: Alzheimer's Society; 2014.
6. Snowdon DA. Healthy aging and dementia: findings from the Nun Study. Ann Intern Med. 2003;139(5_Part_2):450–4.
7. Alzheimer's Society. What is dementia? Factsheet 400LP. London: Alzheimer's Society; 2017. https://www.alzheimers.org.uk/about-dementia/types-dementia/alzheimers-disease. Accessed 30 Jan 2019.
8. National Institute for Clinical Excellence. Dementia: assessment, management and support for people living with dementia and their carers. NICE guideline. London: NICE; 2018. https://www.nice.org.uk/guidance/ng97. Accessed 30 Jan 2019.
9. Savica R, Murray ME, Persson XM, Kantarci K, Parisi JE, Dickson DW, Petersen RC, Ferman TJ, Boeve BF, Mielke MM. Plasma sphingolipid changes with autopsy-confirmed Lewy body or Alzheimer's pathology. Alzheimers Dement (Amst). 2016;3:43–50.
10. McKeith IG, Boeve BF, Dickson DW, Halliday G, Taylor JP, Weintraub D, Aarsland D, Galvin J, Attems J, Ballard CG, Bayston A. Diagnosis and management of dementia with Lewy bodies: fourth consensus report of the DLB Consortium. Neurology. 2017;89(1):88–100.
11. Wilfong L, Edwards NE, Yehle KS, Ross K. Frontotemporal dementia: identification and management. J Nurse Pract. 2016;12(4):277–82.
12. Alzheimer's Research UK. What is frontotemporal dementia? London: Alzheimer's Research UK; 2016. https://www.alzheimersresearchuk.org/about-dementia/types-of-dementia/frontotemporal-dementia/ftdabout/. Accessed 6 Mar 2019
13. Coppus AM, Evenhuis H, Verberne GJ, Visser F, Van Gool P, Eikelenboom P, Van Duijin C. Dementia and mortality in persons with Down's syndrome. J Intellect Disabil Res. 2006;50(10):768–77.
14. Caceres BA, Frank MO, Jun J, Martelly MT, Sadarangani T, De Sales PC. Family caregivers of patients with frontotemporal dementia: an integrative review. Int J Nurs Stud. 2016;55:71–84.
15. Poblador-Plou B, Calderón-Larrañaga A, Marta-Moreno J, Hancco-Saavedra J, Sicras-Mainar A, Soljak M, Prados-Torres A. Comorbidity of dementia: a cross-sectional study of primary care older patients. BMC Psychiatry. 2014;14:84. https://doi.org/10.1186/1471-244X-14-84.

16. Browne J, Edwards DA, Rhodes KM, Brimicombe DJ, Payne A. Association of comorbidity and health service usage among patients with dementia in the UK; a population-based study. MJ Open. 2017;7(3):e012546. https://doi.org/10.1136/bmjopen-2016-012546.
17. Scrutton J, Brancati CU. Dementia and comorbidities; ensuring parity of care. London: The International Longevity Centre; 2016.
18. Husebo BS, Achterberg W, Flo E. Identifying and managing pain in people with Alzheimer's disease and other types of dementia: a systematic review. CNS Drugs. 2016;30(6):481–97.
19. Schofield P. The assessment of pain in older people: UK national guidelines. Age Ageing. 2018;47(Suppl_1):i1–22.
20. Spector A, Orrell M. Using a biopsychosocial model of dementia as a tool to guide clinical practice. Int Psychogeriatr. 2010;22(6):957–65.
21. Kitwood T, Bredin K. Towards a theory of dementia care: personhood and well-being. Ageing Soc. 1992;12(3):269–87.
22. Kitwood TM. Dementia reconsidered: the person comes first. Buckingham: Open University Press; 1997.
23. Kydd A, Sharp B. Palliative vcare and dementia – a time and place? Maturitas. 2016;84:5–10. https://doi.org/10.1016/j.maturitas.2015.10.007.
24. van der Steen JT, Radbruch L, Hertogh CM, de Boer ME, Hughes JC, Larkin P, Francke AL, Jünger S, Gove D, Firth P, Koopmans RT. White paper defining optimal palliative care in older people with dementia: a Delphi study and recommendations from the European Association for Palliative Care. Palliat Med. 2014;28(3):197–209.
25. Voisin T, Vellas B. Diagnosis and treatment of patients with severe Alzheimer's disease. Drugs Ageing. 2009;26(2):135–44.
26. Schafirovits-Morillo L, Suemoto CK. Severe dementia: a review about diagnoses, therapeutic management and ethical issues. Dement Neuropsychol. 2010;4(3):158–64.
27. Lithgow S, Jackson GA, Browne D. Estimating the prevalence of dementia: cognitive screening in Glasgow nursing homes. Int J Geriatr Psychiatry. 2012;27(8):785–91.
28. Alzheimer Scotland. The fair dementia care commission. delivering fair dementia care for people with advanced dementia. Edinburgh: Alzheimer Scotland; 2019. https://www.alzscot.org/assets/0003/2746/McLeish_Report_updated_24.01.19_Web.pdf. Accessed 4 Feb 2019.
29. Hanson E, Hellström A, Sandvide Å, Jackson GA, MacRae R, Waugh A, Abreu W, Tolson D. The extended palliative phase of dementia—an integrative literature review. Dementia. 2019;18(1):108–34.
30. Goodman C, Froggatt K, Amador S, Mathie E, Mayrhofer A. End of life care interventions for people with dementia in care homes: addressing uncertainty within a framework for service delivery and evaluation. BMC Palliat Care. 2015;14(1):42.
31. Homerová I, Waugh A, MacRae R, Sandvide A, Hanson E, Jackson G, Watchman K, Tolson D. Dementia palliare best practice statement. Glasgow: University of the West of Scotland. http://dementia.uws.ac.uk/documents/2015/12/dementia-palliare-best-practice-statement-web.pdf. Accessed 14 Feb 2019.
32. Clare L, Rowlands J, Bruce E, Surr C, Downs M. The experience of living with dementia in residential care: an interpretative phenomenological analysis. The Gerontologist. 2008;48(6):711–20.
33. van der Steen JT, Dekker NL, Gijsberts MJ, Vermeulen LH, Mahler MM. Palliative care for people with dementia in the terminal phase: a mixed-methods qualitative study to inform service development. BMC Palliat Care. 2017;16(1):28.
34. Alzheimer's Disease International. Improving healthcare for people living with dementia coverage, quality and costs now and in the future. World Alzheimer report. London: Alzheimer's Disease International (ADI); 2016.
35. Broady TR, Saich F, Hinton T. Caring for a family member or friend with dementia at the end of life: a scoping review and implications for palliative care practice. Palliat Med. 2018;32(3):643–56.
36. Jones L, Candy B, Davis S, Elliott M, Gola A, Harrington J, Kupeli N, Lord K, Moore K, Scott S, Vickerstaff V. Development of a model for integrated care at the end of life in advanced dementia: a whole systems UK-wide approach. Palliat Med. 2016;30(3):279–95.

37. Arcand M, Brazil K, Nakanishi M, et al. Educating families about end-of-life care in advanced dementia: acceptability of a Canadian family booklet to nurses from Canada, France, and Japan. Int J Palliat Nurs. 2013;19:67–74.
38. Tolson D, Fleming A, Hanson E, Abreu W, Crespo ML, MacRae R, Jackson G, Touzery SH, Routasalo P, Holmerová I. Achieving prudent dementia care (palliare): an international policy and practice imperative. Int J Integr Care. 2016;16(4):18.
39. Singleton J. Head, heart and hands model for transformative learning: place as context for changing sustainability values. J Sustain Edu. 2015;9:1–6.
40. Brown M, Fox H. Care of the adult with dementia. In: Elcock K, Wright W, Newcombe P, Everett F, editors. Essentials of nursing adults. London: SAGE; 2019. p. 359–76.
41. Closs SJ, Dowding D, Allcock N, et al. Towards improved decision support in the assessment and management of pain for people with dementia in hospital: a systematic meta-review and observational study. Southampton: NIHR Journals Library; 2016. https://doi.org/10.3310/hsdr04300. Health Services and Delivery Research, No. 4.30. https://www.ncbi.nlm.nih.gov/books/NBK390792/. Accessed 4 Feb 2019.
42. Husebo BS, Ballard C, Sandvik R, Nilsen OB, Aarsland D. Efficacy of treating pain to reduce behavioural disturbances in residents of nursing homes with dementia: cluster randomised clinical trial. BMJ. 2011;343:d4065.
43. Jablonski RA, Kolanowski AM, Azuero A, Winstead V, Jones-Townsend C, Geisinger ML. Randomised clinical trial: efficacy of strategies to provide oral hygiene activities to nursing home residents with dementia who resist mouth care. Gerontology. 2018;35(4):365–75.
44. Pearson A, Chalmers J. Oral hygiene care for adults with dementia in residential aged care facilities. JBI Reports. 2004;2(3):65–113.
45. Neal N, Catic AG. Feeding issues in advanced dementia. In: Catic AG, editor. Ethical considerations and challenges in geriatrics. Cham: Springer; 2017. https://doi.org/10.1007/978-3-319-44084-2_9.
46. Brown M, McWhinnie H, McAlister and Banks P. Food for thought: enhancing dietary preferences for the person with advanced dementia. Edinburgh: Queens Nursing Institute for Scotland; 2014. https://www.qnis.org.uk/wp-content/uploads/2016/11/Food-for-Thought-Report.pdf. Accessed 2 Feb 2019.
47. van der Steen JT, Smelling HJ, van der Wouden JC, Bruinsma MS, Scholten RJ, Vink AC. Music-based therapeutic interventions for people with dementia. Cochrane Database Syst Rev. 2018:7.
48. Lorusso LN, Bosch SJ. Impact of multisensory environments on behavior for people with dementia: a systematic literature review. The Gerontologist. 2108;58(3):e168–79. https://doi.org/10.1093/geront/gnw168.
49. Tolson D, Watchman K, Richards N, Brown M, Jackson G, Dalrymple A, Henderson J. Enhanced sensory day care: developing a new model of day care for people in the advanced stage of dementia: a pilot study. Glasgow: Alzheimer Scotland; 2015.
50. Stacpoole M, Thompsell A, Hockley J. Toolkit for implementing the Namaste Care programme for people with advanced dementia living in care homes. https://www.stchristophers.org.uk/wp-content/uploads/2016/03/Namaste-Care-Programme-Toolkit-06.04.2016.pdf. Accessed 2 Feb 2019.

Persons with Advanced Heart Failure: A Caregiver-Focused Approach

15

Alexandra Hodson

Contents

15.1	Background	201
	15.1.1 Heart Failure	201
	15.1.2 Advanced Heart Failure	202
	15.1.3 Palliative Approach	203
	15.1.4 Bereavement	204
15.2	Heart Failure in the Community	205
15.3	Practice Implications	207
	15.3.1 Communication with Family Caregivers	207
	15.3.2 Assess the Needs of Family Caregivers	207
	15.3.3 Encourage Family Caregivers to Access Respite Services	208
	15.3.4 Positive Aspects of Family Caregiving	209
	15.3.5 Additional Education and Training	209
15.4	Research Implications	210
15.5	Conclusion	210
References		211

15.1 Background

15.1.1 Heart Failure

Heart failure (HF) is a common chronic disease with current estimates suggesting that 26 million people worldwide have been diagnosed with this condition [1]. HF does not discriminate based on age, although the majority of the population with this disease is considered to be an older adult. Classified as a life-limiting illness, it is typical for half of these persons diagnosed with HF to die within the first 5 years

A. Hodson (✉)
Faculty of Nursing, University of Regina, Saskatoon, SK, Canada
e-mail: alexandra.hodson@uregina.ca

[2]. Healthcare professionals working with this population are therefore required to address issues related to end-of-life and palliative care. Historically in practice, the palliative care needs of persons with HF have not been adequately addressed leading to persons and their caregivers being unaware that death was a possibility. Current practice guidelines suggest that end-of-life discussions should be initiated early in the disease process [3] which is occurring to varying degrees in our current healthcare practice environments; however, much work needs to be done to improve the experience of end of life for persons with HF and their families. In general, persons with HF have unique needs that require adaptation of palliative care services to address these challenges in the advanced stages of their illness.

15.1.2 Advanced Heart Failure

Advanced HF is characterized by periods of acute symptom exacerbation, requiring that persons have assistance with health maintenance and daily symptom management. Advanced HF is commonly defined as a person who meets criteria 3 or 4 of the New York Heart Association which includes persons who experience symptoms related to their disease at rest and with minimal exertion. Persons who meet criteria for advanced HF will experience extreme fatigue, shortness of breath, pain, increased frequency of hospitalizations, and mental health challenges including anxiety and depression [4]. Despite appropriate treatments, these symptoms often persist [2], reducing quality of life for the patient and their family as well as creating an increased need for family support in the home (community) environment.

The disease trajectory of HF is unpredictable, characterized by episodes of acute symptom exacerbation, followed by periods of symptom stability [5]. When a person has a diagnosis of HF, it is hard to predict which symptoms will occur or how long they will live as the disease presentation is unique to each individual. Persons with advanced HF experience end of life in two prominent ways. As represented in the Fig. 15.1 given herein, people with advanced HF may experience a sudden death event. These events can occur anywhere along the continuum, and are represented in Fig. 15.1 by the descending dotted lines. In other cases, persons with advanced HF may undergo a slow decline in heart function with acute periods of symptom exacerbation requiring hospitalization. Persons with advanced HF recover from these episodes but usually do not return to their level of functioning that was present prior to hospitalization.

Recent developments in cardiac care have contributed to an extension of the advanced stages of HF [6]. The trajectory is then further complicated by these medical advances; for example, at some points along the continuum, persons with advanced HF may qualify to have a medical device implanted known as a Left Ventricular Assist Device (LVAD). An LVAD is an electronic device that is surgically implanted in a patient to assist with moving blood effectively through the heart. The device is controlled by an external power supply [7]. Implantation of an LVAD can revert persons with advanced HF to a higher level of heart function which serves to reduce patient symptoms and lengthen life, although at some point, family caregivers

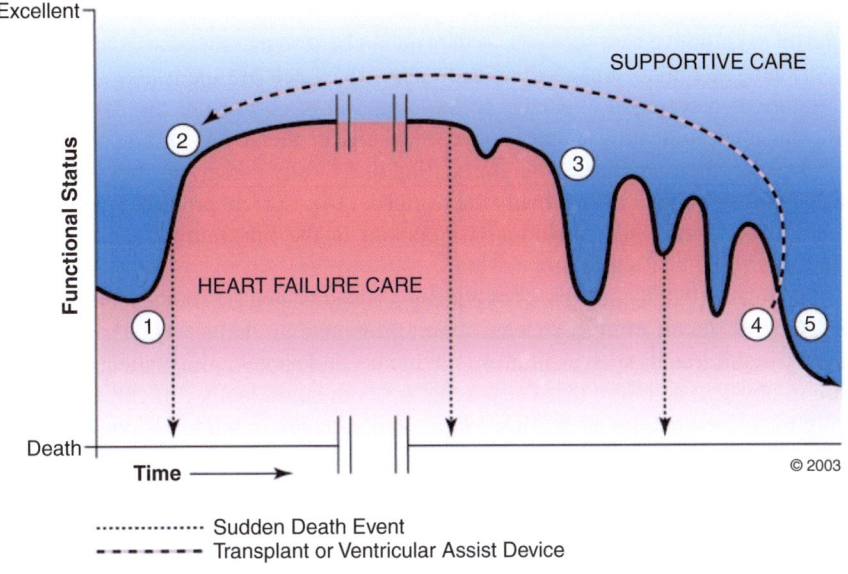

Fig. 15.1 Heart failure disease trajectory (Permission to reproduce) [5]

may have to participate in difficult discussions with healthcare providers on when to deactivate the device [8]. If a person with advanced HF meets specific criteria, they may also qualify for a heart transplant where, if successful, the patient would naturally acquire a marked reduction in symptoms. Given the variability in the disease progression of HF, it is not surprising that there is a possibility for multiple end-of-life scenarios. This unpredictability is complex and may produce anxiety when persons with advanced HF are navigating the healthcare system.

15.1.3 Palliative Approach

High-quality palliative care at end of life is a basic human right for all Canadians [9]; however, current estimates of utilization show that less than 10% of persons with HF receive appropriate end-of-life services [5]. Cancer continues to be the most common illness for referral to palliative care services despite the diagnosis of cancer accounting for only 25% of total deaths in Canada [10]. The unfortunate reality is that for many families impacted by HF, discussions regarding the need to refer to palliative care services are limited [11]; thus, adequate support is often not being provided during this important phase of life. When support is inadequate, patient preferences at end of life are not incorporated into the plan of care and may lead family caregivers to experience remorse about the end-of-life experience [11]. Palliative care services are beneficial as they can help the caregiver and patient, focus on improving quality of life, and address issues that arise as a result of the process of dying [12].

Literature suggests that healthcare professionals tend to feel uncertain about referral to palliative care services, as they do not believe that they have the appropriate training to initiate end-of-life discussions [13]. Lack of time is also cited in the literature as a common challenge to the initiation of end-of-life discussions [13]. Unclear communication about prognosis results in misunderstanding throughout the disease process with the literature citing that family caregivers may not recognize that the patient will eventually die from HF [14]. Current protocol suggests that healthcare professionals should advise persons of the life-limiting nature of their illness early in the disease progression.

The roles of family caregivers of persons with advanced HF include management of complex medication regimens, monitoring patient daily weights, enforcing dietary requirements such as limiting salt intake, and encouraging patient participation in physical activity [15]. These tasks are both emotionally difficult and physically intensive creating a situation where family caregiver burden is common. The way of life for the family caregiver is sometimes described as a constant state of anxiety created by the need to closely monitor the patient for signs and symptoms of HF, even during periods of illness stability [15].

Symptoms experienced in advanced HF also severely limit the patient's ability to assist with things like management of the household resulting in further workload placed on the family caregiver [4]. It is not surprising then that the risk for caregiver burden increases when persons with advanced HF are required to attend multiple medical appointments while receiving conflicting advice on how to effectively provide care or being sent for unnecessary tests [13, 15]. It is important to support the needs of family caregivers, as they play a vital role in promoting health and managing symptoms of persons with advanced HF. When the needs of the family caregiver are not met, they are at increased risk of detrimental mental and physical health outcomes, creating a situation where they have difficulty fulfilling their important role [16]. Consensus exists amongst researchers that many of the needs of persons with advanced HF can be effectively addressed by gaining access to palliative care services [17] thus creating a situation where implementation of palliative services could serve to alleviate or reduce feelings of caregiver burden.

15.1.4 Bereavement

Palliative care services do not cease with death of the patient but instead extend beyond to assist families during the bereavement period [12]. As a person with advanced HF moves toward the end of life, it is important for families to have access to palliative care services that will encourage them to reflect on life experiences, accept death as a likely outcome, as well as focus energies on enjoying their remaining days [18]. Access to palliative care services is known to increase the likelihood that death will be perceived as a peaceful event [19]. A peaceful death has been characterized in the HF literature as a period free of pain and unnecessary treatments and a situation where there is effective communication between a limited number of care providers [11]. Controlling symptoms becomes a priority for end-of-life care, as this contributes to an increase in quality of life [20]. Although a peaceful death is important for the patient, it is also equally important for the family caregiver, as a negative perception of the experience at end of life reduces the family caregiver's ability to cope and has been attributed to increased levels of depression in the bereavement period [11]. In addition, family caregivers who experience emotional distress during bereavement have themselves been shown to have higher mortality rate [21].

Evidence suggests that when death is unanticipated, family caregivers are at an increased risk of having an inability to cope during the bereavement period [22]. This is specifically important to be aware of in relation to the HF population because research suggests family caregivers of persons with HF often retrospectively report that they did not feel prepared for end of life [8]. It is important to be aware that family caregivers of persons with advanced HF who die suddenly are at increased risk for complicated grief, and support for this sub-group should be prioritized. Healthcare professionals responsible for referrals to palliative or hospice services need to be aware of the importance of early access to these services for persons with HF and their family caregivers, preferably at the beginning of the disease trajectory as this can support the development of effective coping skills [23].

15.2 Heart Failure in the Community

A current trend in chronic disease management is the transition from a primarily hospital-based care model to a community-based approach [24] requiring that healthcare professionals need to feel comfortable in their ability to manage complex chronic illness in a community setting. As the Canadian healthcare system shifts client care from the hospital to the community setting [25], there will be an increased need for family members to take on the role of a caregiver; however, this shift in service delivery will be unsustainable if healthcare professionals do not provide support for families undertaking this important role. Family caregivers of persons living with advanced HF have a challenging role with many needs that are unique to the diagnosis of HF. When compared to family caregivers of person in the earlier stages of disease, caregivers of persons with advanced HF demonstrate greater mental health concerns [26]. The remainder of this chapter will focus on the experience of the family caregiver of the individual with advanced HF. The family caregiver is defined in this chapter as any person who is involved in the provision of care to the care recipient, commonly the spouse but could also pertain to other relationships such as the patient's adult child, sibling, or friend.

Viewing the family caregiver in isolation from the patient is impractical as people are highly influenced by the context of their environment [27]. According to family systems theory, the family caregiver and the patient influence the health and wellness of each other [27]. For example, when a family caregiver is unable to perform their role effectively, the literature suggests that hospitalization rates of persons with HF are increased [28]. In the interest of both the patient and the family caregiver, it is important to address the needs of caregivers of persons with advanced HF. Without family caregivers, the additional costs to our healthcare system would be unsustainable and therefore it is important that family caregivers receive professional support in managing their role. Due to budgetary limitations, it is common for much of the professional focus to go to the patient while the family caregiver struggles with few resources.

The role of the caregivers for persons with advanced HF is challenging, characterized by uncertainty, and the difficulty in establishing any sense of normality [15]. Hodson [29] describes the experience of caregiving for persons with advanced HF as a journey in a constant *state of flux*. When interviewed, family caregivers of persons with advanced HF expressed frustration with the limitations imposed on them as a result of the unpredictability of their caregiving role [30]. These limitations can include frequent changes to the plan of care that do not allow the development of consistent daily routines and financial challenges due to costs associated with being users of the healthcare system such as parking and accommodation costs. In addition, family caregivers find it difficult to make plans outside of the home as a result of the fluctuating patient health status, making it hard to determine if the patient will be well enough to leave their home on a specified day. Healthcare professionals must take these limitations into account when developing a plan of care, as well as assess for further challenges that family caregivers may be facing in their daily lives and work to develop family-focused care plans.

For a better understanding of what it might feel like to care for a person with advanced HF, imagine:

> You have just been employed in a position where you do not have the required qualifications. Each day would bring with it a new learning challenge and just as you begin to feel as if you have figured out your role, an additional skill is added to your list of learning requirements. Learning how to perform your new job as caregiver of a person with advanced HF is a process that tests your ability to be flexible while continually being presented with road blocks. This role as caregiver may not have been the path you imagined but you continue to do it because of a sense obligation and in fact, you may be the only potential candidate for the position.

As healthcare professionals, it may be helpful to take time to remember the adjustment that was once required when entering school to train for our profession. Learning required hours of reading and continual practice. Skills did not always come easy and with that, sometimes came anxiety and frustration. Family caregivers are diving head first into a new world where they may be struggling to understand the terminology and do not feel that they have the confidence or the skills to perform the amount and type of care that the healthcare system is expecting of them. It is important to prepare and support family caregivers in their role, making sure to be patient and provide all the needed encouragement along the way. The next section in the chapter will discuss strategies to incorporate into current practice that will enhance the experience for family caregivers of persons with advanced HF.

15.3 Practice Implications

Family caregivers play an invaluable role in providing care to persons with HF and they should be seen as key members of the healthcare team. Healthcare professionals working in direct contact with persons with advanced HF can improve the experience of caregiving immediately by implementing basic changes into their practice. Improving the experience may be as simple as taking the time to talk to the family caregiver, asking for their feedback and incorporating this feedback into the planning process as well as assessing their needs and offering support when required. The following recommendations for practice are based on research specific to the experience of caregiving for persons with advanced HF.

15.3.1 Communication with Family Caregivers

Current Canadian guidelines in HF care have identified incorporating the family caregiver in the plan of care as being essential [31]. In the community, the family caregiver will be responsible for providing much of the care to the individual with advanced HF and exclusion from the process can serve to increase caregiver anxiety and feelings of burden. Healthcare professionals depend on family caregivers to provide the required supports and often the caregivers are more familiar with the patient and their care needs, therefore it is imperative that they be included in the decision-making process if they desire.

When including family caregivers, it is important to avoid using terminology that the caregiver is unfamiliar with, such as medical jargon or acronyms. Family caregivers would also benefit from having one main care provider as the designated contact person. Due to the complexity of care for a patient with advanced HF, the patient may be required to receive care from a variety of professionals such as a cardiologist, nurse practitioner, special care aides, family physician, and/or nurses specialized in chronic disease management. Family caregivers of persons with advanced HF report that they become frustrated with having to communicate with a wide range of healthcare professionals [15]. With the multitude of care providers, there is also a risk for family caregivers to receive conflicting care recommendations. Having one main contact allows for continuity of care between healthcare professionals and fewer communication challenges.

15.3.2 Assess the Needs of Family Caregivers

Family caregivers have a variety of needs that are often neglected. These needs cut across multiple health domains including physical, emotional, social, and spiritual domains. When these needs are effectively being met, family caregivers report a greater ability to manage the daily challenges that are characteristic of caring for an individual with advanced HF [32]. As the patient's abilities decline, the demands of the family caregivers will increase and this may lower their resilience toward being able to recognize and meet their own needs [32]. This is when healthcare professionals can intervene by helping family caregivers to identify which needs are not being adequately addressed and developing a plan that is mutually beneficial for the family caregiver and the patient. Interventions need to be tailored to each individual caregiver situation and their need deficit; some examples of strategies that family caregivers of persons with advanced HF have found valuable to support their own physical and emotional needs include praying, participating in activities related to their ideas of spirituality, becoming physically active, socializing, participating in a hobby, or babysitting grandchildren [15]. In some cases, family caregivers may require referral to outside agencies such as a social worker or mental health nurse for further support to identify strategies for self-care.

Financial needs rate high amongst the concerns for family caregivers of persons with advanced HF [33]. In a study conducted by Kitko and Hupcey [15] with family caregivers of persons with advanced HF, the participants expressed concerns over the inability to meet financial obligations associated with costs such as travel to and from appointments, parking, accommodations when overnight stays are required, and purchasing necessary medications. Lost wages due to having to miss work to attend medical appointments also contributed to feelings of financial uncertainty [34]. Healthcare professionals can serve as a bridge for families to access subsidized programs by being aware of the programs offered in the community and seeking referrals if required.

Family caregivers of persons with advanced HF have a variety of educational needs. A large source of educational needs originates from the necessity to provide *skilled* care to the individual with HF and can include learning how to assess the patient for symptom deterioration, titrate medication doses based on pertinent clinical data, and administering intravenous medications in the home environment [33, 34]. When interviewed, family caregivers of persons with HF highlighted a knowledge deficit related to emergency preparedness, wanting to know what to do if the patient's heart stops beating while at home or if the patient is no longer able to breath [8, 35]. Family caregivers also reported eagerness to mentally prepare for what the end-of-life experience would look like, and whether it would involve any pain or anxiety [8]. Clearly, family caregivers have complex situations that require adequate support from knowledgable healthcare professionals.

15.3.3 Encourage Family Caregivers to Access Respite Services

Family caregivers of persons with advanced HF frequently report a lack of self-care and a tendency to put the needs of the patient before their own [15]. Examples of self-care activites that family caregivers have the potential to neglect include providing their body with adequate nutrients, remembering to take medications, attending medical appointments for their own health needs and getting adequate sleep. Accessing respite services allows family caregivers the opportunity to spend time away from their relative with HF to focus on their own needs. It is common for family caregivers to be resistant to the utilization of respite services unless the symptoms of the individual with HF are stable [15]; therefore, healthcare professionals may need to take time to provide teaching related to the value of seeking respite services as well as assist family caregiver in choosing activities that are meaningful and serve to reduce feelings of burden. Family caregivers also have a tendency to utilize the respite time to meet the needs of the care recipient such as obtaining medications [35]; however, to maintain overall health, it is important for family caregivers to participate in activities unrelated to the patient.

15.3.4 Positive Aspects of Family Caregiving

Although caregiving for persons with advanced HF is challenging, there are positive aspects that tend to be forgotten and need to be brought to the fore. Prioritizing negative associations with caregiving may alter the way the family caregiver perceives their role and does not provide a balanced approach to the caregiving context. Research reveals the positive aspects of family caregiving such as (a) the development of a stronger relationship with the care receiver, (b) increase in personal skills and abilities, (c) an enhanced sense of self, and (d) feelings of personal satisfaction [36]. For example, family caregivers of persons with advanced HF living in the community have been required to learn new skills such as providing daily hygiene care, wound care, assessment techniques and medication management. Family caregivers may also be required to compensate for the patient's inability to assist in the household activities and therefore are required to learn new skills such as how to cook or fix a car [15, 30]. Initially for many family caregivers, these new skills are anxiety provoking. Although once mastered, these tasks have been shown to contribute to an increase in caregiver self-esteem [34]. Family caregivers of persons with advanced HF also report learning strategies to improve mental health such as taking a step back to appreciate the small joys in life and changing their focus to living in the moment [33]. It is important to promote the positive aspects of family caregiving as a means to balance the inevitable negative aspects of the complex caregiving context often associated with HF.

15.3.5 Additional Education and Training

Family caregivers have a desire for open and honest dialogue about death between the patient, caregiver and healthcare professional [15], but these discussions are not always being initiated by healthcare professionals. Family caregivers need to be aware that HF is a life-limiting disease and they require counsel on possible end-of-life scenarios as lack of knowledge in these areas can lead to complicated grief during the bereavement period. To allow for the healthcare professional to adequately address end-of-life concerns, it is important that they feel comfortable discussing the possibilities of death. It may therefore be necessary to seek out further education and training in the area of palliative care for persons with chronic conditions. It may also be necessary to advocate for educational opportunities on topics such as end of life, palliative care, and/or advanced HF in nursing programs or places of work (e.g., home care services).

15.4 Research Implications

The provision of healthcare should be based on research to ensure that professionals are providing strong evidence-based care to patients and their families. From a research perspective, the current understanding of the caregiving experience for persons with advanced HF needs to be expanded. Examples of current gaps that need to be addressed include conducting research within Canada, utilizing participants from different cultural groups, comparing experience by gender, and exploring different relationship structures such as same sex marriages. Future research should also avoid focusing alone on the negative aspects of the caregiving experience. Developing interventions that support the needs of family caregivers of persons with advanced HF should be a priority. Researchers could begin by analyzing the literature to determine which caregiver interventions have been successful in similar population groups such as family caregivers of persons with chronic obstructive pulmonary disorder and test/adapt successful interventions with caregivers of persons with advanced HF. With this research basis, healthcare professionals can develop evidence-based plans of care that are tailored to the unique needs of persons with advanced HF and their family caregivers.

15.5 Conclusion

There is an aspect of uncertainty surrounding the disease trajectory for persons with HF. This life-limiting illness is characterized by periods of stability followed by rapid deteriorations in health status with an unpredictable end-of-life experience. When a patient enters the advanced stage of HF, they will present with symptoms of HF such as shortness of breath, consistently with minimal exertion or when at rest which limits their ability fulfilling their own care needs. This contributes to the added pressure placed on family caregivers of these persons who themselves report high levels of physical and emotional challenges related to their role as caregivers. Persons with HF and their families can benefit from access to palliative care services; however, barriers exist that limit the use in this population.

The experience of caregiving for persons with advanced HF is a journey in a state of flux [29], characterized by the need to adapt each day in response to the inconsistent health status of the patient. Family caregivers often find themselves absorbed in the constant needs of the patient, while forgetting to meet their own needs. Not all reports of caregiving are negative, with some family caregivers reporting that their journey allows them the opportunity to learn new skills and to develop a deeper relationship with the patient. Unfortunately, family caregivers of persons with HF have unique needs that have been neglected in both practice and research. Healthcare professionals must be including family caregivers in the decision-making process, addressing the caregiver's needs (i.e. financial, emotional, spiritual, and physical) and encouraging them to access respite services. To enhance our ability to support the diverse needs of the family caregiver population, it is important to take advantage of educational opportunities to increase comfortability with discussing end-of-life concerns with persons with HF and their families. Family caregivers are depended upon to support the needs of persons with advanced HF in the community and therefore they deserve continued support throughout their caregiving journey.

References

1. Ponikowski P, Anker S, AlHabib K, Cowie M, Force T, Hu S, et al. Heart failure: preventing disease and death worldwide. ESC Heart Fail. 2014;1(1):4–25. https://www.escardio.org/static_file/Escardio/Subspecialty/HFA/WHFA-whitepaper-15-May-14.pdf. Accessed 20 Jan 2019.
2. Hupcey J, Kitko L, Alonso W. Patients' perceptions of illness severity in advanced heart failure. J Hosp Palliat Nurs. 2016;18:110–4. https://doi.org/10.1097/NJH.0000000000000229.
3. Emanuel L, Librach L. Palliative care core skills and clinical competencies. 2nd ed. St. Louis: Elsevier; 2011.
4. Adler E, Goldfinger J, Kalman J, Park M, Meier D. Palliative care in the treatment of advanced heart failure. J Am Heart Assoc. 2009;120:2597–696. https://doi.org/10.1161/circulationaha.109.869123.
5. Goodlin SJ. Palliative care in congestive heart failure. J Am Coll Cardiol. 2009;54:386–96. https://doi.org/10.1016/j.jacc.2009.02.078.
6. Cubbon R, Gale C, Kearney L, Schechter C, Brooksby W, Nolan J, et al. Changing characteristics and mode of death associated with chronic heart failure caused by left ventricular systolic dysfunction: a study across therapeutic eras. Circ Heart Fail. 2011;4:396–403.
7. McCarthy P, Smedira N, Vargo R, Goormastic M, Hobbs R, Starling R, et al. One hundred patients with the heartmate left ventricular assist device: evolving concepts and technology. J Thorac Cardiovasc Surg. 1998;115:904–12.
8. McIlvennan C, Jones J, Allen L, Swetz K, Nowels C, Matlock D. Bereaved caregiver perspectives on the end-of-life experience of patients with a left ventricular assist device. JAMA Intern Med. 2016;176:534–8.
9. Stajduhar K. Chronic illness, palliative care, and the problematic nature of dying. Can J Nurs Res. 2011;43:7–15.
10. Parliament of Canada. Quality end-of-life care: the right of every Canadian. Ottawa, ON: Parliament of Canada; 2000. http://www.parl.gc.ca/Content/SEN/Committee/362/upda/rep/repfinjun00-e.htm Accessed January 27 2019.
11. Small N, Barnes S, Gott M, Payne S, Parker C, Seamark D, et al. Dying, death and bereavement: a qualitative study of the views of carers of people with heart failure in the UK. BMC Palliat Care. 2009;8. doi:https://doi.org/10.1186/1472-684X-8-6.
12. Canadian Hospice Palliative Care Association. 2013. A model to guide hospice palliative care. Based on the national principles and norms of practice . http://www.chpca.net/media/319547/norms-of-practice-eng-web.pdf. Accessed 19 Jan 2019.
13. Browne S, Macdonald S, May CR, Macleod U, Mair FS. Patient, carer and professional perspectives on barriers and facilitators to quality care in advanced heart failure. PLoS One. 2014;9:1–8.
14. Ivany E. Understanding palliative care needs in heart failure. Br J Card Nurs. 2015;10:348–53.
15. Kitko LA, Hupcey JE. The work of spousal caregiving of older adults with end-stage heart failure. J Gerontol Nurs. 2013;39:40–7.
16. Evangelistaa LS, Stromberg A, Dionne-Odom JN. An integrated review of interventions to improve psychological outcomes in caregivers of patients with heart failure. Curr Opin Support Palliat Care. 2016;10:25–31.
17. Bowers MT. Managing patients with heart failure. J Nurse Pract. 2013;9:634–42.
18. McWilliam CL, Ward-Griffin C, Oudshoorn A, Krestick E. Living while dying/dying while living: older clients' sociocultural experience of home-based palliative care. J Hosp Palliat Nurs. 2008;10:338–49.

19. Boucher J, Bova C, Sullivan-Bolyai S, Theroux R, Klar R, Terrien J, et al. Next-of-kin's perspective of end-of-life care. J Hosp Palliat Nurs. 2010;12:41–50.
20. Arnold JMO, Liu P, Demers C, Dorian P, Giannetti N, Haddad H, et al. Canadian Cardiovascular Society consensus conference recommendations on heart failure 2006: diagnosis and management. Can J Cardiol. 2006;22:23–45. https://doi.org/10.1016/s0828-282x(06)70237-9.
21. Stroebe M, Schut H, Stroebe W. Health outcomes of bereavement. Lancet. 2007;370:1960–73.
22. Shah S, Carey I, Harris T, DeWilde S, Victor C, Cook D. The effect of unexpected bereavement on mortality in older couples. Am J Public Health. 2013;103:1140–5. https://doi.org/10.2105/AJPH.2012.301050.
23. Howlett J, Morrin L, Fortin M, Heckman G, Strachan PH, Suskin N, et al. End-of-life planning in heart failure: it should be the end of the beginning. Can J Cardiol. 2010;26:135–41. https://doi.org/10.1016/s0828-282x(10)70351-2.
24. Hayes S, Peloquin S, Howlett J, Harkness K, Giannetti N, Rancourt C, et al. A qualitative study of the current state of heart failure community care in Canada: what can we learn for the future? BMC Health Serv Res. 2015;15:290. https://doi.org/10.1186/s12913-015-0955-4.
25. Public Health Agency of Canada. Preventing chronic disease strategic plan 2013–2016: Canadian living healthier and more productive lives. Ottawa, ON: Public Health Agency of Canada; 2013. http://publications.gc.ca/collections/collection_2014/aspc-phac/HP35-39-2013-eng.pdf. Accessed 19 Jan 2019.
26. Saunders M. Perspectives from family caregivers receiving home nursing support. Home Healthc Nurs. 2012;30:82–90.
27. Wright L, Leahey M. Nurses and families: a guide to family assessment and intervention. 6th ed. Philadelphia, PA: FA Davis Company; 2013.
28. Aggarwal B, Pender A, Mosca L, Mochari-Greenberger H. Factors associated with medication adherence among heart failure patients and their caregivers. J Nurs Edu Pract. 2015;5:22–7. https://doi.org/10.5430/jnep.v5n3p22.
29. Hodson A. The experience of caregiving for persons with advanced heart failure: An integrative review. Master's thesis. 2017. University of Saskatchewan. Saskatoon, Saskatchewan, Canada. https://harvest.usask.ca/bitstream/handle/10388/7783/HODSON-THESIS-2017.pdf?sequence=1&isAllowed=y. Accessed 7 Mar 2019.
30. Aldred H, Gott M, Gariballa S. Advanced heart failure: impact on older patients and informal carers. J Adv Nurs. 2005;49:116–24.
31. Howlett J, Chan M, Ezekowitz JA, Harkness K, Heckman GAM, Kouz S, et al. The Canadian Cardiovascular Society heart failure companion: bridging guidelines to your practice. Can J Cardiol. 2016;32:296–310. https://doi.org/10.1016/j.cjca.2015.06.019.
32. Furlong K, Wuest J. Self-care behaviors of spouses caring for significant others with Alzheimer's disease: the emergence of self-care worthiness as a salient condition. Qual Health Res. 2008;18:1662–72. https://doi.org/10.1177/1049732308327158.
33. Scott L. Technological caregiving: a qualitative perspective. Home Health Care Manag Pract. 2001;13:227–35.
34. Hupcey J, Fenstermacher K, Kitko L, Fogg J. Palliative needs of spousal caregivers of patients with heart failure followed up at specialized heart failure centers. J Hosp Palliat Nurs. 2011;13:142–50.
35. Braannstrom M, Ekman I, Boman K, Strandberg G. Being a close relative of a person with severe, chronic heart failure in palliative advanced home care: a comfort but also a strain. Scand J Caring Sci. 2007;21:338–4.
36. Peacock S, Forbes D, Markle-Reid M, Hawranik P, et al. The positive aspects of the journey with dementia: using a strengths-based perspective to reveal opportunities. J Appl Gerontol. 2010;29:640–59.

Development of a Model to Guide Conversations About Internet Use in Cancer Experiences: Applications for Hospice and Palliative Care

16

Kristen R. Haase

Contents

16.1	Method..	214
16.2	Findings..	215
16.3	The Model...	216
16.4	Discussion...	219
	16.4.1 Practice Implications..	219
	16.4.2 Educational Implications...	220
	16.4.3 Research Implications...	220
16.5	Conclusions...	221
References..		221

Cancer is a global health concern and primarily a disease of older adults. In Canada, one in two people can expect a diagnosis of cancer in their lifetime, and 70% of those diagnoses currently occur in those over age 70 years of age [1]. A diagnosis of cancer has physical and psychosocial implications, related to the challenges of mentally processing a potentially life-limiting illness and coping with the effects of surgical or pharmacological treatments [2]. Many people with cancer report health information as a key support at the time of diagnosis and beyond. Health information assists people at the time of diagnosis as they choose treatments, make decisions about courses of therapy, and transition to survivorship or palliative care [3].

As the internet has become more freely accessible—current estimates indicate that ~90% of Canadians have access [4]—it has become increasingly common for people seeking health information to use the internet [5, 6]. Although healthcare

K. R. Haase (✉)
College of Nursing, University of Saskatchewan, Saskatoon, SK, Canada

Saskatchewan Centre for Patient-Oriented Research, Saskatoon, SK, Canada
e-mail: Kristen.haase@usask.ca

© Springer Nature Switzerland AG 2019
L. Holtslander et al. (eds.), *Hospice Palliative Home Care and Bereavement Support*, https://doi.org/10.1007/978-3-030-19535-9_16

professionals are still the number one source of information preferred by patients, the internet eclipses their accessibility. The internet is a quick and easy means to locate health information and is relatively unfettered, meaning that it is accessible at any time and there are no gatekeepers; this is as a clear advantage over healthcare professionals for health information.

People of all ages with cancer are increasingly using the internet for cancer-related information. Even older adults, who have historically been considered internet and technology *laggards*, have changing attitudes and behaviours towards technology with adults over age 65 reporting growing internet use [7]. This requires us to think about the role the internet can play in patient experiences with cancer, and what, if any, role healthcare professionals play in drawing on this growing source of information.

Older adults with cancer and other chronic diseases are more likely to need hospice palliative care than other age groups [8]. Despite cancer being a disease of the aged, there has been little focus on the physical, psychosocial, and survivorship needs of older adults with cancer, often due to ageist perceptions that older adults with cancer would forgo treatment or be more likely to choose less aggressive treatment options [9, 10]. Older adults have also been excluded from many studies due to the complexity of their health related to existence of multiple chronic conditions (also called multimorbidity), frailty, and functional decline [11]. Thus, despite cancer being a disease of older adults, there is still limited research to support older adults and clinicians working with older adults with cancer. However, in the context of growing reliance on internet information by all age groups, there is a need to understand how older adults with cancer can be supported as they use internet resources to manage their cancer diagnosis across all stages of the cancer trajectory, including palliative care.

In this chapter, I will draw on a recent study on use of the internet for cancer-related information to manage cancer experiences. I will present a research-derived model that can be used by clinicians to have conversations about internet information use. This model was developed based on the accounts of people with cancer but can serve as a useful framework for discussions of internet information for people with other life-limiting illness who also may be facing the end of life and have difficult decisions to make.

16.1 Method

This study was guided by an interpretive descriptive mixed methods approach [12, 13]. The main findings of this study have been published elsewhere [14–16], thus I will provide only a brief overview of methods.

Using an embedded concurrent design, the dominant qualitative research methodology was complemented by a supplementary quantitative approach (QUAL + quan) [17]. Several data sources were used, including: (1) a sample of commonly searched cancer websites; (2) interviews with people newly diagnosed with cancer; (3) interviews and focus groups with healthcare professionals in cancer care; and (4) feedback from peers, experts, and clinicians. The study was conducted at a University-affiliated cancer treatment centre in Western Canada, and approved by the relevant research ethics board.

16.2 Findings

From the multiple data sources collected, we gained an understanding of how people with cancer used cancer-related internet information to manage their cancer experiences. These findings are very relevant to those with other diseases, and may be particularly useful for clinicians in palliative and hospice care, as they work with people and their families at the end of life. Preceding the model and discussion of its applicability to hospice and palliative care settings, I will present a brief summary of the findings, as they provide context for the development of the model.

In the qualitative review of websites, we explored the online milieu in an effort to understand the types of cancer information and content available, and what patients find when seeking information on the internet. Findings from this review enable an understanding of the types of cancer content and information that an individual can expect to find when they search online for cancer information using common search terms (cancer, cancer treatment, breast cancer, lung cancer, etc.). The most abundant information is biomedical and empirical information about diagnosis, types of treatment and related effects, and medical management of cancer. This is vital information as patients make sense of any illness. Despite an abundance of information about physical management of cancer, there was limited information to support other aspects of management. For example, information addressing strategies towards self-management of illness and treatment side effects, contextual factors, death and dying, and existential challenges. These findings are significant as they raise questions and concerns about the information that people with cancer and other illnesses find when searching independently for information, especially about end of life, including hospice and palliative care information. These findings also give a sense of where clinicians need to bolster information.

In our interviews with patients, we explored how cancer-related internet information shaped their cancer experiences, and how it informed interactions with healthcare professionals and healthcare services. Participants described that from the time of diagnosis, patients found cancer-related internet information as their most important source of information, next to their healthcare professional. Patients felt that cancer-related internet information complemented the information provided by their healthcare professional and allowed them to have a better understanding of complex cancer and medical information. Many patients described a staged approach to cancer-related internet information use. First, they would obtain information from their healthcare professional, and then they would consult the internet—at their own pace and on their own terms—to gain a comprehensive understanding of their diagnosis. Patients also described using the internet to manage their symptoms and to assist them as they navigated the complexities of the healthcare system. The internet was used to guide decision-making, particularly when two or more choices were available to the patient. Clearly, the internet played a crucial role in multiple facets of patients' understanding of their diagnosis and the cancer experience.

Healthcare professional participants acknowledged that many of their patients rely on the internet to understand and process their diagnosis. For instance, upon receiving their diagnosis, patients would go to the internet to learn about their illness and to process information provided by their healthcare professional. Healthcare professionals identified two transitions where they felt information was needed to bridge the gap between cancer care and primary care: first, when entering cancer care at the time of diagnosis and, second, when discharged from cancer care back into the care of the primary physician. Healthcare professionals found that patients often experienced undue stress and anxiety around these times, and likely relied more on the internet to process their concerns in the absence of ideal healthcare professional or other support. However, healthcare professionals postulated that, even once in the cancer care system, patients may feel unsure about asking certain questions and, moreover, that clinic conditions do not always permit engaging with all patients.

Although healthcare professionals acknowledged and supported patient use of the internet, they also indicated associated challenges. Participants expressed concern about patients accessing information that they were ill-equipped to understand or that was wholly inaccurate. Healthcare professionals described that even when patients found what they called "good quality" information, they were skeptical that the average patient (i.e. with no prior medical knowledge) would be able to parse through that information and identify what was applicable to their specific diagnosis. The case of Complementary and Alternative Medicine (CAM) was also cited as a main topic of internet information that patients shared with healthcare professionals that generated concerns for healthcare professionals.

This data is important in and of itself and presents conclusions for nursing students and healthcare professionals to reflect upon. When triangulated with the findings from the additional data sources, these findings pose thought-provoking directions for future research and nursing practice, including hospice and palliative care within the context of cancer in older adults.

16.3 The Model

Drawing on the findings discussed above, I created the following approach to begin conversations about cancer-related internet information use: Ask, Listen, Engage, Reflect/Reorient, and Time (ALERT) (Fig. 16.1). This approach and the requisite nursing strategies described below are within the scope of practice of nurses and most healthcare professionals and are relevant to other domains of healthcare where patients use online information for self-management and to guide their use of healthcare services. In the following, I will discuss the components of the model, with discussion of its application in hospice and palliative care settings.

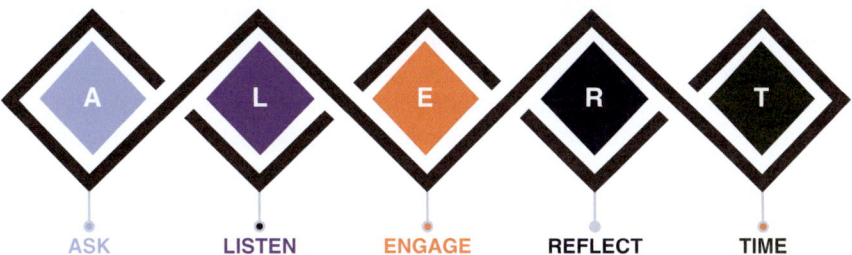

Fig. 16.1 Alert model

1. ***Ask*** patients and their families about their use of internet information and whether this is a source of information they rely on. Although some professional sources encourage patients to start this conversation, patient participants in this study clearly felt that they wanted healthcare professionals to broach this topic first. As one clinician stated, *When I do ask patients and their families about what websites they are looking at, it really gives me a lot of insight into what they're thinking, and what I need to address* (oncologist). Furthermore, providers seemed to feel that having this conversation, regardless of what patients told them, was a good way to initiate an important discussion and understand patient questions about their illness and what they wanted to know. Asking relates to assessment, which is the first step of the nursing process and the foundation of clinical reasoning in nursing [18].

    Within the context of the study findings, particularly the website review, wherein there was an absence of information about death or dying, broaching said conversations may be especially helpful to patients and families. Past research reiterates the importance of these conversations, for example, in one study, people at the end of life who underwent treatment for cancer expressed regret because they did not understand what treatment would entail, and felt that their end-of-life care did not fit their needs [19]. Initiating these conversations on information seeking may also open discussions about end of life, and because online information is lacking in this domain, it is doubly worthwhile to intervene. This is especially relevant in community-based palliative and hospice settings where most people are looking for ways to access information and support from home.

2. ***Listen*** to what your patient tells you. Listening and the accompanying non-verbal skills are an essential component of the patient–nurse relationship [20]. Active listening skills allow nurses to understand their patients' information needs and permit the patient time to share their needs or what they have already found on the internet. Using therapeutic silence has also been lauded as an important tool for nurses to encourage patients sharing, particularly at end of life [21]. As one participant found, listening to the patient's real concern is important, as things are not always what they seem: *'they say "I've read on the internet that this will, totally prevent my nausea".' They're not just saying that; they're saying, "I don't want to throw up". "'I'm mortally afraid of having to puke my*

way through the day' like it's different". It's more personal than the questions appear when they're being asked' (Pharmacist).

Past research on conversations around end-of-life care demonstrate that patients sometimes feel nurses demonstrate an *unwillingness to listen* [22]. This reiterates the importance of both initiating these conversations, and then being open to listen and process the questions and consequences of what patients are asking, rather than rushing to speak or instruct patients on what to do. Again, if asking patients about information found on the internet or other information preferences opens up an opportunity to hear a person's concerns, we must in fact listen to these concerns.

3. ***Engage*** with your patient. As laid out by best practice guidelines, engage your patient to establish a therapeutic partnership, ensure that they feel comfortable sharing, and ensure they understand your desire for them to have the best possible information [23]. Developing rapport and dialogue with the patient, rather than viewing patient interactions as a simple linear transaction, creates opportunities for patients to feel like empowered partners rather than passive subjects [24]. In the context of hospice and palliative care or end of life, there is a need to be present and accommodating around sensitive existential conversations [21]. Strang and colleagues talk about the process of these conversations on sensitive topics evolving over time through a process, which includes opening conversations, presence, sensitivity, and using both words and silence therapeutically [21]. Particularly in hospice and palliative care, where relationships may extend over time, this process of engagement may extend for weeks or months, rather than days.

4. ***Reorient*** or reflect on what patients share with you. Nurses put forward the idea of reorienting and reflecting what patients tell them as a means of affirmation. The nurse, having heard what information the patient has found, identifies their concern and, if necessary, redirects them to different or better internet information. One nurse described this in the context of really hearing what the patient is saying, understanding their concern within the context of that therapeutic relationships, and then helping the patient to address their issue or concern, with better information: *Most often they just want us to say "you should do this" or "you should do that". But it's not that easy. Then they have the influences of these blogs or this (internet) information that isn't from reputable sources. That's where I've had – not issues, but – kind of having to re-orient their thinking after they've been exposed to that* (Nurse). This intervention positions nurses to acknowledge patient resourcefulness as a strength, thereby validating their information-seeking efforts [25]. By reflecting, nurses can also take the empirically focused internet information and put it into a holistic context.

5. ***Time and timing*** refers to the importance of incorporating discussions of internet information throughout the nurse–patient relationship and cancer/illness trajectory. Many healthcare professional participants identified a reluctance to engage in discussions about internet information at the first meeting with a patient for lack of rapport, whereas others expressed that there is no perfect time. However, patients may pass through the care of a palliative care nurse or nursing

student in a matter of one or two visits, and thus healthcare professionals need to capitalize on the opportunity to address patient concerns at every visit and in every interaction [26]. The notion of 'Time' should be a reminder that every time patients interact with their nurses, nurses can use ALERT. Nurses also mentioned that many patients used their phone or iPad to pass the time, which can also serve as a prompt to have discussions about patient information needs and internet-related questions.

Time is also relevant in the context of understanding the constraints related to initiating difficult conversations. Many studies have found that nurses feel they lack the time and the organizational structures to initiate sensitive conversations about end of life [27, 28]. However, this lack of 'appropriate' time may then lead to avoiding the conversations altogether, which has the potential to lead to a lack of timely hospice and palliative care. Following the aforementioned approach to time conversations about internet information across the cancer/illness trajectory may mitigate concerns related to missing important conversations, or patients being blindsided.

16.4 Discussion

The ALERT approach is a unique research-derived model that can help to facilitate discussions with patients using internet information during a cancer or life-limiting diagnosis, and also when in hospice, or palliative home care. This model and its implementation in hospice palliative care and end-of-life care settings have implications for practice, research, and education.

16.4.1 Practice Implications

The ALERT model starts with the nurse asking the patient about their use of internet resources and permitting exploration from that starting point, rather than placing the burden of initiating these conversations on patients. Second, the website analysis indicated that internet information on death and dying is not readily accessible or apparent when searching for cancer information. Thus, using the ALERT model may provide some insight into gaps in information, particularly when a person has a received a terminal or life-limiting diagnosis and has been looking for information on palliation. Nurses can also reflect and reorient the concerns of the patient by listening to the information they have uncovered and putting it into a holistic context.

In hospice and palliative care contexts, there are numerous opportunities for the ALERT model to inform practice. For example, past research on internet use in hospice has found that patients, caregivers, and healthcare professionals are looking online for information to support their end-of-life needs [29]. Nurses can use ALERT in practice as a means of framing discussions of internet use with hospice users, thereby supporting their information seeking.

16.4.2 Educational Implications

Nursing education needs to be dynamic and responsive to the changing landscape of healthcare and society in general [30]. As such, nursing curriculum experts advocate that nursing curriculum should be: (1) context-relevant, (2) evidence-informed, and (3) unified [31]; therefore, there is a need to keep current our understandings of the best ways to communicate information, and engage with patients.

Although technology and informatics in nursing education are a growing area of curriculum focus, the emphasis typically rests on the use of electronic health records, nurse-centred applications, and integration of high- or medium-fidelity simulation teaching approaches [32, 33]. However, there remains an opportunity to act on patients' use of technology and encourage future nurses to incorporate this into their practice. Because our study found that internet use allows patients to feel a sense of control, autonomy, and greater ability to manage their illness, it is important for health professional students to have an awareness of the empowering impact of information. This is important because of a documented tension amongst healthcare professionals around patients' use of the internet [16]. We can address these tensions in our nursing curriculum, thereby preparing students as they may encounter these dilemmas in their own practice. For instance, developing case studies on the issue of patient-sought internet information may allow nursing students to reflect upon how they would respond, and how they will approach this in practice. This is especially relevant in the context of hospice and palliative care, where knowledge of a *good death* may have important implications for patients and their families and of which newly trained health professionals should have an awareness. As such, nursing students would benefit from the ALERT model discussed above, as a simple tool easily applied in clinical practice. Together, these actions in nursing curriculum can prepare a future generation of nurses to be more equipped to approach patients' self-sought internet information.

16.4.3 Research Implications

There is much research being conducted in the field of health informatics and about how mobile health (mhealth) and wired devices can impact care. There is also growing research in how interventions tailored to support self-management needs can bolster quality of life and empower people to manage their own health conditions, which relates to enhancing a quality end-of-life experience. There is, however, limited research on interventions for specific population that may be less likely to use technology, including older adults, new Canadians, and people for whom English is not a first language. Meeting the needs of these population will require rethinking and reframing how technology is designed, who uses technology, and, perhaps, require changes in both stereotypes and perspectives, all of which can be established through future research.

16.5 Conclusions

Given the increase in internet use amongst older adults with cancer, there is a growing need to recognize the implications of this information source. How we situate this ALERT in practice and what we do as nurses to encourage or facilitate patient's own information seeking may impact their illness experiences. The ALERT model discussed in this study may serve as one useful model to frame these discussions, empowering both nurses and patients as they discuss internet information use. The ALERT model is even more important in the palliative context as information on death and dying is scarce online, and thus patients and their families will benefit from the support of their nurse as they endeavour to find and understand the best possible information, at such an important time.

Acknowledgements This research was funded by a grant from the Canadian Association of Nurses in Oncology. I would like to gratefully acknowledge the patients and healthcare professionals who took part in this research and gave freely of their time. I would also like to acknowledge Drs. Roanne Thomas, Wendy Gifford, Lorraine Holtslander and Dave Holmes for their generous contributions to the evolution and development of this work.

References

1. Canadian Cancer Society. Canadian cancer statistics. Toronto, ON: Canadian Cancer Society; 2018.
2. Bultz BD, Carlson LE. Emotional distress: the sixth vital sign-future directions in cancer care. Psycho-Oncology. 2006;15(2):93–5.
3. Matsuyama RK, Kuhn LA, Molisani A, Wilson-Genderson MC. Cancer patients' information needs the first nine months after diagnosis. Patient Edu Counsel. 2013;90(1):96–102.
4. IWS. Internet World Stats: usage and population statistics. 2019. http://www.internetworldstats.com
5. Shea-Budgell MA, Kostaras X, Myhill KP, Hagen NA. Information needs and sources of information for patients during cancer follow-up. Curr Oncol. 2014;21(4):165–73.
6. Greer JA, Amoyal N, Nisotel L, Fishbein JN, MacDonald J, Stagl J, et al. A systematic review of adherence to oral antineoplastic therapies. Oncologist. 2016;21(3):354–76.
7. Perrin A. Social media usage. Washington, DC: Pew Research Center; 2015.
8. Statistics Canada. Population projections for Canada, provinces and territories – 2009–2036: Statistics Canada. http://www.statcan.gc.ca/daily-quotidien/100526/dq100526b-eng.htm
9. Hurria A, Naylor M, Cohen HJ. Improving the quality of cancer care in an aging population: recommendations from an IOM report. JAMA. 2013;310(17):1795–6.
10. Hurria A, Mohile SG, Dale W. Research priorities in geriatric oncology: addressing the needs of an aging population. J Natl Compr Canc Netw. 2012;10(2):286–8.
11. Wildiers H, Heeren P, Puts M, Topinkova E, Janssen-Heijnen ML, Extermann M, et al. International Society of Geriatric Oncology consensus on geriatric assessment in older patients with cancer. J Clin Oncol. 2014;32(24):2595.
12. Thorne S. Interpretive description. Walnut Creek, CA: Left Coast Press; 2016.
13. Cresswell JW. Basic features of mixed methods research. A concise introduction to mixed methods research. Thousand Oaks, CA: SAGE; 2014. p. 1–9.
14. Haase KR, Thomas R, Gifford W, Holtslander L. Managing cancer experiences: an interpretive description study of internet information use. Cancer Nurs. 2018. https://doi.org/10.1097/NCC.0000000000000619.

15. Haase KR, Thomas R, Gifford W, Holtslander L. Ways of knowing on the internet: a qualitative review of cancer websites from a critical nursing perspective. Nurs Inq. 2018;25(3).
16. Haase KR, Thomas R, Gifford W, Holtslander L. Healthcare professional views on the intersection of patient internet use, relationships, and health service use in cancer care. Eur J Cancer Care. 2018.
17. Cresswell JW, Plano Clark VL. Designing and conducting mixed methods research. Thousand Oaks, CA: Sage; 2011.
18. Alfaro-LeFevre R. Overview of nursing process, clinical reasoning, and nursing practice today. Applying nursing process: the foundation for clinical reasoning. Philadelphia, PA: Lippincott Williams & Wilkins; 2014. p. 1–45.
19. Scott IA, Mitchell GK, Reymond E, Daly MP. Difficult but necessary conversations—the case for advance care planning. Med J Austr. 2013;199:4.
20. McCabe C, Timmins F. Communication skills. Communication skills for nursing practice. Basingstoke: Palgrave Macmillan; 2013. p. 71–92.
21. Strang S, Henoch I, Danielson E, Browall M, Melin-Johansson C. Communication about existential issues with patients close to death—nurses' reflections on content, process and meaning. Psycho-Oncology. 2014;23(5):4.
22. Clover A, Browne J, McErlain P, Vandenberg B. Patient approaches to clinical conversations in the palliative care setting. J Adv Nurs. 2004;48(4):8.
23. Registered Nurses Association of Ontario. Facilitating client centred learning: clinical best practice guidelines 2012. Toronto, ON: Registered Nurses Association of Ontario. http://rnao.ca/sites/rnao-ca/files/BPG_CCL_2012_FA.pdf.
24. Sanford RC. Caring through relation and dialogue: a nursing perspective for patient education. Adv Nurs Sci. 2000;22(3):1–15.
25. Feeley N, Gottlieb L. Nursing approaches for working with family strengths and resources. J Fam Nurs. 2000;16(3):9–24.
26. Thomas-MacLean RL, Hack TF, Kwan W, Towers A, Miedema B, Tilley A. Arm morbidity and disability after breast cancer: new directions for care. Oncol Nurs Forum. 2008;35(1):65–71.
27. Clarke A, Ross H. Influences on nurses' communications with older people at the end of life: perceptions and experiences of nurses working in palliative care and general medicine. Int J Older People Nurs. 2006;1(1):9.
28. McDonnell M, Johnson G, Gallagher A, McGlade K. Palliative care in district general hospitals: the nurse's perspective. Int J Palliat Nurs. 2002;8:6.
29. Willis L, Demiris G, Oliver DP. Internet use by hospice families and providers: a review. J Med Syst. 2007;31(2):4.
30. Jensen R, Meyer L, Sternberger C. Three technological enhancements in nursing education: informatics instruction, personal response systems, and human patient simulation. Nurs Edu Pract. 2009;9(2):86–90.
31. Iwasiw CL, Goldenberg D, Andrusyszyn M. Creation of an evidence-informed, context-relevant, unified curriculum. Curriculum development in nursing education. Burlington, MA: Jones & Bartlett Publishers; 2014.
32. Ehnfors M, Grobe SJ. Nursing curriculum and continuing education: future directions. Int J Med Inform. 2004;73(7):591–8.
33. Ruchala PL. Curriculum development and approval processes in changing educational environments. In: Keating SB, editor. Curriculum development and evaluation in nursing. New York, NY: Springer; 2014. p. 33–47.

Long-Term Care

17

Genevieve Thompson and Shelley Peacock

> *You matter because you are you, and you matter to the end of your life.*
> –Dame Cicely Saunders

Contents

17.1	Long-Term Care...	224
	17.1.1 Community-Based Long-Term Care..	224
	17.1.2 Facility-Based Long-Term Care..	225
17.2	The Role of Palliative Care in Long-Term Care..	226
	17.2.1 Delivery of Palliative Care in Long-Term Care..	227
	17.2.2 Moving Forward: An Integrated Approach to Palliative Care....................	229
	17.2.3 Promising Practices...	230
17.3	Implications for Practice, Policy, and Education...	232
17.4	Conclusions...	233
References...		233

The purpose of this chapter is to present how palliative care in the community is offered in the long-term care setting, specifically in residential long-term care homes. The chapter will begin with a discussion of the concept of long-term care, followed by the role of palliative care in residential long-term care home

G. Thompson (✉)
College of Nursing, Helen Glass Centre for Nursing, University of Manitoba, Winnipeg, MB, Canada
e-mail: genevieve.thompson@umanitoba.ca

S. Peacock
College of Nursing, University of Saskatchewan, Saskatoon, SK, Canada
e-mail: shelley.peacock@usask.ca

© Springer Nature Switzerland AG 2019
L. Holtslander et al. (eds.), *Hospice Palliative Home Care and Bereavement Support*, https://doi.org/10.1007/978-3-030-19535-9_17

settings, the challenges to implementing palliative care, examining what a palliative approach to care involves, and will conclude with a discussion of promising practices in this important area, along with implications for education and policy.

17.1 Long-Term Care

Long-term care is a term that incorporates a variety of services that are required for the physical, social, and psychological needs of persons who are not able to function independently [1]. In the 1960s, the term "long-term care" tended to refer to *nursing homes* that provided care to persons who could no longer live in their own home [2]. The view of *institutional* care is strongly associated with the concept of long-term care, yet it is important to note that long-term care services are also provided in the community. It can be useful to consider long-term care across a continuum that includes living in one's own home with minimal assistance from both family/friends and formal care providers as one end of the spectrum versus those more vulnerable persons requiring 24-h care provided in a skilled facility as the other end [3]. The transition over the spectrum of long-term care can advance as a person ages and chronic conditions progress, resulting in increased dependence and reliance on others to perform activities of daily living. Over the long-term care continuum, a variety of services are available.

17.1.1 Community-Based Long-Term Care

The delivery of community-based long-term care is intended as a smooth transition among various types of interventions and services (i.e., preventative, acute, rehabilitative, and supportive) based on the unique and individual needs of persons. Ideally, long-term care services are offered such that they enable persons to remain in their own home for as long as possible [4] as this is what most people desire. The types of services offered include: (a) nursing care; (b) personal support such as self-directed care, housekeeping, or meal preparation; (c) respite or day programs; (d) palliative care; (e) rehabilitative care, such as occupational or physical therapy; and (f) providing necessary medical equipment and supplies [5].

Long-term care services in the community are typically delivered in the form of *home care*, the demand for which is increasing. To meet this demand, home care services have moved to supporting patients with more pressing needs by means of post-acute or short-term (nursing) care, leaving less resources for persons requiring long-term (more socially-based) support [4]. The result of this move has meant that family carers are increasingly responsible for providing long-term care in the community. Home and community-based services are intended to be a support for persons who do not yet qualify for admission to a residential long-term care home, often with the intent to delay this admission for as long as possible.

17.1.2 Facility-Based Long-Term Care

Long-term care services provided in a residential setting are the most concentrated type of service delivery on the long-term care continuum. The most common types of shared, residential dwellings include and are referred to in Canada as: (a) assisted living centers, (b) nursing homes, and (c) chronic and long-term care hospitals. For our purposes, we will use the term residential long-term care home. The goal of these dwellings is to maintain an optimum level of functioning for persons requiring this necessary support and that the services are consistently delivered with basic human rights and dignity in mind [1]. The transition and decision to move from one's own home to a shared dwelling can be made for various reasons. Lack of availability of willing family carers, failing health, frailty, and concerns for safety are all motivating factors for admitting persons to settings that are able to provide 24-h, intensive supportive services [3].

Persons living in residential long-term care homes require significant assistance with physical care that is usually provided by unregulated healthcare providers [6], while the emotional, cognitive, social, psychological, and spiritual needs of residents may be more challenging to address. Nurses (i.e., registered nurses, registered psychiatric nurses, or licensed practical nurses) have significant leadership roles in residential long-term care homes; this role is increasingly important, given the complexity of the care that is now required to be delivered in most facilities [2].

It is important to bear in mind that persons living (and dying) in residential long-term care homes tend to be some of the most vulnerable persons compared to those persons that live in the community [7]. For example, persons living with dementia often present with functional limitations and significant cognitive impairment that can cause a burden for family carers and that precipitate the need for residential long-term care home admission. Research demonstrates that the prevalence of dementia among long-term care residents may be as high as 95% [7].

According to the World Health Organization (WHO), there is a universal problem in how to meet the increasing demands for long-term care [8]. Changing family demographics, aging populations, and women undertaking paid work contribute to the shifts in social structures that lead to an increasing need for greater long-term care services. Development of appropriate long-term care services needs to be based on partnerships with institutions, communities, families, and other care partners, as well as the responsibility of government [1]. Many persons are living longer and with more complex chronic conditions, and a significant concern is that not enough has been done to organize and prepare for the future need for increased long-term care services, including residential settings. It is expected that by 2020, up to as many as 40% of all people who are permanent residents in residential long-term care homes in the United States will die there [9]; this number is closer to 70% of Canadian residents [10]. To ensure that these individuals receive high quality care at the end of their lives, adopting a palliative approach to care is critical. Indeed, some would even argue that it is a fundamental human right [11]. The remainder of this chapter will focus on palliative care as it is delivered in the community among residential long-term care homes.

17.2 The Role of Palliative Care in Long-Term Care

Palliative care is a philosophy of care that is rooted in the notion that all persons are deserving of a good death and that persons should live well until they die. At its core, palliative care aims to improve the quality of life for people living with life-limiting illness, through the early identification, assessment, and treatment of pain, as well as other physical, emotional, cognitive, social, psychological, and spiritual needs; supports decision-making and engaging in goals of care discussion; and ensures that people and their family are at the center of care [12]. According to the WHO [12], palliative care:

1. Affirms life and regards death as a normal process.
2. Intends to neither hasten nor postpone death.
3. Ideally, should guide care practices from the time of diagnosis of any life-limiting illness (e.g., dementia, chronic obstructive pulmonary disease, or congestive heart failure), through to bereavement care for family members.

There is increasing recognition that palliative care is a vital and integral part of all clinical practice, regardless of illness, its stage of progression, or the context in which the care is provided [13]. An important consideration is nomenclature; while often end-of-life care is frequently used interchangeably with palliative care, end-of-life care is time-bound with a typical care trajectory of weeks, days, or even hours of life [14]. In this respect, end-of-life care is an important part of the broader umbrella mandate of palliative care.

There have been several national and international organizations that have advocated that the palliative care philosophy should guide care practices within residential long-term care homes, owing to the significant needs presented by many residents. The presence of multiple comorbidities, a gradual process of general deterioration, and increasing frailty contribute to the complexity of care within this population [15]. Research into the levels of distress experienced by frail long-term care residents is growing. The incidence of depressive syndromes in this population is high, with a recent literature review reporting the prevalence of depression ranging from 24% to 82% [16]. Worsening general health and a lack of emotional and social support are factors associated with depression among residential long-term care residents [17].

Recent research into the level of pain experienced daily by residents of long-term care indicates that approximately 60% of residents with cognitive impairment experience either consistent low or mild pain in their last six months of life, and about 34% experience either high or increasing pain levels during this time frame [18]. This finding of persistent pain over consecutive, regular assessments, and that pain increases significantly over the last weeks of life has been documented by others [19, 20]. In their paper examining symptom burden, Hoben and colleagues [21] identified that urinary and fecal incontinence along with responsive behaviors (e.g., restlessness, calling out, etc.) were the three most prevalent symptoms experienced by residential long-term care home residents near the end of life. Cognitively intact long-term care home residents are at risk of other poor psychosocial outcomes, contributing to existential suffering and a fractured sense of dignity that includes but is not limited to loneliness and feelings of hopelessness [22].

Further literature examining dying in residential long-term care homes documents that residents experience poorly managed symptoms, may undergo questionable or unnecessary interventions, lack an advance care plan, and die in isolation, coupled with their family members receiving little in the way of support [23]. Several large studies have indicated that in the final weeks of life, many long-term care home residents are hospitalized and receive burdensome or potentially unnecessary treatments [21, 24]. These findings are troubling in that many of these factors constitute or can contribute to a "bad death" from the perspective of residents, family members, and healthcare providers alike. Additionally, these factors may result in suffering and a decreased quality of life in the final months and weeks before death. Though the proportion of residential long-term care home residents who have completed advance directives has risen dramatically in the preceding decades, the most common advance directives were *do not resuscitate* orders and living wills and do not document preferences regarding limiting aggressive interventions or desired comfort measures [25]. Towsley, Hirschman and Madden [26] characterize end-of-life care communication in residential long-term care homes as "missed conversations;" rarely were care residents' or family members' preferences elicited nor was information regarding preferences for code status, hospitalization, completing an advance directive, or other measures to bring about comfort at life's end discussed. More work needs to be done to address these missing preferences in order to support a good death for individuals, free of unwanted, perhaps even unnecessary, aggressive interventions.

17.2.1 Delivery of Palliative Care in Long-Term Care

Many have attributed the problems of integrating the palliative care philosophy to the care setting due to the socio-medical-cultural context of residential long-term care [14]. Examining the historical development of residential long-term care in tandem with the social, medical, and regulatory context in which care is provided, sheds light on how the medical model has come to dominate the care approach in residential long-term care homes today and has subsequently shaped the adoption of palliative care in this setting [14]. Indeed, the medical model, with its focus on cure, restoration, and rehabilitation, quite simply creates barriers to the delivery of high-quality palliative care. Within the medical model view, implementing palliative care can occur only when curative options have failed and therefore the individual is identified as needing to shift to palliative care. In viewing palliative care through this lens, a dichotomy between curative/restorative care and palliative care is created which presupposes that the person has "failed" at treatment/rehabilitation and perpetuates the idea that palliative care is only offered when no other options for care exists (see Fig. 17.1). In many instances, the delivery of palliative care in residential long-term care homes has been hampered by the perception that only those

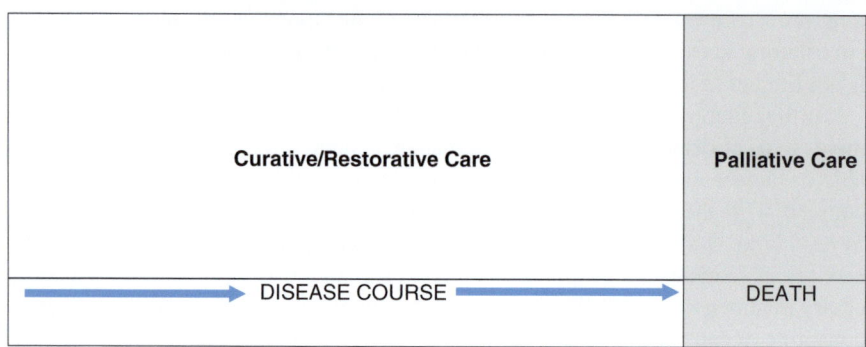

Fig. 17.1 Old model of palliative care. Source: Author adapted from the Canadian Hospice Palliative Care Association and Lynn [28]

residents who are actively dying are eligible for this type of care [14]. In their recent study, Sussman and colleagues [27] identified the palliative care approach being in philosophical alignment as providing comfort to those actively dying residents and their families.

A second challenge within this context is the perception that accurate prognosis is critical when trying to establish which residents in long-term care homes would benefit from palliative care [14]. In examining research on illness trajectories, Lunney et al. [29] noted four trajectories of dying: (a) sudden death, (b) terminal illness, (c) organ failure, and (d) frailty. The majority of residents in long-term care homes can be classified in the frailty trajectory; in other words, those on a trajectory of "steady prolonged dwindling" with no discernable end stage which would signal an appropriate shift to palliative care. It is important to bear in mind that each trajectory is distinct and presents unique challenges in recognizing when palliative care should be implemented. However, if we take the view that we need to establish the precise moment in a resident's illness trajectory to broach discussions regarding palliative care, we fail to capitalize on the benefits of early adoption of palliative care. Rather, adopting the approach as advocated by Bern-Klung [30] that we need to change our mindset from trying to decide who is "dying" to asking ourselves, "who could benefit from palliative care?" is a critical shift required in residential long-term care homes. Some have advocated that residential long-term care homes should be viewed as primarily a hospice setting; a care setting that is guided by the palliative approach from the day of admission with an emphasis on thriving until the end [31]. Adopting such a focus could ultimately benefit all residents as the philosophy of palliative care, with its emphasis on psychosocial needs, could increase quality of life and quality of care [30].

In light of the inherent challenges of providing palliative care in residential long-term care homes, a number of palliative care delivery models have been developed in order to enhance the quality of palliative care for residents. These models include specialized palliative care units located within residential long-term care homes [23, 32]; external hospice-nursing home partnerships [32]; and palliative care consulting services [23, 32].

The hospice model, which is primarily a service delivery model found in the United States, enrolls residents who are identified as having six months of life or less to live, and who elect to forego disease-directed treatments and acute hospitalization, onto their services [33]. This model employs healthcare providers with specialized palliative care training to deliver or augment current care. Positive resident outcomes have been espoused, particularly when hospice services have been implemented in the long-term care home setting, including: (a) decreased hospitalizations in the final 30 days of life; (b) improved pain assessment and management; (c) decreased use of physical restraints; (d) residents less likely to receive intravenous/parenteral feedings; (e) residents less likely to receive medications by means of intravenous or intramuscular injections; and (f) residents less likely to have feeding tubes in place [34, 35]. However, literature examining referral to hospice care in the United States indicates that the timing of referrals to hospice care, and specifically late hospice referrals or underuse of hospice in long-term care is problematic [36]. This delay can result in a very short time period the resident is actually enrolled to receive hospice services, thereby reducing the positive impact this type of care may have on their dying process, a similar outcome to when we only view residents who are actively dying as eligible for palliative care.

In order to overcome some of the challenges and limitations as previously outlined, the palliative care consulting service model is not limited to those who are actively dying. Rather, Ersek and Wilson [23] posit that palliative care consulting services are advantageous within the residential long-term care home setting as they can be made available to all residents and are not limited to the imminently dying. Additionally, palliative care consulting services strive to enhance the structures and processes of the home's environment in order to facilitate the uptake of evidence-based palliative care knowledge into practice [23] to the benefit of all residents not just those actively dying. A limitation, however, still exists with this model in that it requires significant resources and availability of specialists in palliative care: two factors that are lacking in the Canadian landscape (see Quality End-of-Life Care Coalition [37]). It also presupposes that the needs of residents require care beyond the scope and skill of residential long-term care home staff. Evidence suggests that while the educational preparation of current residential long-term care staff may be lacking in palliative care knowledge [38] with training in the core principles of palliative care including pain and symptom management, many of needs of long-term care home residents can be adequately met by "generalists" often within a new paradigm of a palliative approach to care.

17.2.2 Moving Forward: An Integrated Approach to Palliative Care

The model espoused as particularly relevant to individuals living in residential long-term care homes is a *palliative approach* to care. Conceptualized as adapting and integrating the core principles and values from palliative care such as a focus on the quality of life of the person, patient and family-centered care, and impeccable pain and symptom management into the care received by persons who have life-limiting conditions, the palliative approach to care can be implemented alongside chronic disease management [39], thereby benefitting all residents. In this way, the palliative approach moves away from dichotomizing care and forcing individuals to choose between "curative" versus "comfort" to a holistic partnership whereby palliative care is offered with acute/curative/restorative management. As the person's needs change over time, palliative care takes a more prominent role as the curative intent declines [39].

The palliative approach was first described by Kristjanson and colleagues [40] as an approach to care for those with advancing chronic illness who may not require specialized palliative care services, such as hospice services, yet would benefit from care providers who espouse an open and positive attitude toward death and dying. In this approach, all care providers are equipped with the tools for the prevention and relief of suffering through early identification, assessment and treatment of physical, emotional, cognitive, psychosocial, spiritual and existential problems. Sawatzky and colleagues [41] have further identified three key themes relevant to a palliative approach to care including: (1) an upstream orientation to ensure that the needs of individuals with a life-limiting condition and their family are addressed early on (e.g., from time of diagnosis); (2) the adaption of palliative care knowledge and expertise to the specific needs of the population in question; and (3) the integration and conceptualization of the palliative approach into various facets of the healthcare system (e.g., delivered in every setting of care). To this effect, promising practices which foster care models for implementing the palliative approach in residential long-term care homes have emerged in the last several years.

17.2.3 Promising Practices

Within the Canadian landscape, access to specialized palliative care experts or hospice models of care is greatly limited. The *Quality End-of-Life Care Coalition of Canada* [42] reports that for the average Canadian experiencing a life-limiting illness, only 15% have access to specialized care. We can only postulate that the number is even lower for those in residential long-term care homes. To overcome this barrier, models advocating for the implementation of the palliative approach to care that foster the development of in-house expertise within residential long-term care settings have emerged. In Canada, Kelley and colleagues [43] first developed a framework for residential long-term care homes that established the key components of a palliative approach for this care setting. This model noted the importance of clinical, educational, and policy interventions along with the creation of community partnerships to support palliative care in residential long-term care homes (see Fig. 17.2). This model recognized the significant role that healthcare aides (also known as nursing care aides in some jurisdictions) play in residential long-term care homes, and therefore an important consideration when implementing a palliative approach is to provide educational preparation for healthcare aides, along with the professional facility staff.

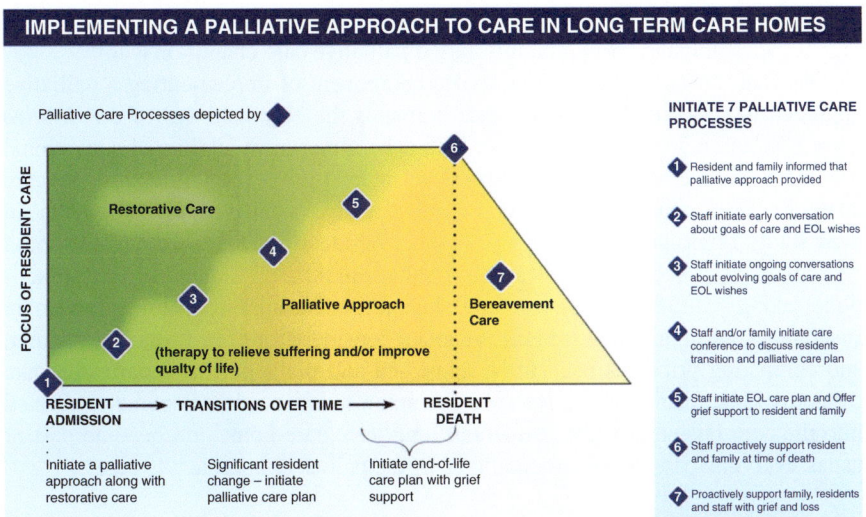

Fig. 17.2 Palliative care in residential long-term care homes. Source: Kelley et al. [43]

A novel means of providing this education are the *Comfort Care Rounds*; a strategy for addressing the palliative and end-of-life care educational and support needs within a residential long-term care home [44]. Creating a forum for staff and volunteers to engage in discussions regarding palliative and end-of-life care, these sessions are typically led by a trained palliative care expert who may start by reviewing recent resident deaths and then asking a series of questions to tailor the rounds to the attendees' learning and reflection needs [44]. Rounds may be delivered in a more formal setting such as a conference room or as a huddle on a residential care unit. Regardless of the venue, the goal is to foster discussion, reflection, correct misconceptions or provide suggestions for evidence-based practices through education, and provide emotional support.

To overcome the challenges of poor communication regarding resident and family care preferences, Parker and colleagues [45] developed guidelines for palliative care case conferences in residential long-term care homes, which were further adopted and refined as part of the *Strengthening a Palliative Approach in Long-term Care* (SPA-LTC) project [46]; a research project that builds and expands the work first established by Kelley and colleagues [43]. This conference, coined the *Family Care Conference*, is triggered by declining resident health status as measured by the palliative performance scale, and are focused on eliciting the values, wishes, and preferences for care near the end of life. Using an interdisciplinary team approach, residents (if they are able) and their family members, complete a form prior to the meeting to stimulate reflection and guide discussion [47]. A tangible care plan is developed in this discussion. Emerging evidence indicates that these structured family care conferences enhance end-of-life communication, particularly as it related to physical and spiritual care [48]. These regular resident and family meetings are critical to quality care as indicated by the palliative care practice guidelines and standards for nursing homes [49]. One key aspect of ensuring these regular meetings is the establishment of a facility-based palliative care champion team.

The final attribute identified as a core component of implementing a palliative approach in residential long-term care homes is the establishment of a *Palliative Care Champion Team*. Comprised of staff who either have additional educational training in palliative care and/or express an interest in the area, the palliative care champion team aims at developing on-site capacity for the palliative approach. In their study, Temkin-Greener and colleagues [49] identified that a core team should be comprised of social work, healthcare aides, nursing, physician, or nurse practitioner along with therapy, dietary and chaplaincy if available. In order to remain sustainable, administrative support, financial considerations, turnover and staffing, and competing priorities need to be appraised and plans put in place to mitigate concerns [33]. Ideally, palliative care champion teams need to become integrated into the core business of the residential long-term care home and become part of usual, everyday care; a fundamental goal of the palliative approach to care.

17.3 Implications for Practice, Policy, and Education

In moving toward the adoption of a palliative approach to residential long-term care, a fundamental shift in the way we embrace this topic is required; registered nurses with expertise in palliative care are in a unique position to champion this approach in residential long-term care homes. Individuals no longer become "palliative" nor are they told, "nothing more can be done" when restorative or curative care options diminish. Death is not viewed as a failure; however, it is the failure to provide the optimal environment which addresses the physical, emotional, cognitive, social, psychological, and spiritual needs of residential care home residents, which becomes unacceptable. Some of these changes will require revising regulatory policies that restrict risk or view normal changes in residents as they approach the end of life as poor quality indicators. For example, policies around nutrition may need to be altered as weight loss is a predictable and normal experience in those who are dying. Policies that are risk adverse and limit food choices, rather than allowing residents to "eat for comfort" need to be broached. Practices and policies will move toward early conversations around advance care planning that are inclusive of residents, to discuss their values, wishes, and preferences for quality care as they approach the end of their life. Indeed, we must treat the communication skills required to hold these conversations in the same vein as skills such as cardio-pulmonary resuscitation—a skill that requires training and ongoing certification in order to foster expertise.

In a palliative approach, we would educate nursing students and registered nurses who practice in this environment, around the core principles, necessary skills, and values of palliative care. Education and training on pain and symptom management, psychosocial support, and spiritual care are required. Steps to educate providers on ways to simultaneously address restorative and palliative care needs are required, as is how to augment the provision of palliative care in residential long-term care homes over time. This will require assisting healthcare providers, like registered nurses, to shift their views from seeing death and dying as failure, to one that normalizes dying and fosters the support needed to assist residents to live well until the end.

17.4 Conclusions

This chapter included discussion of long-term care in terms of what services are offered over the continuum of care, with a focus on residential long-term care homes in order to support discussion of palliative care delivery specific to these homes. An important consideration is that palliative care as a *philosophy of care* is of benefit to all residents, whether they are actively dying or not. The chapter presented the framework of Kelley et al. [43] and further developed by Kaasalainen and colleagues [46], as an example (from Canada) of how to espouse a palliative approach in residential long-term care homes. Much more needs to be done to change and improve practice in residential long-term care homes to incorporate the important aspects of a palliative approach in order to benefit as many residents as possible and ultimately achieve the value of each individual as noted by Dame Cecily Saunders.

References

1. Beard J, Officer A, Arujo de Caravalho I, Sadana R, Pot A, Michel JP, et al. The world report on ageing and health: a policy framework for healthy ageing. Lancet. 2016;387:2145–54. https://doi.org/10.1016/S0140-6736(15)00516-4.
2. Miller CA. Health care settings for older adults. In: Miller C, editor. Nursing for wellness in older adults. 7th ed. New York, NY: Wolters Kluwer; 2015. p. 80–97.
3. Kramer-Kile M, Osuji J, Larsen P, Lubkin I. Chronic illness in Canada: impact and intervention. Burlington: Jones and Bartlett Learning; 2014.
4. Levine C, Halper D, Peist A, Gould D. Bridging troubled waters: family caregivers, transitions, and long-term care. Health Aff. 2010;29:116–24. https://doi.org/10.1377/hlthaff.2009.0520.
5. MacAdam M. Moving toward health service integration: provincial progress in system change for seniors. Ottawa, ON: Canadian Policy Research Networks; 2009. http://www.cprn.org/documents/51302_EN.pdf. Accessed 12 Feb 2019.
6. Canadian Healthcare Association. New directions for facility-based long-term care. Ottawa, ON: Canadian Healthcare Association; 2009. https://www.advantageontario.ca/oanhssdocs/Issue_Positions/External_Resources/Sept2009_New_Directions_for_Facility_Based_LTC.pdf. Accessed 12 Feb 2019.
7. Seitz D, Purandare N, Conn D. Prevalence of psychiatric disorder among older adults in long-term care homes: a systematic review. Int Psychogeriatr. 2010;22:1025–19. https://doi.org/10.1017/S1041610210000608.
8. World Health Organization. Ethical choices in long-term care: what does justice require? Geneva: WHO; 2002. www.who.int/chp/knowledge/publications/ethical_choices.pdf?ua=1. Accessed 12 Feb 2019.
9. Centre to Advance Palliative Care. Improving palliative care in nursing homes. New York, NY: Centre to Advance Palliative Care; 2008. https://media.capc.org/filer_public/c7/37/c737e095-72a6-476a-abd1-445aad8a91f5/3123_1606_nursinghomereport-rev.pdf. Accessed 12 Feb 2019.

10. Menec VH, Nowicki S, Blandford A, Veselyuk D. Hospitalizations at the end of life among long-term care residents. J Gerontol A Biol Sci Med Sci. 2009;64(3):395–402. https://doi.org/10.1093/gerona/gln034.
11. Brennan F. Palliative care as an international human right. J Pain Symptom Manag. 2007;33:494–9. https://doi.org/10.1016/j.jpainsymman.2007.02.022.
12. World Health Organization. Palliative care for older people: better practices. Copenhagen: Regional Health Office for Europe; 2011. http://www.euro.who.int/_data/assets/pdf_file/0017/143153/e95052.pdf. Accessed 12 Feb 2019.
13. Luddington L, Cox S, Higginson I, Livesley B. The need for palliative care for patients with non-cancer diseases: a review of the evidence. Int J Palliat Nurs. 2001;7(5):221–6. https://doi.org/10.12968/ijpn.2001.7.5.12635.
14. Thompson S, Oliver DP. A new model for long-term care: balancing palliative and restorative care delivery. J Hous Elderly. 2008;22(3):169–94. https://doi.org/10.1080/02763890802232014.
15. Covinsky KE, Eng C, Lui LY, Sands LP, Yaffe K. The last 2 years of life: functional trajectories of frail older people. J Am Geriatr Soc. 2003;51(4):492–8.
16. Drageset J, Eide GE, Ranhoff AH. Anxiety and depression among nursing home residents without cognitive impairment. Scand J Caring Sci. 2013;27(4):872–81. https://doi.org/10.1111/j.1471-6712.2012.01095.x.
17. Barca ML, Selbaek G, Laks J, Engedal K. Factors associated with depression in Norwegian nursing homes. Int J Geriatr Psychiatry. 2009;24(4):417–25. https://doi.org/10.1002/gps.2139.
18. Thompson GN, Doupe M, Reid C, Baumbusch J, Estabrooks CA. Pain trajectories of nursing home residents nearing death. J Am Med Dir Assoc. 2017;18(8):700–6. https://doi.org/10.1016/j.jamda.2017.03.002.
19. Estabrooks CA, Hoben M, Poss JW, Chamberlain SA, Thompson GN, Silvius JL, Norton P. Dying in a nursing home: treatable symptom burden and its link to modifiable features of work context. J Am Med Dir Assoc. 2015;16(6):515–20. https://doi.org/10.1016/j.jamda.2015.02.007.
20. Hendriks SA, Smalbrugge M, Galindo-Garre F, Hertogh CM, van der Steen JT. From admission to death: prevalence and course of pain, agitation, and shortness of breath, and treatment of these symptoms in nursing home residents with dementia. J Am Med Dir Assoc. 2015;16(6):475–81. https://doi.org/10.1016/j.jamda.2014.12.016.
21. Hoben M, Chamberlain SA, Knopp-Sihota JA, Poss JW, Thompson GN, Estabrooks CA. Impact of symptoms and care practices on nursing home residents at the end of life: a rating by front-line care providers. J Am Med Dir Assoc. 2016;17(2):155–61. https://doi.org/10.1016/j.jamda.2015.11.002.
22. Drageset J, Kirkevold M, Espehaug B. Loneliness and social support among nursing home residents without cognitive impairment: a questionnaire survey. Int J Nurs Stud. 2011;48(5):611–9. https://doi.org/10.1016/j.ijnurstu.2010.09.008.
23. Ersek M, Wilson SA. The challenges and opportunities in providing end-of-life care in nursing homes. J Palliat Med. 2003;6(1):45–57. https://doi.org/10.1089/10966210360510118.
24. Ersek M, Carpenter JG. Geriatric palliative care in long-term care settings with a focus on nursing homes. J Palliat Med. 2013;16(10):1180–7. https://doi.org/10.1089/jpm.2013.9474.
25. Levy CR, Fish R, Kramer A. Do-not-resuscitate and do-not-hospitalize directives of persons admitted to skilled nursing facilities under the Medicare benefit. J Am Geriatr Soc. 2005;53(12):2060–8. https://doi.org/10.1111/j.1532-5415.2005.00523.x.
26. Towsley GL, Hirschman KB, Madden C. Conversations about end of life: perspectives of nursing home residents, family, and staff. J Palliat Med. 2015;18(5):1–8. https://doi.org/10.1089/jpm.2014.0316.
27. Sussman T, Kaasalainen S, Mintzberg S, Sinclair S, Young L, Ploeg J, et al. Broadening end-of-life comfort to improve palliative care practices in long term care. Can J Aging. 2017;36(3):306–17. https://doi.org/10.1017/S0714980817000253.
28. Lynn J. Living long in fragile health: the new demographics shape end of life care. Hastings Cent Rep. 2005;Spec No:S14–8.

29. Lunney JR, Lynn J, Hogan C. Profiles of older medicare decedents. J Am Geriatr Soc. 2002;50(6):1108–12.
30. Bern-Klug M. Transforming palliative care in nursing homes: the social work role. New York, NY: Columbia University Press; 2010.
31. Engle VF. Care of the living, care of the dying: reconceptualising nursing home care. J Am Geriatr Soc. 1998;46(9):1172–4. https://doi.org/10.1111/j.1532-5415.1998.tb06663.x.
32. Carlson MD, Lim B, Meier DE. Strategies and innovative models for delivering palliative care in nursing homes. J Am Med Dir Assoc. 2011;12(2):91–8. https://doi.org/10.1016/j.jamda.2010.07.016.
33. Norton SA, Ladwig S, Caprio TV, Quill TE, Temkin-Greener H. Staff experiences forming and sustaining palliative care teams in nursing homes. Gerontologist. 2018;58:e218–25. https://doi.org/10.1093/geront/gnx201.
34. Cimino NM, McPherson ML. Evaluating the impact of palliative or hospice care provided in nursing homes. J Gerontol Nurs. 2014;40:10–4. https://doi.org/10.3928/00989134-20140909-01.
35. Stevenson DG, Bramson JS. Hospice care in the nursing home setting: a review of the literature. J Pain Symptom Manag. 2009;38:440–51. https://doi.org/10.1016/j.jpainsymman.2009.05.006.
36. Munn JC. Telling the story: perceptions of hospice in long-term care. Am J Hosp Palliat Care. 2012;29(3):201–9. https://doi.org/10.1177/1049909111421340.
37. Quality End-of-Life Care Coalition of Canada. Blueprint for action 2010–2020. Ottawa, ON: Quality End-of-Life Care Coalition of Canada; 2010. http://www.qelccc.ca/media/3743/blueprint_for_action_2010_to_2020_april_2010.pdf. Accessed 12 Feb 2019.
38. Unroe KT, Cagle JG, Lane KA, Callahan CM, Miller SC. Nursing home staff palliative care knowledge and practices: results of a large survey of frontline workers. J Pain Symptom Manag. 2015;50(5):622–9. https://doi.org/10.1016/j.jpainsymman.2015.06.006.
39. Sawatzky R, Porterfield P, Roberts D, Lee J, Liang L, Reimer-Kirkham S, et al. Embedding a palliative approach in nursing care delivery: an integrated knowledge synthesis. Adv Nurs Sci. 2017;40(3):263–79. https://doi.org/10.1097/ANS.0000000000000163.
40. Kristjanson L, Toye C, Dawson S. New dimensions in palliative care: a palliative approach to neurodegenerative diseases and final illness in older people. Med J Aust. 2003;179(6 Suppl):S41–3. https://doi.org/10.5694/j.1326-5377.2003.tb05578.x.
41. Sawatzky R, Porterfield P, Lee J, Dixon D, Lounsbury K, Pesut B, et al. Conceptual foundations of a palliative approach: a knowledge synthesis. BMC Palliat Care. 2016;15(1):5. https://doi.org/10.1186/s12904-016-0076-9.
42. Canadian Hospice Palliative Care Association. A model to guide hospice palliative care: based on national principles and norms of practice. Ottawa, ON: Canadian Hospice Palliative Care Association; 2013. http://www.chpca.net/media/319547/norms-of-practice-eng-web.pdf. Accessed 12 Feb 2019.
43. Kelley ML, et al. Quality palliative care in long-term care. Tools and resources for organizational change. Thunder Bay, ON: Palliative Alliance; 2017. http://www.palliativealliance.ca. Accessed 12 Feb 2019.
44. Wickson-Griffiths A, Kaasalainen S, Brazil K, McAiney C, Crawshaw D, Turner M, et al. Comfort care rounds: a staff capacity-building initiative in long-term care homes. J Gerontol Nurs. 2015;40(1):42–8. https://doi.org/10.3928/00989134-20140611-01.
45. Parker D, Clifton K, Tuckett A, Walker H, Reymond E, Prior T, et al. Palliative care case conferences in long-term care: views of family members. Int J Older People Nursing. 2016;11(2):140–8. https://doi.org/10.1111/opn.12105.
46. Kaasalainen S, Sussman T, Neves P, Papaioannou A. Strengthening a palliative approach in long-term care (SPA-LTC): a new program to improve quality of living and dying for residents and their family members. J Am Med Dir Assoc. 2016;17(3):B21.
47. Parker D, Hughes K. Comprehensive evidence-based palliative approach in residential aged care: executive summary. Canberra, ACT: Australian Government Department of Health and Aging; 2010. https://www.caresearch.com.au/Caresearch/Portals/0/Documents/WhatisPalliativeCare/Other%20National/cebparac/Cebparac_Three_page_summary.pdf. Accessed 12 Feb 2019.

48. Durepos P, Kaasalainen S, Sussman T, Parker D, Brazil K, Mintzberg S, et al. Family care conferences in long-term care: exploring content and processes in end-of-life communication. Palliat Support Care. 2018;16:590–601. https://doi.org/10.1017/S1478951517000773.
49. Temkin-Greener H, Ladwig S, Caprio T, Norton S, Quill T, Olsan T, et al. Developing palliative care practice guidelines and standards for nursing home-based palliative care teams: a Delphi study. J Am Med Dir Assoc. 2015;16(1):86.e1–7. https://doi.org/10.1016/j.jamda.2014.10.013.

When Home Is a Prison: Exploring the Complexities of Palliative Care for Incarcerated Persons

18

Meridith Burles and Cindy Peternelj-Taylor

Contents

18.1	Introduction	237
18.2	Background	238
18.3	Theoretical and Conceptual Considerations	239
18.4	Nursing in Correctional Environments: A Model for Care	240
18.5	The Correctional Client and Palliative Care	241
18.6	The Nurse–Client Relationship	242
	18.6.1 Supportive Interventions	243
18.7	Professional Role Development	244
	18.7.1 Professional Identity	244
	18.7.2 Continuing Education and Specialized Training	244
18.8	Treatment Setting	245
	18.8.1 Generalized Care	246
	18.8.2 In-Prison Palliative Care	246
18.9	Societal Norms	247
18.10	The Need for Nursing Research	249
18.11	Closing Thoughts	249
References		250

18.1 Introduction

As the number of incarcerated persons increases worldwide, the demand for healthcare in correctional settings is high. In particular, there has been a significant shift in the demographics of correctional populations in recent decades, with older individuals making up a substantial number of the total population of incarcerated persons [1–3]. In Canada, individuals who are 50 years of age or older are the fastest

M. Burles (✉) · C. Peternelj-Taylor
College of Nursing, University of Saskatchewan, Saskatoon, SK, Canada
e-mail: meridith.burles@usask.ca; cindy.peternelj-taylor@usask.ca

© Springer Nature Switzerland AG 2019
L. Holtslander et al. (eds.), *Hospice Palliative Home Care and Bereavement Support*, https://doi.org/10.1007/978-3-030-19535-9_18

growing cohort of the correctional population [4], a trend that is also seen in other Western nations including the United States [5] the United Kingdom [6], and Australia [7]. Referred to as "prison boomers" [8], the health challenges experienced by this cohort are typically much worse than their chronological age would suggest, and more typical of a chronologically much older population [8, 9]. As a result, many incarcerated persons age in place and face the prospect of dying while serving time, resulting in a "double burden" that includes withholding their freedom and access to health services [10].

In this chapter, we seek to outline key considerations for nursing related to palliative care within correctional settings and identify strategies that registered nurses might adopt to enhance the effectiveness of palliative care provision for this vulnerable population. We begin with an overview of background literature and the human rights approach that aims to guide correctional healthcare practice, followed by consideration of various relational and contextual factors that influence palliative care with respect to a model of care for registered nurses working in correctional environments [11].

18.2 Background

Given the increasing number of aging and infirm incarcerated persons, improvements are greatly needed to address the demand for correctional healthcare services and ensure adequate care and support are available to this population who are frequently affected by, or at risk for a variety of physical and mental health conditions. This moral responsibility is underscored by the United Nations Standard Minimum Rules for the Treatment of Prisoners, called the *Mandela Rules*. The Mandela Rules reinforce that access to healthcare, which mirrors professional and community standards, is a right that should be ensured for those who are incarcerated [12]. Despite such rules regarding access and minimum standards of care, older incarcerated persons are especially at risk of having unmet health needs due to educational, resource, and infrastructure limitations. Specifically, correctional healthcare providers are often professionally ill-equipped to address the complex health needs of aging incarcerated persons including acute and long-term health concerns, and palliative and end-of-life care. Healthcare providers often experience limited support for their professional roles, as they struggle to provide care that is inadequately resourced and are frequently challenged by their knowledge deficits related to palliative care provision within the confines of a prison environment [13]. The infrastructure of correctional institutions is also rarely suitable for aging, infirm, and dying persons because they were not designed for this population [14, 15]. Sadly, moral and ethical dilemmas about whether incarcerated persons deserve compassionate care influence healthcare funding and delivery [13, 16]. Therefore, despite recognition of the inadequacy of services for aging and dying incarcerated persons, the contentious nature of correctional healthcare continues to deter increased capacity and resource allocation.

Given the inadequacy of correctional settings for addressing the complex health needs of dying incarcerated persons, there has been a move to advocate for compassionate release. Although legally permissible under various jurisdictional laws and acts, such practices are not common in Canada and the United States due to safety concerns and societal beliefs that dying incarcerated persons should not be given scarce beds in community long-term care facilities [10, 15, 17]. The process of applying for compassionate release is time consuming, resource intense, and requires interdisciplinary collaboration and coordination. Even when approved, incarcerated persons may be estranged from their families, lack appropriate support networks, or resources in the community may not be available in many cases [17, 18]. As an alternative, some correctional institutions are addressing the growing need to care for the dying through the establishment of palliative care units within the secure environment [19, 20]. Such facilities remain the exception, rather than the norm, and additional efforts are needed to ensure access to appropriate palliative care within correctional settings through the establishment of correctional palliative care programs, or via compassionate release programs in order to access long-term care facilities and community palliative care programs.

Registered nurses play an important role in the delivery of palliative care within the healthcare system broadly but are particularly significant to provision of such care via generalized and specialized care programs within correctional settings. Foremost, registered nurses are responsible for direct healthcare delivery through their engagement with ill persons who are incarcerated. Additionally, they interact and collaborate with other healthcare providers and correctional staff and have significant influence within interdisciplinary care teams. However, it is important to recognize that such nursing care takes place within a context that is influenced by interpersonal, institutional, societal factors, which are further outlined below with respect to the model for nursing care in correctional environments [11].

18.3 Theoretical and Conceptual Considerations

The significance of being able to access appropriate palliative care services for incarcerated persons is underscored by human rights and social justice approaches that define healthcare as a right [12]. Specifically, it is important to recognize that incarceration is the punishment for crimes committed, and not the withholding of basic necessities such as healthcare [15, 17, 21]. Furthermore, many persons who find themselves dying while incarcerated, have not been sentenced to life in prison, but must face this possibility, particularly when they are sentenced as older adults, given lengthy sentences, or experience significant decline in their health due to the exacerbation of chronic health concerns and limited access to quality correctional health services [10]. However, as Rich and Ashby [22] explain, incarcerated persons tend to be "banished to the outer bounds of society and social consciousness, ...and few would think of employing compassion when it comes to criminals" (p. 271). Therefore, challenging such views in order to fulfill human rights and ensure humane and compassionate palliative care services for incarcerated persons is complicated.

Nursing practice within a correctional context is especially complex because it brings together the "coupling of two contradictory socio professional mandates: to punish and to provide care" ([23], p. 3). Jails, prisons, and correctional facilities provide social necessities and social goods. These environments meet their social necessity mandate through social control of those in their care. The protection of the community at large is perceived as a direct consequence of the processes of confinement and control. These same settings also provide social goods in the form of healthcare to those who are confined. In essence, correctional nurses are charged with the dilemma of providing social good (health care) within institutions dedicated to the provision of social necessities (confinement) [24–26]. This coexistence of social control and nursing care creates a paradox for registered nurses and other healthcare providers [23, 24], one that is laden with clinical issues and moral dilemmas not commonly encountered in more traditional healthcare settings. It is within this paradox that the competing demands for custody and caring are embraced and registered nurses navigate their professional roles.

The World Palliative Care Alliance [27] has emphasized that the right to healthcare should include access to effective care for those with life limiting illnesses across the illness trajectory. From this perspective, lack of access to appropriate palliative care services for incarcerated persons is inhumane, as suffering may be prolonged unnecessarily [2]. Such a custodial focus on punishment that underscores incarceration is contradictory to the principles of palliative care, specifically the emphasis on holistic, compassionate, patient- and family-centered care [28]. Thus, it is important to consider the rights of incarcerated persons and the intentions of detainment in order to ensure access to appropriate care. While debates about correctional healthcare persist, and until more formalized procedures and programs become established on a global scale, there is a need for guidance for registered nurses and other healthcare providers who seek to adopt best practices for palliative care within correctional settings.

18.4 Nursing in Correctional Environments: A Model for Care

Registered nurses working with incarcerated persons will find a familiar nursing role, one that is "like 'stepping through the looking glass'—everything is the same, yet different" ([29], p. 54). To illustrate the intricate nature of providing care for this population, a model of care, originally developed to provide a framework for teaching forensic nursing in secure environments [11], was adapted for use in the correctional milieu. The components of the *Nursing in Correctional Environments: A Model for Care* [11] highlight the contextual and clinical practice issues affecting the articulation of a professional nursing role in the provision of care to incarcerated persons. As shown in Fig. 18.1, the components of the model are comprehensive in nature, and include *the incarcerated client, the nurse–client relationship, professional role development, the treatment setting,* and *societal norms*. While each component of the model is discussed separately in the following sections, the components are both interactive and dynamic, and take into consideration individual circumstances, as well as the nature and limitations of the setting in which nursing practice takes place. Depending on how the role of the nurse is defined, it may be that not all

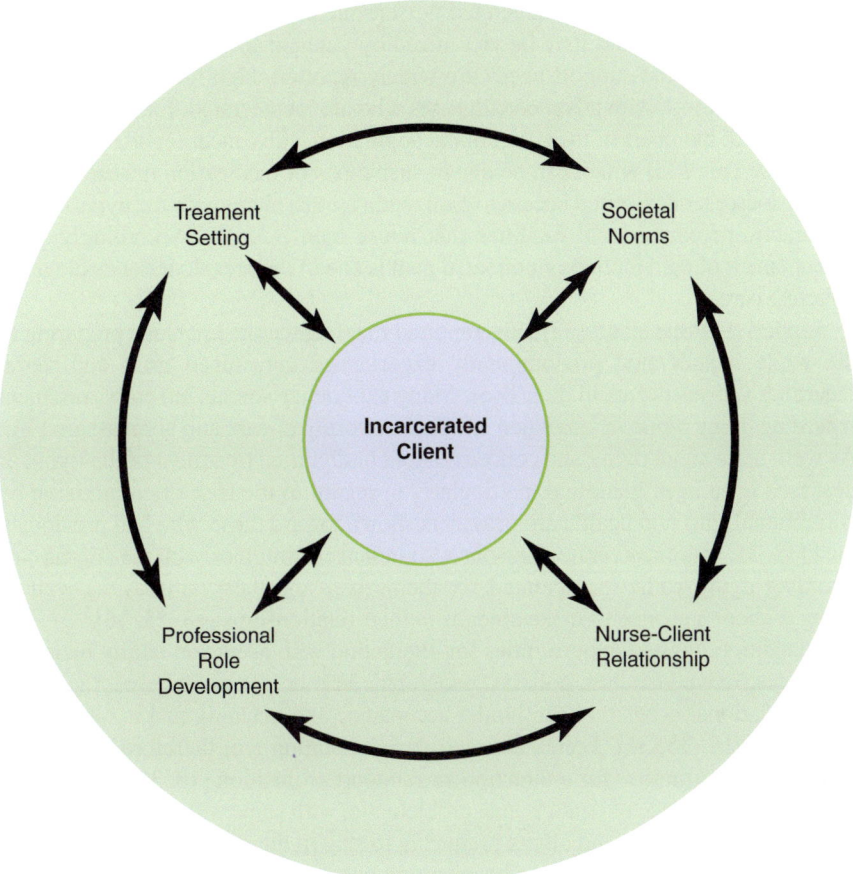

Fig. 18.1 Nursing in correctional environments: a model for care. Source: Adapted from Peternelj-Taylor © 2004

correctional nurses will engage fully with each component of the model of care. However, the model mirrors the nature and scope of contemporary correctional nursing in Canada and abroad [25].

18.5 The Correctional Client and Palliative Care

The need for improved palliative care for correctional populations is raised in existing research that examines incarcerated persons' perspectives and experiences. The comparatively poor health of incarcerated persons is well documented, with estimates that their health resembles that of someone significantly older, and premature death from illness is common [28, 30]. Many are affected by infectious diseases and chronic illnesses that often become terminal including dementia and cancer [15].

Even so, aging and infirm incarcerated persons are still expected to follow typical correctional routines and may be victimized by younger incarcerated persons [15, 31]. Unmet care and support needs are widely reported, highlighting the stressful reality facing those with advanced illnesses who are incarcerated. Existing research indicates that members of the correctional population with cancer reported untreated and severe pain [28] which can be due to suspicions of medication misuse, insufficient resources, and limited access to pain medications, along with the hypermasculine nature of correctional facilities that house men [15, 32]. Accordingly, poor management of pain including untreated pain is one of the prevalent issues plaguing effective care.

Sanders and Stensland [33] have reported that incarcerated persons preparing to die while incarcerated predominantly experienced unresolved grief and regret regarding various events in their lives. Many experience shame and embarrassment regarding dying while incarcerated and feel unworthy of care and compassion [34]. As well, fears about dying and concerns about undignified treatment of the dying or deceased have been identified, particularly in regard to the lack of compassion by correctional staff and healthcare providers shown toward those who had previously died [18, 35, 36]. Incarcerated persons also indicated struggles with the stigma surrounding dying while incarcerated for themselves and their families, as well as dying without a chance to make amends in their relationships [18, 35, 36].

In addition, limited opportunities for interaction with peers and family members due to restrictive visitation policies, geographic barriers, or estrangement generate unmet relational needs that can hinder acceptance and meaning making at the end of life [17, 18, 35, 36]. Loneliness and social isolation are, therefore, prominent given few opportunities for interaction and support acquisition [18, 36, 37]. Lack of control over the place of death is also problematic, with some wanting to die outside of correctional settings and others preferring to stay in their regular unit rather than being transferred to a medical or hospice unit away from peers [33]. This research demonstrates the complexities that dying while incarcerated generates, including the resulting personal and interpersonal tensions that are generated and difficult to manage.

18.6 The Nurse–Client Relationship

Nursing by its very nature is relational; it is through the nurse–client relationship that nurses gain a deeper understanding and appreciation of the human condition. In the correctional milieu, the ability to establish and maintain a therapeutic relationship with incarcerated persons is among the most important competencies required by correctional nurses [24, 25]. The registered nurse's ability to provide competent and ethical palliative care can be compromised by animosity and the stigma surrounding crime, criminality, as well as societal perceptions that those who are incarcerated are undeserving of palliative care [16]. Engagement in a therapeutic relationship with an incarcerated person facing death can be especially difficult for registered nurses when the client has been convicted of committing a morally reprehensible act; such a client may "evoke feelings of disgust, repulsion, and fear" ([38], p. 153).

Registered nurses, however, can demonstrate compassion and empathy in their interactions with dying incarcerated persons [13, 36, 39], while also acting in accordance with institutional guidelines. Although demonstrating respect for those who are incarcerated can be difficult within institutional spaces [13], their detainment does not justify inhumane treatment or withholding of appropriate services, and healthcare providers need to be able to see the person as a person and not the crime that they committed [24]. Unfortunately, acrimonious relationships between prisoners and correctional staff often shape all aspects of prison life. Such relationships are often based on mutual mistrust and an absence of empathy which can carry over to relationships with healthcare providers. Healthcare providers can be criticized by correctional staff for acting compassionately toward prisoners, whereas discussions of palliative care might be met with suspicion by prisoners who equate such care with withdrawal of treatment [36, 40, 41].

Dignity in dying for incarcerated persons is related to autonomy and involvement in decision-making, as well as self-respect, modesty, and privacy [15]. While opportunities for autonomy can be challenging for those who are incarcerated, participation in end-of-life care decision-making can be facilitated by registered nurses and other healthcare providers. For instance, Enders et al. [42] emphasize the need to broach advanced care directives with incarcerated persons with compromised health by first providing them with basic information about health and healthcare. It is important, however, to recognize that such conversations often occur within a context of mistrust that characterizes the correctional setting [33, 41]. Furthermore, some incarcerated persons will lack knowledge of their condition and the objectives of palliative care, or cognitive capacity to participate in decision-making [32, 42]. As such great sensitivity and empathy are needed to facilitate such conversations.

18.6.1 Supportive Interventions

A key component of registered nurses' provision of palliative care for dying persons can include supporting meaning-making and addressing relational needs. Doing so can be difficult because dying while incarcerated is often experienced in terms of fear, grief, and guilt [33, 35], and few opportunities for interaction with others beyond healthcare providers exists [36]. Sanders and Stensland [33] reported that seeking to identify a purpose to their lives was a central component of incarcerated persons' preparation for death. For some of the participants in their study, spirituality offered a sense of purpose and way of finding meaning in their life and impending death. Other participants located their sense of purpose in service and giving back to others, which allowed them to attach meaning to their lives while incarcerated. O'Connor [39] emphasizes the importance of mental healthcare and person-centered interventions, and the need to integrate these into the correctional setting to assist incarcerated persons with management of existential and relational concerns. For instance, life review and legacy-making activities are proposed as tools for promoting hope and coping with dying, as well as engagement in cultural and religious practices [35, 39]. These findings highlight areas in which nurses can support dying incarcerated persons as they near the end of life. For example, registered nurses can facilitate the process of finding purpose and meaning for those nearing the end of life or connect dying incarcerated persons with family members and other support providers who can assist with these processes, such as religious counsellors.

18.7 Professional Role Development

Historically, role development for correctional nurses has been difficult, owing to the myth that registered nurses who work in prisons are "second-class nurses" unable to secure employment elsewhere [26]. During this time of a global nursing shortage, recruitment and retention of registered nurses to correctional environments can be particularly challenging for prison and correctional administrators. Given the breadth and scope of nursing within correctional settings, and the increasing need for correctional nurses to provide palliative and end-of-life care, it is clear that correctional nurses are specialists in their own right.

18.7.1 Professional Identity

The role of registered nurses as moral agents in their work with incarcerated persons is one of the greatest challenges that nurses experience when working in correctional environments. Remaining true to their professional nursing roles and avoiding being seduced or co-opted into assuming custodial roles, where expectations and responsibilities seem more clearly defined, can be especially challenging [25, 26, 29, 43]. Registered nurses practicing in correctional environments must have a strong nursing identity in order to maintain their professional authority and responsibility, without succumbing to the temptation to align themselves with the correctional staff.

18.7.2 Continuing Education and Specialized Training

Continuing professional development for registered nurses who practice within correctional environments is critical, as it reinforces the therapeutic identity of nurses, emphasizes specialized skill development, assists with nursing policy development, and contributes to recruitment and retention in this specialized area of practice [25, 44]. Howe and Scott [45] have emphasized the importance of education in end-of-life care for registered nurses working in corrections to ensure appropriate knowledge, skills, and awareness of issues related to care for the dying while incarcerated.

While additional education and skill development is critical for registered nurses and other healthcare providers, these authors also highlighted the importance of providing correctional officers with information to increase their understanding of palliative and end-of-life care needs required of aged, infirm, and dying incarcerated persons. Turner et al. [46] also identified a need for staff training and support, for both healthcare and custodial staff. These authors believe that enhanced awareness, education, and support for managing anticipated deaths are central to promoting effective palliative care.

The Canadian Nurses Association certification in Hospice Palliative Care Nursing is a nationally recognized nursing specialty credential for registered nurses (see https://www.cna-aiic.ca/en/certification). While this certification is not specific to nursing practice in corrections, certification focuses on core skills and competencies required of palliative care regardless of the setting in which nursing practice takes place, thus providing direction in meeting the unique needs of correctional nurses working with palliative incarcerated persons. Furthermore, collaborating with community-based palliative care nurses and healthcare providers can enrich the correctional nurse's practice, provide professional support, confirm the standard of care, and together explore problem solving of issues unique to the correctional milieu [46].

18.8 Treatment Setting

Correctional settings are extreme environments in which to deliver healthcare. Specifically, the interpersonal climate and organizational culture are mired by the emphasis on power and control over incarcerated persons which is established through the physical and interpersonal environments [23, 24]. Such environments greatly impact healthcare providers' roles and practices and pose significant challenges to the provision of care that are not present in other care settings. With respect to palliative care provision, healthcare providers are particularly disadvantaged and must negotiate limited access to appropriate resources within unsuitable infrastructures [14, 47].

However, as noted previously, compassionate release of incarcerated persons is not common due to the stigma surrounding incarcerated persons, safety concerns, and the persistently high demand for long-term or palliative care facilities among community members [40, 44]. The opportunity for compassionate release exists in law in most western countries; such practices can ensure access to appropriate care. However, there are various complexities related to organizing such transfers or release within a short time frame that hinder its successful execution including a lack of family support and resources [10, 17, 18, 48]. As such, the demand for palliative care within correctional settings may not decrease in the near future, as shifts in societal views and increased coordination with community-based organizations are likely to take time.

18.8.1 Generalized Care

Above all, most correctional settings are ill-equipped to meet the needs of aging and ill persons because they were designed for a younger population [14, 15]. In addition, primary care services might be the extent of what is provided within a correctional healthcare unit, and specialist services such as palliative care are often limited [10, 18, 36]. Limited access to pain medication, healthcare supplies, and other resources can therefore pose a problem to effective care delivery [28, 36], as can demands for health services that outweigh providers' capacity [13]. Furthermore, the need to attend to security above health issues also complicates palliative care delivery [28, 45].

While there has been much attention given to how to best adapt to meet the increasing demand for palliative care within correctional settings in recent years, many policies and programs draw upon guidelines emerging from the United States, a forerunner in this area. Specifically, the guiding responsive action in corrections end-of-life (GRACE) project concluded that palliative principles should be integrated into correctional settings, although adaptations might be necessary. For example, efforts should focus on involvement of family members (when possible), modification of correctional regulations to ensure comfort measures and effective pain management, and collaboration across disciplines [49]. In the Canadian context, Correctional Service Canada [50] developed *Hospice Palliative Care Guidelines* to guide palliative care provision within correctional settings based upon national principles and norms [51]. Despite these guidelines, formalized evidence regarding how these are actualized in practice is limited, and the development and implementation of a palliative care agenda remains in its infancy. Similarly, the United Kingdom also has yet to establish a national strategy to inform correctional palliative care, as they continue to focus on transfer for care or compassionate release when possible [32]. However, this inaction will become increasingly problematic as demand increases and healthcare providers struggle to overcome barriers to effective care.

18.8.2 In-Prison Palliative Care

Given the challenges arising for palliative care provision within generalized health services, some correctional settings primarily in the United States have ensured access to end-of-life care through the development of their own palliative care programs that are designed to be similar to community programs [20]. For example, the Louisiana State Penitentiary hospice program at Angola is a widely recognized example [52]. This program, and others like it, involve other incarcerated persons as peer caregivers, who are trained prior to engaging in hands-on care activities under the supervision of a correctional hospice team [36, 47]. Peer caregiving is viewed as essential to effective and high quality care within correctional settings because peers can empathize with the dying person and invest more time than healthcare providers [53].

A great deal of coordination with correctional staff and amongst the hospice team is required to ensure effective palliative care; this is supported by commitment to patient-centered care, security, safety, respect, adaptability, and a sense of responsibility to uphold standards of care [53]. Accordingly, such programs and end-of-life care initiatives are complex to implement and require system-wide buy-in [54]. Specifically, dedication on the part of correctional administrators, staff, healthcare providers, and peer caregivers is required. In Canada, guidelines have been developed by Correctional Service Canada [50], but there is little to no published evidence of how they are being implemented, the quality of care being received, or specific challenges to palliative care provision.

Such efforts to provide palliative care within correctional settings have been found to have positive benefits for the dying and incarcerated persons more generally, as well as for correctional staff and healthcare providers. Specifically, research that has examined various aspects of correctional palliative care programs has shown that their existence generated increased respect, dignity, and compassion between correctional staff and incarcerated persons [55]. In addition, incarcerated persons who participated in peer caregiving viewed their roles as contributing to improved dying experiences [56]. Furthermore, peer caregivers reported positive outcomes for their own well-being, including enhanced self-esteem and self-worth, as well as a greater sense of caring and compassion [57]. The atmosphere of correctional settings was also benefited by existence of the hospice program, with reports of more humane, caring, and compassionate interactions between incarcerated persons and staff and healthcare providers [47, 55]. The cost-effective nature of such programs has also been reported [36], bolstering the positive benefits.

Within correctional palliative care programs, registered nurses play a central role in overseeing the care of peer caregivers and assume responsibility for ensuring the provision of appropriate care [47]. Namely, registered nurses are crucial to interprofessional collaborations, and can act as liaisons between different members of the care team. In addition, fostering collaborations with community-based palliative care specialists and hospice staff can also yield benefits to all involved [46, 58]. Loeb et al. [48] emphasizes that such collaborations and efforts to ensure appropriate training of all involved can help to overcome barriers to palliative care provision arising from the complexity of the correctional environment. Registered nurses may also find themselves playing a supportive role to peer caregivers facing distress due to exposure to the deaths of their peers. Encouraging the development of resilience and coping strategies in grieving peer caregivers is, thus, important to maintenance of peer caregivers within the hospice program [56]. Loeb et al. [47] suggest that ensuring time for peer caregivers to memorialize the deceased peer is valuable, as is the availability of grief counseling and educational opportunities.

18.9 Societal Norms

Registered nurses can and do play an important role within the delivery of palliative and hospice care to dying incarcerated persons. However, as noted earlier, it is imperative to recognize that this care takes place within a broader societal context. Humane care is defined by society, including the public, politicians, and the media.

Rich and Ashby [22] declare "with some exceptions, it appears that the nonincarcerated world spends little time, if any at all, thinking about how prisoners are treated, whether during detainment or incarceration, (or) after release" (p. 269). However, when the issue of correctional healthcare is raised, immense social and political animosities emerge, and dying incarcerated persons receive little public sympathy [16, 44]. As Novek [59] passionately argues, incarceration imposes a pariah status on persons, regardless of the severity of the crimes committed, and without consideration of social inequalities that precede criminality. Thus, the immense stigma surrounding certain offences, particularly those that are violent or sexual in nature, produces a lack of public sympathy for all who are incarcerated [10]. Such a sentiment contributes to incarcerated persons being devalued and framed as undeserving of care [21].

Although beliefs that incarcerated persons do not deserve healthcare contravenes their human rights [12], they continue to influence the organization of corrections and resource allocation. Namely, the degrading and dehumanizing treatment of incarcerated persons has been made worse by longer sentencing practices and neoliberal policies that both directly and indirectly affect corrections, including insufficient funding generally and for healthcare in many countries [10, 13]. On the other hand, the continual expansion of correctional facilities reveals society's preference for incarcerating the marginalized, and widespread failure to address the complex factors that contribute to crime, criminality, and incarceration in the first place. Specifically, it can be more popular to fund correctional institutions and programs than strategies to deal with poverty, homelessness, mental illness, and substance misuse disorders. As such, there is a need to improve access to healthcare services for vulnerable and marginalized groups. Such interventions should be founded on the conviction that caring for marginalized individuals, including incarcerated persons, is the moral and appropriate thing to do [24, 44].

Accordingly, social and political beliefs and resultant policies regarding incarcerated persons create various challenges for palliative care provision, in addition to the complexities related to security, training, and infrastructure considerations. However, ensuring access to palliative care for dying incarcerated persons must be considered within the broader context of human rights and social policy, with palliative care being guaranteed through correctional programs or transfer to the community. Failing to do so violates provision of basic necessities and the basic ethic of care that underscores nursing and healthcare [15, 21]. As such, conscious efforts are needed toward ethical caring for dying incarcerated persons, and to raise awareness of the rights to healthcare that this population possesses, and to shift societal norms. On the other hand, it has also been argued that ensuring access to palliative care in corrections is not the answer; rather, greater efforts are needed to more fully embrace compassionate release through the transfer of incarcerated persons into the community at the end of life [15]. Therefore, the nature of care for dying incarcerated persons will need to continue to evolve with such debates. Regrettably, the release of offenders is often viewed as politically unwise, fiscally questionable, and philosophically unpalatable [60]. Rich and Ashby [22] have concluded that:

Most people, in Western countries anyway, live in this dichotomized world where good people in society are protected, often inadequately as they would see it, by a justice system that keeps offenders locked up away from them....Those who have never visited a prison say it is too soft. Politicians know that there are no votes in prison reforms, and justice must be tough (p. 271).

18.10 The Need for Nursing Research

There is an immense need for research that explores the experiences of dying incarcerated persons, and those of healthcare providers and staff associated with their care. In particular, few studies have been conducted that privileges the firsthand perspective of aging and dying persons who reside in correctional settings [18, 33, 35, 36], and such research is particularly needed outside of the United States. In addition, while some research has focused on those directly involved with hospice care programs in correctional settings, greater attention should be paid to registered nurses' experiences and understandings of palliative, hospice, and end-of-life care provision of incarcerated persons, and especially of working collaboratively with other healthcare providers and peer caregivers. Such research can contribute to evidence-informed practice and policies. Innovative approaches to research would be particularly valuable, such as patient-oriented approaches that seek to engage aging incarcerated persons, peer caregivers, healthcare providers, and decision-makers as members of the research team, enabling those with direct knowledge to identify priorities and set the research agenda. Findings from such research can be utilized by knowledge users and decision-makers. Furthermore, evaluation of existing guidelines and programs is also essential to determine efficacy of healthcare provision, best practices, and areas for improvement, as the scant studies that have sought to do so have served to inform expanded efforts in other correctional settings [20, 53].

18.11 Closing Thoughts

In this in-depth consideration of palliative care for incarcerated persons, we have outlined factors contributing to the demand for access to such care due to the increasing numbers of aging and infirm persons residing in correctional settings, as well as the complexities that exist for registered nurses and other healthcare providers. Namely, nursing within correctional environments occurs within the context of interactional, institutional, and sociopolitical features that are unique to correctional settings. These features contribute to barriers that plague delivery of adequate, effective, and ethical care for those who are dying. Accordingly, awareness of the model of care for nursing in correctional environments provides a foundation for nurses to successfully navigate the myriad of challenges specific to caring for this highly stigmatized and vulnerable population. When home is a prison, addressing the palliative care needs of incarcerated persons is morally and professionally the right thing to do.

References

1. Hayes AJ, Burns A, Turnbull P, Shaw JJ. The health and social needs of older male prisoners. Int J Geriatr Psychiatry. 2012;27(11):1099–166.
2. Human Rights Watch. Old behind bars: the aging prison population in the United States. New York, NY: Human Rights Watch; 2012. http://www.hrw.org/sites/default/files/reports/usprisons0112webwcover_0.pdf
3. Office of the Correctional Investigator. Annual report 2017–2018 (Cat. No. PS100). Ottawa, ON: Her Majesty the Queen in Right of Canada; 2018. http://www.oci-bec.gc.ca/cnt/rpt/pdf/annrpt/annrpt20172018-eng.pdf
4. Reitano J. Adult correctional statistics in Canada, 2015/2016. Juristat (No. 85-002-X). Ottawa, ON: Canadian Centre for Justice Statistics; 2017.
5. Carson EA, Sabol WJ. Aging of the state prison population, 1993–2013. Special report. Washington, DC: Bureau of Justice Statistics, U.S. Department of Justice; 2016. https://www.bjs.gov/content/pub/pdf/aspp9313.pdf
6. House of Commons Library. Briefing paper. Number SN/SG/04334. London: UK Prison Population Statistics; 2017.
7. Stevens BA, Shaw R, Bewert P, Salt M, Alexander R, Gee BL. Systematic review of aged care interventions for older prisoners. Australas J Ageing. 2017. https://doi.org/10.1111/ajag.12484.
8. Psick Z, Ahalt C, Brown RT, Simon J. Prison boomers: policy implications of aging prison populations. Int J Prison Health. 2017;13(1):57–63. https://doi.org/10.1108/IJPH-09-2016-0053/.
9. Fazel S, Hope T, O'Donnell I, Piper M, Jacoby R. Health of elderly male prisoners: worse than the general population, worse than younger prisoners. Age Ageing. 2001;30(5):403–7.
10. Turner M, Peacock M, Payne S, Fletcher A, Froggatt K. Ageing and dying in the contemporary neoliberal prison system: exploring the 'double burden' for older prisoners. Soc Sci Med. 2018;212:161–1-67. https://doi.org/10.1016/j.socscimed.2018.07.009.
11. Peternelj-Taylor C. NURS 486: forensic nursing in secure environments. Saskatoon, SK: College of Nursing, University of Saskatchewan; 2004.
12. United Nations General Assembly. Resolution adopted by the General Assembly on 17 December 2015. United Nations standard minimum rules for the treatment of prisoners (the Nelson Mandela rules) 2016. https://undocs.org/A/RES/70/175
13. Brown M. Empathy and punishment. Punishment Soc. 2012;14(4):383–401.
14. Beckett J, Peternelj-Taylor C, Johnson R. Growing old in the correctional system. J Psychosoc Nurs Ment Health Serv. 2003;41(9):12–8.
15. Zinger I, Landry M-C. Aging and dyign in prison: an investigation into the experiences of older individuals in federal custody. 2019. http://www.oci-bec.gc.ca/cnt/rpt/pdf/oth-aut/oth-aut20190228-eng.pdf
16. Burles M, Peternelj-Taylor C, Holtslander L. A 'good death' for all? Examining issues for palliative care in correctional settings. Mortality. 2016;21(2):93–111.
17. Office of the Correctional Investigator. Annual report of the Office of the Correctional Investigator 2016–2017. (No. PS100). Ottawa, ON: Her Majesty the Queen in Right of Canada; 2018.
18. Aday R, Wahindin A. Older prisoners' experiences of death, dying and grief behind bars. Howard J Crim Just. 2016;55(3):312–27.
19. Evans C, Herzog R, Tillman T. The Louisiana State Penetentiary: Angola prison hospice. J Palliat Med. 2002;5(4):553–8.
20. Hoffman HC, Dickinson GE. Characteristics of prison hospice programs in the United States. Am J Hosp Palliat Med. 2011;28(4):245–52.
21. Maeve K, Vaughn M. Nursing with prisoners: the practice of caring forensic nursing or penal harm nursing? Adv Nurs Sci. 2001;24(2):47–65.
22. Rich LE, Ashby MA. Crime and punishment, rehabilitation or revenge: bioethics for prisoners? J Bioeth Inq. 2014;11(3):269–74.

23. Holmes D. Governing the captives: forensic psychiatric nursing in corrections. Perspect Psychiatr Care. 2005;41(1):3–13.
24. Peternelj-Taylor C. An exploration of othering in forensic psychiatric and correctional nursing. Can J Nurs Res. 2004;36(4):130–46.
25. Peternelj-Taylor C. Care of persons under forensic purview. In W Austin, D Kunyk, CA Peternelj-Taylor, MA Boyd. Psychiatric & mental health nursing for Canadian practice, 4 2019 Philadelphia, PA, Wolters Kluwer 919–934
26. Peternelj-Taylor C, Johnson R. Serving time: Psychiatric mental health nursing in corrections. J Psychosoc Nurs Ment Health Serv. 1995;33(8):12–9.
27. World Palliative Care Alliance. Global atlas of palliative care at the end of life. London: World Palliative Care Alliance; 2014.
28. Maschi T, Marmo S, Han J. Palliative and end-of-life care in prisons: a content analysis of the literature. Int J Prison Health. 2014;10(3):172–97.
29. Smith S. Stepping through the looking glass: Professional autonomy in correctional nursing. Correct Today. 2005;70:54–6.
30. Fazel S, Baillargeon J. The health of prisoners. Lancet. 2011;377:956–65.
31. Bedard R, Metzger L, Williams B. Ageing prisoners: an introduction to geriatric health-care challenges in correctional facilities. Int Rev Red Cross. 2016;98(903):917–39.
32. Stone K, Papadopoulos I, Kelly D. Establishing hospice care for prison populations: an integrative review assessing the UK and the USA perspective. Palliat Med. 2012;26:969–78.
33. Sanders S, Stensland M. Preparing to die behind bars: the journey of male inmates with terminal health conditions. J Correct Health Care. 2018;24(3):232–42.
34. Handtke V, Wangmo T. Ageing prisoners' views on death and dying: contemplating end-of-life in prison. Bioeth Inq. 2014;11:373–86.
35. Aday RH. Aging prisoners' concerns toward dying in prison. Omega. 2006;52(3):199–216.
36. Loeb SJ, Penrod J, McGhan G, Kitt-Lewis E, Hollenbeak C. Who wants to die in here? Perspectives of prisoners with chronic conditions. J Hosp Palliat Care Nurs. 2014;16(3):173–81.
37. Linder JF, Meyers FJ. Palliative care for prison inmates: "don't let me die in prison". J Am Med Assoc. 2007;296(8):894–901.
38. Jacob JD, Gagnon M, Holmes D. Nursing so-called monsters: on the importance of abjection and fear in forensic psychiatric nursing. J Forensic Nurs. 2009;5(3):153–61.
39. O'Connor MF. Finding boundaries inside prison walls: case study of a terminally ill inmate. Death Stud. 2004;28:63–76.
40. Williams BA, Sudore RL, Greifinger R, Morrison RS. Balancing punishment and compassion for seriously ill prisoners. Ann Intern Med. 2011;155(2):122–7.
41. Wion RK, Loeb SJ. End-of-life care behind bars: a systematic review. Am J Nurs. 2016;116(3):24–36.
42. Enders SR, Paterniti DA, Meyers FJ. An approach to develop effective health care decision making for women in prison. J Palliat Med. 2005;8(2):432–9.
43. Holmes D. Nursing in corrections: lessons from France. J Forensic Nurs. 2007;3(3–4):126–31.
44. Peternelj-Taylor C, Woods P. Correctional health. In: Stamler LL, Yiu L, Dosani A, Etowa J, Van Daalen-Smith C, editors. Community health nursing: a Canadian perspective. 5th ed. North York, ON: Pearson Canada Inc; 2019. p. 471–88.
45. Howe JB, Scott G. Educating prison staff in the principles of end of life care. Int J Palliat Nurs. 2012;18:391–5.
46. Turner M, Payne S, Barbarachild Z. Care or custody? An evaluation of palliative care in prisons in north west England. Palliat Med. 2011;25(4):370–7.
47. Loeb SJ, Hollenbeak CS, Penrod J, Smith CA, Kitt-Lewis E, Crouse SB. Care and companionship in an isolating environment. J Forensic Nurs. 2013;9(1):35–44.
48. Office of the Correctional Investigator. Annual report of the Office of the Correctional Investigator 2012–2013. (No. PS100-2013E-PDF). Ottawa, ON: Her Majesty the Queen in Right of Canada; 2013.
49. Ratcliff M, Craig E. The GRACE project. Guiding end-of-life in corrections 1998–2001. J Palliat Med. 2004;7(2):373–9.

50. Correctional Service Canada. Hospice palliative care guidelines for Correctional Services Canada. Ottawa, ON: Correctional Service Canada; 2009.
51. Ferris F, Balfour H, Bowen K, Farley J, Hardwick M, Lamontange C, et al. A model to guide patient and family care: based on nationally accepted principles and norms of practice. J Pain Symp Manag. 2002;24(2):106–23.
52. Tillman T. Hospice in prison: the Louisiana State Penitentiary hospice program. J Palliat Med. 2000;3:513–24.
53. Cloyes KG, Rosenkranz SJ, Berry PH, Supiano KP, Routlt M, Shannon-Dorcy K, Llanque SM. Essential elements of an effective prison hospice program. Am J Hosp Palliat Care. 2016;33(4):390–402.
54. Loeb SJ, Wion RK, Penrod J, McGhan G, Kitt-Lewis E, Hollenbeak CS. A toolkit for enhancing end-of-life care: an examination of implementation and impact. Prison J. 2018;98(1):104–18.
55. Wright KN, Bernstein L. Creating decent prisons: a serendipitous finding about prison hospice. J Offender Rehabil. 2007;44(4):1–16.
56. Supiano KP, Cloyes KG, Berry PH. The grief experience of prison inmate hospice volunteer caregivers. J Soc Work End Life Palliat Care. 2014;10(1):80–94.
57. Yampolskaya S, Winston N. Hospice care in prison: general principles and outcomes. Am J Hosp Palliat Med. 2003;20(4):290–6.
58. Loeb SJ, Penrod J, Hollenbeak CS, Smith CA. End-of-life care and barriers for female inmates. J Obstetr Gynecol Neonat Nurs. 2011;40(4):477–85.
59. Novek E. The color of hell: reframing race and justice in the age of mass incarceration. Atl J Commun. 2014;22:1–4.
60. Chiu T. It's about time. Aging prisoners, increasing costs and geriatric release. New York, NY: Vera Institute of Justice; 2010. https://storage.googleapis.com/vera-web-assets/downloads/Publications/its-about-time-aging-prisoners-increasing-costs-and-geriatric-release/legacy_downloads/Its-about-time-aging-prisoners-increasing-costs-and-geriatric-release.pdf

Pediatric Palliative and Hospice Care in Canada

19

Jill M. G. Bally, Nicole R. Smith, and Meridith Burles

Contents

19.1	Introduction...	253
19.2	Family Experiences and Need for Specialized Care.....................................	254
19.3	Pediatric Hospice Palliative Care in Canada..	256
	19.3.1 Definition and Philosophy..	256
	19.3.2 Illnesses Requiring Pediatric Hospice Palliative Care....................	257
19.4	What Does Pediatric Hospice Palliative Care Look Like in Practice?...........	258
	19.4.1 Settings...	258
	19.4.2 Interdisciplinary Teams...	259
	19.4.3 Comprehensive Care...	260
19.5	Indigenous Perspectives in Canada..	262
19.6	Implications for Nursing Practice, Education, and Research........................	263
	19.6.1 Practice...	263
	19.6.2 Education..	265
	19.6.3 Research...	265
19.7	Conclusion...	266
References..		267

19.1 Introduction

The term *palliative care* can often evoke an image of a person who is bedridden, aging, and at the end of their life with no remaining treatment options. A young child and their family do not typically spring to mind. However, in Canada, it is estimated that approximately 2400 infants, children, and young adolescents are diagnosed with, and die annually due to, serious illness [1]. Serious illnesses such as life-threatening (LTIs) and life-limiting illnesses (LLIs) include cancerous tumors

---

J. M. G. Bally (✉) · N. R. Smith · M. Burles
College of Nursing, University of Saskatchewan, Saskatoon, SK, Canada
e-mail: jill.bally@usask.ca; n.r.smith@usask.ca; meridith.burles@usask.ca

and blood-related cancers, congenital malformations and disorders, and genetic abnormalities. Despite the general misconception of palliative care being a service delivered only to adults, infants, children, and adolescents account for a sector of our population that may require advanced and specialized care. There has been documented evidence that children with LTIs and LLIs would greatly benefit with access to pediatric hospice palliative care [2, 3].

While the number of pediatric diagnoses requiring pediatric hospice care may seem small, when faced with serious illness and the possibility of a child's death, a family undergoes many uncertainties and traumatic experiences. The expected normal order of life is significantly disrupted and a diagnosis of an LTI or LLI can greatly alter family functioning and overall well-being. The importance of addressing a child and their family members' physical, emotional, cultural, spiritual, and psychosocial needs has been well documented in pediatric hospice palliative care research, yet access to support in these areas is inconsistent and unclear [4, 5].

Children who have LTIs and LLIs often require the use of pediatric hospice palliative care starting at the time of diagnosis [5, 6]. Having specialized supportive care can greatly improve the quality of life of both the child and their entire family, ease overall suffering, enhance functioning, and support family growth in all dimensions of well-being [4, 5, 7, 8]. Despite the growing knowledge and research in pediatric palliative care that advocates for formal programs for this unique and vulnerable population, organized interdisciplinary pediatric hospice palliative care for families is limited in many parts of the world, including Canada [6, 7, 9]. Globally, the number of well-developed pediatric hospice palliative care programs are minimal and tend to be found only in highly populated areas [10, 11]. This remains true for Canadian families as the majority of formal pediatric hospice palliative care services and programs in Canada are hospital based, offered through tertiary healthcare centers in major cities. However, there are a growing number of free-standing hospices for infants, children, and adolescents impacted by LTIs and LLIs across Canada.

To provide additional information about the content presented above, this chapter will explore the family experiences when a child is diagnosed with and in treatment for an LTI or LLI, the main tenets of pediatric hospice palliative care, and nursing practice in Canadian pediatric hospice palliative care. The chapter will conclude with a unique commentary on considerations related to Canadian Indigenous perspectives and implications for practice, education, and research. This chapter will help registered nurses and nursing students to better understand palliative and hospice care in pediatrics, related nursing care, and the need for education and research with the aim of enhancing care for infants, children, and families impacted by LTIs and LLIs.

19.2 Family Experiences and Need for Specialized Care

In Canada and many parts of the world, medical advances have reduced pediatric mortality rates, and have also enhanced survival rates resulting in an increase in the number of children and families living with grave illnesses. These families face persistent stress in adapting to related life-threatening challenges as they proceed through uncertain transitions due to illness [12, 13]. The impact on children with LTIs or LLIs and their families is significant [14, 15]. Siden et al. [11] stated that children with progressive metabolic, neurological, or chromosomal conditions and their families anticipate an unknown lifespan, endure unstable and often painful symptoms, and cope with unpredictable emotional and spiritual crises as the condition progresses along an uncertain trajectory, often toward death [11, 16]. Similarly, the Canadian Psychology Association (2009) has suggested that the death of a child is viewed as outside the natural order of life because typically children represent hope, energy, and health [12]. Therefore, when a child is diagnosed with an LTI or LLI, a family's faith, hope, and belief and trust in the future can be extensively compromised and even shattered.

Although some reports have found that parental caregivers of children with chronic illnesses fare well, much of the related scientific literature described parents who are adversely affected by the demands of caregiving [13, 14, 17–19]. The shock at the time of diagnosis, repeated threats to the life of the child, lengthy and intensive treatment, and financial burden, all place significant strain on the parents of these children. In turn, the health and well-being of parental caregivers are frequently diminished [20, 21], family roles and functioning shift [21], and quality of life may suffer [22, 23]. Parents have described their experiences in various ways, all depicting their uncertain, unknown, and turbulent lives, for example, stating it is like "running down a blind alley in the dark, just so scared all the time" [17], "navigating uncharted territory" [13], and it is like "the bottom drops out of your world" [18].

While many parents experience challenging and complex emotions, feelings, and thoughts, many parents contend that hope is one of the only resources left when they hear their child's life-limiting or life-threatening diagnosis and ultimately transition to lengthy treatment options. Parents describe hope as supportive, critical, and empowering [19–21], and felt that hope supports the wide array of caregiving activities in which they participate. Specifically, parents have defined hope as "an essential, powerful, deliberate, life-sustaining, dynamic, cyclical process that is anchored in time, and is both calming and strengthening, and provides inner guidance through the challenging experience of preparing for the worst and hoping for the best" [19]. Other parents described hope as tenuous and tenacious, easy and difficult, the shifting focus of hope, but most concur that its importance and presence remained constant, even with lingering despair [21, 22]. As such, hope provided parents with the strength to endure the constant vacillation between preparing for the death and fighting for the survival of their infant, child, or adolescent and their family life [19].

Given the above-mentioned complex, traumatic, and unrelenting experiences, many studies have indicated that pediatric family caregivers report the need for specialized comprehensive health care [3, 20, 24–27]. The kind of supportive care required for children with LTIs and LLIs and their families does not stop at treatment, reduced morbidity and mortality, nor with the quality and dignity of life of the child. Instead, the goal for effective, holistic treatment is comprehensive health care that includes all family members, particularly, informal family caregivers [2, 10,

28–31]. This complex and yet comprehensive care is challenging and demands a unique, collaborative team approach [23–26].

19.3 Pediatric Hospice Palliative Care in Canada

The intent of pediatric hospice palliative care practice is to relieve the pain and suffering of children and their families, and to enhance their quality and dignity of life with the ultimate, underlying goal of equitable and effective supportive care. Specifically, pediatric palliative care is achieved through universal principles set out by WHO (1998), some of which include focusing on pain and symptom relief; offering a support system to families to assist with coping during the child's illness; providing this care in conjunction with other therapies beginning with diagnosis, extending throughout the illness, and into bereavement if needed; and utilizing a team approach to care for, and support patients and their families [10]. The care of such children and their family members can be provided by healthcare models with individualization of each program to address and recognize available resources, community characteristics, and appropriate cultural considerations.

Specifically in Canada, the expressions "palliative care" and "hospice care" are often used interchangeably and both refer to a specific approach to care. However, some people use hospice care to describe care that takes place in the community instead of in hospitals. To differentiate, the terms are used differently in the United States. For example, while both palliative care and hospice care provide comfort, palliative care often begins at the time of diagnosis and parallel to treatment. On the other hand, hospice care tends to start after treatment has been stopped and when death is imminent [24]. Furthermore, there is no national palliative care program or strategy in Canada, and instead, there are a variety of partners, specialists, and organizations with responsibilities aimed at best serving the population such as the federal government, Health Canada, Indigenous Services Canada, Canadian Hospice and Palliative Care Association, the Public Health Agency of Canada, Canadian Hospice Palliative Care Association Pediatric Interest Group, and many more [25]. However, in 2017, the Canadian government passed into law an Act providing for the development of a framework on palliative care in Canada which was completed in 2018. The framework titled *The Framework on Palliative Care in Canada* is intended to provide "a collective vision for palliative care aiming to ensure Canadians have the best possible quality of life, right up to the end of life" ([25] p. 18).

19.3.1 Definition and Philosophy

A specific definition of pediatric hospice palliative care is difficult to capture succinctly as it encompasses all aspects of care for an ill child and their family. Specifically, pediatric hospice palliative care is both a philosophy and a delivery model of specialized care focusing on total comprehensive care for infants, children, and adolescents and their families across the illness trajectory and into bereavement [4]. However, it is generally agreed that pediatric hospice palliative care is an approach that improves the quality of life and death of patients and their families facing challenges associated with LTIs and LLIs, through the prevention and relief of suffering by means of early identification, assessment, and treatment of pain and other symptoms, physical, psychosocial, and spiritual dimensions of health [26]. It is a holistic approach that focuses on families and children, guiding them through living, dying, grieving processes, and bereavement [4]. There is no time limit or specific age to consider when providing pediatric hospice palliative care and this care should be implemented early in diagnoses, not only when treatment has failed or death is near [26]. Those specializing in pediatric hospice palliative care recognize that children living with LTIs and LLIs require a special approach unique to their age, development, illness, and family [4] that can only be reasonably met with the integration of a trained interdisciplinary team and experienced community organizations. Unlike adults, children will understand their illnesses and death dependent on their age and development. Their ability to cope and communicate will vary and healthcare providers must be prepared to support children and families at all stages of life [4]. Pediatric hospice palliative care providers also recognize that children cannot advocate for themselves in many circumstances and parental caregivers are often burdened with making decisions that have potential to greatly alter their health status [4]. In addition, pediatric hospice palliative care also recognized the impact LTI and LLIs have on siblings.

Grounded in similar guiding principles as adult hospice palliative care, pediatric hospice palliative care advocates for a philosophy that maximizes quality and dignity of life and comfort, even in the likelihood of death. It expands further to focus within a cultural context on relieving the physical, social, psychological, and spiritual suffering experienced by children and their families. Pediatric hospice palliative care recognizes that the entire family unit is affected by a child's illness, and will therefore, require unique and individualized care. Each family's journey will be different and each family will react and require support specific to their own circumstances. Pediatric hospice palliative care providers understand this need and concentrate on helping families to stay connected and to maintain hope, no matter the outcome [4].

19.3.2 Illnesses Requiring Pediatric Hospice Palliative Care

Often children and their families who access pediatric hospice palliative care have been diagnosed with an LTI or LLI. These conditions include illnesses where no reasonable hope of a cure exists, or where curative treatment may be feasible but can also fail. Examples include (a) cancer and irreversible failures of the heart, liver, or kidney; (b) conditions where premature death is inevitable such as cystic fibrosis and Duchenne muscular dystrophy; (c) progressive conditions without curative treatment options such as Batten disease and mucopolysaccharidoses; and (d) irreversible but nonprogressive conditions causing severe disability susceptible to health complications and likelihood of premature death such as severe cerebral palsy, multiple disabilities, and including those that may occur following brain or spinal cord injury, complex healthcare needs, and high risk of an unpredictable life-threatening event or episode [2]. It should be noted that many of the children who require support from pediatric hospice palliative care have been diagnosed with illnesses that occur rarely or occur only in childhood. This can increase the sense of isolation and lack of visible supports for caregivers and family members. Understanding a family's personal journey adds to the unique supportive care they require [4].

19.4 What Does Pediatric Hospice Palliative Care Look Like in Practice?

Pediatric hospice palliative care is optimized for children with suspected or diagnosed LTIs and LLIs and their families when services are integrated early and in conjunction with therapeutic care, and then continued throughout the illness duration, end of life, and bereavement [27, 28, 31]. Pediatric hospice palliative care is the right of every infant, child, or adolescent and their family across the illness trajectory, within healthcare and community settings [2, 10, 27]. Such efforts to support children and their families can enhance holistic care, including improved symptom management, communication, and quality and dignity of life and death [26, 27]. Pediatric hospice palliative care requires coordinated planning and delivery by those formalized caregivers who are knowledgeable about the foundation, philosophy, principles, and standards of practice for care. However, there are many existing challenges and gaps which preempt the implementation of integrated services in many Canadian areas and which need to be mitigated including geographical barriers, economic limitations within the healthcare system, limited continuing education for healthcare providers, and lack of recognition and late implementation of specialized hospice palliative care [26, 29]. Thus, given the challenges related to, and dearth of organizations and institutions providing specialized hospice palliative care for the pediatric population across Canada, health care often falls upon nurses and other healthcare professionals who do not have advanced education and skills enhancement. Regardless, registered nurses are an integral part of providing holistic, comprehensive care to infants, children, and adolescents who are diagnosed with and treated for LTIs and LLIs and are effective members of existing hospice palliative care teams [29]. As such, a beginning awareness of some of the key principles and activities related to pediatric hospice palliative care is important to develop understanding and comfort in providing care to children and families impacted by LTIs and LLIs across all settings.

19.4.1 Settings

Pediatric hospice palliative care is delivered in hospitals, outpatient departments, the community, home, and hospice settings [30], and in both urban and rural settings. Some tertiary care hospital centers offer specialized hospice palliative care to children and families across Canada. Additionally, there are community services which support care to pediatric patients and families in the home setting such as private nursing services, provincially funded home care services, and medical respite. These community supports and organizations play a significant role in supporting parental caregivers to help with completing daily tasks and fulfilling a functional family life. Beginning in the early 1980s in the United Kingdom, free-standing hospice settings were first developed, and have since become more commonplace in other countries including Canada. The free-standing hospice approach was designed to provide services such as respite, specialized end-of-life care, symptom management, and bereavement services [30], and are typically nonprofit community-based services.

In Canada, when formally available, pediatric hospice palliative care focuses on an integrated approach in which hospital, community, and free-standing hospice care are blended to offer choice and comprehensive hospice palliative care to infants, children, and adolescents with LTIs and LLIs and their families [9, 30]. This integrated approach can link together various organizations and opportunities to provide support to families both in and out of the hospital by providing food, shelter, respite, transportation, emotional, spiritual, cultural, medical, and social care. In other cases, when formal specialized care is not available, supportive care is, of course, provided, and frequently takes place in tertiary care centers by a team of practitioners who do not necessarily have specialized advanced education and skills enhancement in pediatric hospice palliative care [30].

19.4.2 Interdisciplinary Teams

Well-integrated expert interdisciplinary teams are central to pediatric hospice palliative care and are patient and family centered. Care teams comprised a variety of healthcare providers including the patient/client/resident, family members, palliative care physicians, pediatricians, nurses, recreation therapists, play therapists, music therapists, grief counselors, social workers, chaplains, schoolteachers, special education assistants, as well as volunteers, and support staff. Together, the specialized teams establish and effectively communicate diagnosis and prognosis (as best as can be done), realistic goals of care, assess needs of the child and the family, provide symptom management, advance care planning, and grief and bereavement care [29]. Team membership may vary and is determined by the services required to address the infant, child, or adolescent, and their family's identified challenges, expectations, wishes, and opportunities. Regardless, the team comes together in order to successfully put the plan of care into action. Each team member has effective communication and advocacy skills, critical problem-solving abilities, knowledge of cultural safety practices, and participates in collaborative healthcare practice. The interdisciplinary team is also knowledgeable about available healthcare services in their community and the needs of infants, children, and adolescents nearing end of life and their families.

19.4.3 Comprehensive Care

Registered nurses play a critical role in the interdisciplinary team who cares for infants, children, and adolescents who have been diagnosed with LTIs and LLIs and their families. Often, nurses are responsible for patient- and family-centered care 24 hours a day, 7 days a week, every day of the year, and as such, provide comprehensive and holistic assessments, carry out an organized ever evolving plan of care accounting for all domains of health (physical, psychosocial, developmental, spiritual, cultural), participate in advanced care planning, end-of-life care, and take part in care during bereavement [4, 31].

Family functioning not only can be disrupted when a child is diagnosed with an LTI or LLI [3, 7], but can also be maintained or reestablished through flexibility in roles, communication, emotion management, and teamwork, all of which promote individual-level adaptation and this supportive care is a significant aspect of the nurse's role [4, 31]. Patient- and family-centered nursing is an approach used in pediatric hospice palliative care that views the family as the unit of care, recognizes that illness impacts families' lives and relationships, and values a strength-based approach, information sharing, respect, participation, and collaboration [32]. For example, a child or adolescent and their family have the right to information about illness, diagnosis, prognosis, and treatment options that is age-appropriate. When information is shared, children and adolescents along with their family members are engaged and empowered and become part of the ongoing and ever evolving decision-making process.

A plan of care based on ongoing comprehensive assessments is an important aspect of pediatric hospice palliative care and is done in collaboration with the patient/client/resident, family, and healthcare team members. Specifically, nurses consider the developmental age of the child and developmental stage of the family, while accounting for the sociocultural context within which the family exists. The ongoing assessment and consistent evaluation includes careful attention to the *physical dimension* of health including pain and symptom management with the goal of reducing or mitigating illness and pharmacological side effects. Additionally, alternative and complementary treatment options can be explored with the child, adolescent, and their family members. The nurse also includes an assessment of the *psychosocial dimension* of health, "and takes into account the emotional, cognitive, and behavioral impact of the illness, and each family member's personality, coping strategies, and past experiences" ([4] p. 19). Nurses collaborate with all team members, and may integrate supportive care from psychologists, social workers, teachers or tutors, and psychiatrists, for example, and consider a variety of aspects of wellness such as anxiety, depression, hope, self-efficacy, distress, and feelings of uncertainty [3, 7]. Nurses also share responsibility in ensuring children and adolescents, and their families have opportunities to make meaning of their experiences and participate in celebrating milestones and momentous occasions, storytelling, art making, creative writing, music therapy, and many other growth-enhancing, family-building opportunities [3, 4, 7]. The *spiritual dimension* of health is an important part of a nurse's assessment and includes ongoing evaluation and consideration of diverse spiritual expectations, needs, and how these may support and inform, or conflict with treatment options and goals. Understanding and supporting the incorporation of spiritual beliefs and traditions is critical to providing comprehensive care. Overall, the nurse's assessment is ongoing and based on age-appropriate and valid evidence-informed assessment tools, and carried out in conjunction with consistent evaluation of family needs, responses, and satisfaction.

Registered nurses are well prepared to support advanced care planning which should be initiated as soon as possible, once a child, adolescent, and their family is ready. Advance care planning goes beyond the typical care plan and focuses on what will be done and what will not be done in regard to both short- and long-term supportive care goals [33]. Families should be provided with frequent opportunities to talk about their needs, wishes, hopes, fears, and expectations in relation to end of life, and preparing for dying and death. This kind of assessment and discussion specifically pertains to "withholding or withdrawing life sustaining treatment, resuscitation, preferred location of death, tissue and organ donation, plans for the child's belongings" ([6] p. 18), and will also include planning for funeral arrangements, celebration of life, and any other realities important to those involved. Families should be encouraged to include or connect with those who help to inform their decision making and who may be of support and comfort such as other family members, friends, spiritual and cultural leaders, and additional healthcare providers. Ongoing discussion and reevaluation of the advance care plan is essential, and the use of an institutional checklist is advised and helpful for both the healthcare team and the family [33].

End-of-life and bereavement supportive care are responsibilities of nurses as part of the interdisciplinary pediatric hospice palliative care team. End-of-life care is provided in partnership with the family and based on past communication with family members and current circumstances. Nurses identify and focus on "the family's strengths; mobilizing personal, family, social and community resources; and providing emotional, practical, social and spiritual support (not treatment) for people experiencing grief and bereavement" ([31] p. 27). Acknowledgment of the child's death is done in an empathetic and compassionate manner and matters related to the death are supported. Families are provided with opportunities for formalized grief support and bereavement care which involves those who the family requests including cultural and spiritual leaders, family members, friends, and others who have expertise in grief counseling and bereavement care.

Additionally, nurses are in an optimal position to integrate cultural and spiritual traditions and ceremonies deemed necessary by the family. Access to continued grief counseling and ongoing bereavement care by the care team, including the nurse(s) who worked closely with the family, is imperative to holisitic care [31]. During the bereavement period, it is not uncommon for the pediatric hospice palliative care team including nurses to be involved in activities such as birthday celebrations, anniversaries of the death, and other traditional ceremonies. During bereavement, the nurse's ongoing assessment is critical as is ensuring families have knowledge of, and access to "a variety of supports and resources to address the ongoing physical, emotional and spiritual needs associated with loss and grief" ([31] p. 29).

19.5 Indigenous Perspectives in Canada

According to the 2016 Census, almost 5% of the population in Canada identify as Indigenous [34]. In Canada, there is no universal Indigenous culture, and different groups possess diverse beliefs and practices [35, 36]. However, some Indigenous cultures share similar views on well-being, such as a holistic approach that attends to physical, emotional, mental, and spiritual dimensions and use of natural medicines along with ceremonies [37]. Such conceptions of well-being may revolve around balance between the four dimensions, and among individuals, communities, the environment, and spirit worlds [38]. It is important to acknowledge that such beliefs differ from those that dominate the Western biomedical approach adopted in Canadian health care. For nurses, recognition of, and effort to understand, Indigenous cultural views of health, healing, life, and death [39] are therefore necessary to promote culturally safe, holistic care and support.

Many Indigenous cultures value children immensely because they represent the future and cultural continuity [40]. Historically, children were raised by parents, grandparents, and extended family [38], and women were highly valued within their communities [41]. However, colonization and its persistent effects on Indigenous peoples have resulted in intergenerational trauma, cultural dispossession, discrimination, gender inequality, and disrupted family and kinship networks [39]. As such, families take many forms and differ in the degree to which they engage with Indigenous culture [35]. Many Indigenous people have also faced personal and intergenerational traumas that can impose lasting impacts on their well-being and coping abilities [42]. Awareness of, and sensitivity to, the potential impacts of colonization, past traumas, and diversity in cultural beliefs and practices are crucial to the delivery of culturally safe health care and support [39], especially for families of children with LTIs and LLIs [35]. As outlined in the Truth and Reconciliation Commission of Canada's recommendations, strategies to overcome health inequities should include recognition and integration of Indigenous healing practices into health care [43], as well as efforts toward reestablishing Indigenous peoples' self-determination and culture through decolonization [43]. While there is ample evidence that culture is a key component of holistic care, healthcare interactions, and end-of-life care [35, 39], there remains a need for greater attention to cultural and spiritual beliefs within existing healthcare and support services.

In addition, Indigenous peoples in Canada and elsewhere face persistent health disparities and suffer a greater disease burden as a result of colonization, intergenerational trauma, and cultural dispossession [37]. Socioeconomic disadvantages, marginalization, and systemic discrimination perpetuate health inequities, along with disparities related to other social determinants [38, 43]. With respect to Indigenous children's health and well-being, existing data show immense disparities between Indigenous and non-Indigenous infants and children [40, 44]. Notably, there are different rates of birth complications, many common childhood diseases, acute and chronic conditions, and exposure to contaminants [37]. Although research data are limited, Indigenous children also face worse outcomes of some LTIs and LLIs, such as lower cancer survival rates compared to non-Indigenous children

[45]. Thus, many Indigenous infants, children, and adolescents will require pediatric palliative or oncology care for an LTI and LLI during their lifetime.

Meanwhile, Indigenous families experience various barriers to healthcare access. Foremost, the rural or remote location in which many Indigenous families reside in Canada poses geographical barriers. For example, approximately 70,000 people live in northern rural and remote areas in Saskatchewan, 46% of which live on First Nations reserves [36]. Limited access to healthcare services within these communities results in residents having to travel to unfamiliar urban centers for care [44, 46], raising issues related to transportation, socioeconomic, and cultural factors [47]. Distress arises from, and can be exacerbated when Indigenous people must leave their communities to receive care in an urban center away from support networks [36, 37].

Accordingly, some rural and remote Indigenous people might delay help seeking for medical conditions to avoid leaving their community [48]. Furthermore, historical treatment, oppressive government policies, and sociopolitical disadvantages and discrimination contribute to unequal patient–provider relationships which produce feelings of powerlessness and mistrust for many Indigenous people [44]. Differences between the conventional (Western) approach to healthcare and traditional cultural practices can produce tension, particularly related to palliative care [35]. Difficult interactions can also arise from a lack of respect, cultural responsiveness, and continuity of care, and issues related to language and communication style [46]. Thus, Indigenous families face several barriers that hinder the chance of receiving culturally sensitive and safe health care and support. It is important that additional attention be paid to these issues in education and research in order to restore respectful relationships based on mutual understanding [43] and inform effective comprehensive nursing education and practice.

19.6 Implications for Nursing Practice, Education, and Research

Given the increasing evidence demonstrating the benefits of pediatric hospice palliative care for infants, children, and adolescents who are impacted by LTIs and LLIs and their families, it is critical to broaden existing knowledge of nursing education at all levels, skill enhancement, access, and acceptance of this specialized care. There are many existing opportunities for nursing education, policy development, and revisions to staffing and systems of health care in hospital and community settings. Attending to these opportunities creates critical opportunities for future research focusing on improving and expanding pediatric hospice palliative care.

19.6.1 Practice

Pediatric hospice palliative care is currently delivered in many different settings across Canada. Whether or not a formal program exists, registered nurses providing pediatric hospice palliative care must understand the complex needs of families who have children diagnosed with LTIs or LLIs [7]. Researchers and care providers advocate that pediatric hospice palliative care should be delivered in all settings where children are cared for and funding for specialized teams made available in every hospital [14]. Ideally, access to pediatric hospice palliative care should be readily available to all Canadians, no matter their geographic location. Having access to a highly trained interdisciplinary pediatric hospice palliative care team would provide a strong support network for parental caregivers to access [14]. Furthermore, there needs to be strong partnerships between hospitals and community hospices in order to enhance the continuum of care. This would empower parental caregivers to feel confident in choosing what setting their child should receive care in that is best for their family.

Registered nurses have many opportunities to enhance the experience of families accessing pediatric hospice palliative care. Initial steps for HCPs could include coordinating care with other specialties, and preparing meaningful verbal and written information on diagnoses and available hospital and community resources. Parental caregivers may benefit from having a prepared booklet to walk them through some expected events in the child's life, how to navigate the healthcare system (who to call, where to go if sick) and what resources they can access for financial, emotional, or social support [7].

Nurses can also act as the team leader in interdisciplinary teams and be the care coordinator for families. They can advocate for families to meet with the palliative care team at the time of diagnoses so that care preferences and emotional support can be implemented early [7]. Utilizing family nursing theories, nurses can take on a leadership role by assessing the needs of the family. The assessment can be supported by administering scales of hope, self-efficacy, distress, and depression to inform providing interventions for those at most risk. Nurses can advocate for parental self-care strategies including mindfulness activities, yoga, adult coloring, physical activity, and journaling [7]. Additional opportunities for nurses' involvement include distributing medical information in a manner that is unique and appropriate to each family situation. Nurses should advocate for the provision of basic needs for family caregivers and can further empower parents by helping them to celebrate everyday victories with their child [7]. Furthermore, pediatric nurses can focus on connecting families to other families and available community supports or respite programs.

There are multiple ways that nurses can integrate a holistic approach to care for families with children who have LTIs and LLIs at both micro- and macro levels. Healthcare professionals should consider taking additional training in pediatric hospice palliative care as a way to strengthen the quality of care they provide [4, 5, 7]. Having this knowledge will better prepare nurses to improve family outcomes and will increase their hope; an essential component needed for family members to journey through an uncertain and isolating time in their lives.

19.6.2 Education

Healthcare providers and parental caregivers generally agree that additional training in pediatric hospice palliative care is essential to providing timely and holistic care to families and children with LLIs or LTIs [5, 7]. For nurses, this education can take place before graduation and should continue to evolve alongside practical experience. Starting at the undergraduate level, nursing education should standardly incorporate hospice palliative care into undergraduate and graduate curriculum. A formal integration of hospice palliative care should be threaded through all years of education. This includes theory courses, clinical settings, and simulation courses. Educators can refer to competencies outlined by the Canadian Association Schools of Nursing when integrating pediatric hospice palliative care into their teaching, and students can use these as a guideline to assess their knowledge and comfort level in this area [49].

The importance of assessing and caring for families in pediatric hospice palliative care has been well documented, so the need for formal education and training in family nursing theories and family-centered care is significant. Starting at the undergraduate level, nursing students should be exposed to implementing family nursing theories into their clinical practice. Early understanding of family assessment tools and theories will foster a family-centered practice and integration of family nursing into curriculums will produce nurses who advocate for family-centered facilities.

In addition to undergraduate and graduate nursing education, formal training for end-of-life care is paramount for healthcare providers to feel confident in the delivery of a pediatric hospice palliative care program [8]. Specific training in pediatric hospice palliative and end-of-life care will also enhance patient experiences. The duration of training sessions will vary, though any additional exposure and formal education on pediatric hospice palliative care will benefit not only families, but also the healthcare providers [5]. This could be short onsite education sessions, or additional certification in pediatric hospice palliative care. No matter the time or route, education in pediatric hospice palliative care should be continuing, evolving, and ongoing throughout the career of any pediatric nurse who cares for children with LTIs or LLIs.

19.6.3 Research

After the overview of pediatric hospice palliative care outlined in this chapter, it is clear there are remaining opportunities for research in this area. There are many gaps in delivery of care and the need to evaluate current practices is essential.

As access to pediatric hospice palliative care programs expand, so does the need to measure and evaluate the impact of these programs. At a practical level, increasing and best utilizing resources to deliver programs in smaller centers should be considered. What training and interdisciplinary team members are needed to provide a pediatric palliative hospice care programs across Canada? How can we connect current programs and formalize the delivery of care? Furthermore, how can we connect families with, and best utilize our community supports as part of a pediatric palliative hospice care program? Many programs exist in hospitals and communities in isolation from one another and connecting these resources will improve family experiences. Only in the past decade has networking increased between care providers and research expanding across sites with efforts such as PedPalASCNET and PACT Research, Canadian research groups focused on pediatric hospice palliative care research.

Research can also be directed to inquire how best to meet the needs of families. This may be done through implementing supportive tools such as booklets or apps that intend to guide families in their journeys to maintain hope. Questions remain regarding what parental caregivers need to be supported in their lived hope experience and in what part of the caregiving experience do they need the most support (diagnosis, in hospital, at home).

Furthermore, inadequate efforts have been made to address health and social inequities, and the numerous factors that contribute to poor health in Indigenous children and their families. Efforts are needed to improve understanding of the needs of Indigenous families of children with LTIs and LLIs to minimize the challenges they face when navigating their child's care and to overcome systemic barriers. Thus, engagement of Indigenous peoples in patient-oriented or participatory action research is critical to generate knowledge of family experiences including identification of priorities for culturally safe, family-centered health care and support. Access to appropriate services can ensure that Indigenous families' diverse psychosocial needs are met, and family well-being is promoted.

It is clear there are many gaps in research that exist for children and their families and it is exciting to realize the many research opportunities that remain in pediatric hospice palliative care. We have only just begun to understand this unique population and their diverse needs. With an open and empathetic approach, well-developed research in this area has the potential to change the lives of not only infants, children, and adolescents diagnosed with LTIs or LLIs, but also their families and the communities who support them.

19.7 Conclusion

This chapter provided an introduction to pediatric hospice palliative care in Canada, a relatively new and growing supportive healthcare option for infants, children, and adolescents who have been diagnosed with an LTI or LLI and their families. Pediatric hospice palliative care was introduced as both a philosophy and a formal, organized, and integrated supportive care model, often provided by a specialized interdisciplinary team of healthcare providers. Pediatric hospice palliative care is of most benefit when introduced early or as soon as a diagnosis is made, and when it continues through end of life and includes bereavement care. In this chapter, a review of the practical approach that a registered nurse may use as part of the interdisciplinary team was provided with concrete examples of strategies to include in providing holistic and comprehensive assessments and plan of care. A unique perspective was included on the state of health and illness of, and access to supportive care for Canadian Indigenous populations. While there is enthusiasm about the growing programs, organizations, care facilities, and research, there is also a call for additional action in order to provide pediatric hospice palliative care to the right infant, child, and adolescent and their family, in the right place, at the right time, and for the appropriate length of time. A number of exciting opportunities for continued development in education, research, and evidence informed practice were presented in this chapter that we hope become part of the impetus for improved pediatric hospice palliative care, not only in Canada but globally.

References

1. Statistics Canada. Leading causes of death of children and youth, by age group, 2006 to 2008: CANSIM tables 102-0561 and 102-0562. Ottawa, ON: Statistics Canada; 2016. http://www.statcan.gc.ca/pub/84f0209x/84f0209x2005000-eng.pdf
2. Together for Short Lives (2019). Help for professionals: definitions. . http://www.togetherforshortlives.org.uk/professionals/childrens_palliative_care_essentials/definitions
3. Bally JM, Smith NR, Holtslander L, Duncan V, Hodgson-Viden H, Mpofu C, Zimmer M. A metasynthesis: uncovering what is known about the experiences of families with children who have life-limiting and life-threatening illnesses. J Pediatr Nurs. 2018;38:88–98.
4. Canadian Hospice Palliative Care Association (CHPCA). Pediatric hospice palliative care: guiding principles and norms of practice. Ottawa, ON: CHPCA; 2006.
5. Vesel T, Beveridge C. From fear to confidence: changing providers' attitudes about pediatric palliative and hospice care. J Pain Symptom Manag. 2018;56(2):205–12.
6. Beaune L, Nicholas D, Bruce-Barrett C, Rapoport D, Cadell S, Ing S. Caring for children with life threatening illnesses: a guide to pandemic planning for paediatric care. Ottawa, ON: CHPCA; 2015.
7. Smith NR, Bally JM, Holtslander L, Peacock S, Spurr S, Hodgson-Viden H, Mpofu C, Zimmer M. Supporting parental caregivers of children living with life-threatening or life-limiting illnesses: a Delphi study. J Spec Pediatr Nurs. 2018;23(4):e12226.
8. Wolfe J, Hinds P, Sourkes B. Textbook of interdisciplinary pediatric palliative care. Amsterdam: Expert Consult Premium Edition-Enhanced Online Features and Print. Elsevier Health Sciences; 2011.
9. Widger K, Davies D, Rapoport A, Vadeboncoeur C, Liben S, Sarpal A, Stenekes S, Cyr C, Daoust L, Grégoire MC, Robertson M. Pediatric palliative care in Canada in 2012: a cross-sectional descriptive study. CMAJ Open. 2016;4(4):E562.
10. World Health Organization. Cancer pain relief and palliative care in children. Geneva: WHO; 1998. https://apps.who.int/iris/bitstream/handle/10665/42001/9241545127.pdf?sequence=1&isAllowed=y. Accessed 5 Jan 2019.
11. Siden H, Steele R, Brant R, Cadell S, Davies B, Straatman L, Widger K, Andrews GS. Designing and implementing a longitudinal study of children with neurological, genetic, or metabolic conditions: charting the territory. BMC Pediatr. 2010;10:67–78.

12. Canadian Psychological Association. Psychology works fact sheet: pediatric palliative care. Ottawa, ON: Canadian Psychological Association; 2009. http://www.cpa.ca/docs/File/Publications/FactSheets/PsychologyWorksFactSheet_PediatricPalliativeCare.pdf. Accessed 5 Jan 2019.
13. Steele RG. Trajectory of certain death at an unknown time: children with neurodegenerative life-threatening illnesses. Can J Nurs Res Arch. 2016;32(3):49–67.
14. Whiting M. Children with disability and complex health needs: the impact on family life: analysis of interviews with parents identified time pressures, the need for carers to adopt multiple roles and being a 'disabled family' as major influences on their lives, as Mark Whiting reports. Nurs Child Young People. 2014;26(3):26–30.
15. Pelentsov LJ, Laws TA, Esterman AJ. The supportive care needs of parents caring for a child with a rare disease: a scoping review. Disabil Health J. 2015;8(4):475–91.
16. Eiser C, Eiser R, Stride C. Quality of life in children with newly diagnosed cancer and their mothers. Health Qual Life Outcomes. 2005;3:29. Retrieved November 8, 2009, from http://www.hqlo.com/content/3/1/29
17. Clarke JN. Mother's home healthcare: emotion work when a child has cancer. Cancer Nurs. 2006;29(1):58–65.
18. Young B, Dixon-Woods M, Findlay M, Heney D. Parenting in a crisis: conceptualising mothers of children with cancer. Soc Sci Med. 2002;55(10):1835–47.
19. Bally JM, Duggleby W, Holtslander L, Mpofu C, Spurr S, Thomas R, Wright K. Keeping hope possible: a grounded theory study of the hope experience of parental caregivers who have children in treatment for cancer. Cancer Nurs. 2014;37(5):363–72.
20. Kylma J, Juvakk T. Hope in parents of adolescents with cancer: Factors endangering and engendering parental hope. Eur J Oncol Nurs. 2007;11(3):262–71.
21. Angstrom-Brannstrom C, Norberg A, Strandberg G, Soderberg A, Dalqvist V. Parents' experiences of what comforts them when their child is suffering from cancer. J Pediatr Oncol Nurs. 2010;27(5):266–75.
22. Kars MC, Grypdonck MH, Beishuizen A, Meijer-van den Bergh EM, van Delden JJ. Factors influencing parental readiness to let their child with cancer die. Pediatr Blood Cancer. 2010;54:1000–8.
23. Faull C, De Caestecker S, Nicholson A, Black F, editors. Handbook of palliative care. Hoboken, NJ: John Wiley & Sons; 2012.
24. Canadian Hospice Palliative Care Association. Fact sheet: hospice palliative care in Canada. Ottawa, ON: Canadian Hospice and Palliative Care Association; 2017.
25. Health Canada. Framework on palliative care in Canada. 2018. https://www.canada.ca/content/dam/hc-sc/documents/services/health-care-system/reports-publications/palliative-care/framework-palliative-care-canada/framework-palliative-care-canada.pdf. Accessed 29 Mar 2019.
26. Alliance, Worldwide Palliative Care, and World Health Organization. Global atlas of palliative care at the end of life. London: Worldwide Palliative Care Alliance; 2014.
27. Kaye EC, Rubenstein J, Levine D, Baker JN, Dabbs D, Friebert SA. Pediatric palliative care in the community. CA Cancer J Clin. 2015;65:315–33.
28. Rempel GR, Ravindran V, Rogers LG, Magill-Evans J. Parenting under pressure: a grounded theory of parenting young children with life-threatening congenital heart disease. J Adv Nurs. 2012;69(3):619–30. https://doi.org/10.1111/j.1365-2648.2012.06044.x.
29. Docherty SL, Thaxton C, Allison C, Barfield RC, Tamburro RF. The nursing dimension of providing palliative care to children and adolescents with cancer. Clin Med Insights. 2012;6:CMPed-S8208.
30. Siden H, Chavoshi N, Harvey B, Parker A, Miller T. Characteristics of a pediatric hospice palliative care program over 15 years. Pediatrics. 2014;134(3):e765–72.
31. Canadian Hospice Palliative Care Association. The pan-Canadian gold standard for palliative home care: toward equitable access to high quality hospice palliative and end-of-life care at home. Ottawa, ON: Canadian Hospice Palliative Care Association; 2006.

32. Johnson BH, Abraham MR. Partnering with patients, residents, and families: a resource for leaders of hospitals, ambulatory care settings, and long-term care communities. Bethesda, MD: Institute for Patient- and Family-Centered Care; 2012.
33. Wiebe A, Young B. Parent perspectives from a neonatal intensive care unit: a missing piece of the culturally congruent care puzzle. J Transcult Nurs. 2011;22(1):77–82.
34. Statistics Canada. Aboriginal peoples in Canada: key results from the 2016 census. Ottawa, ON: Statistics Canada; 2017. https://www150.statcan.gc.ca/n1/en/daily-quotidien/171025/dq171025a-eng.pdf?st=HU7CPedU. Accessed 5 Sept 2018.
35. Cacciatore J. Appropriate bereavement practice after the death of a Native American child. Fam Soc. 2008;90(1):46–50.
36. Irvine J, Quinn B, Stockdale D. Northern Saskatchewan health indicators report 2011. La Ronge, SK: Population Health Unit, Athabasca Health Authority and Keewatin Yatthé and Mamawetan Churchill River Regional Health Authorities; 2011.
37. Postl B, Cook C, Moffatt M. Aboriginal child health and the social determinants: why are these children so disadvantaged? Health Care Q. 2010;14(Special Issue):42–51.
38. King M, Smith A, Gracey M. Indigenous health part 2: the underlying causes of the health gap. Lancet. 2009;374(9683):76–85.
39. Browne AJ, Varcoe C. Critical cultural perspectives and health care involving Aboriginal peoples. Contemp Nurse. 2006;22(2):155–68. https://doi.org/10.5172/conu.2006.22.2.155.
40. Greenwood ML, de Leeuw SN. Social determinants of health and the future well-being of aboriginal children in Canada. Paediatr Child Health. 2012;17(7):381–4.
41. Craig P, Dieppe P, Macintyre S, Michie S, Nazareth I, Petticrew M. Developing and evaluating complex interventions: the new Medical Research Council guidance. BMJ. 2008;337:a1655.
42. Canadian Centre on Substance Abuse. The essentials of… series: trauma-informed care. Ottawa, ON: Canadian Centre on Substance Abuse; 2014. http://www.ccsa.ca/Resource%20Library/CCSA-Trauma-informed-Care-Toolkit-2014-en.pdf#search=all%28trauma-informed%29. Accessed 2 Mar 2019.
43. Truth and Reconciliation Commission of Canada. (2015). Truth and Reconciliation Commission of Canada: calls to action. https://nctr.ca/assets/reports/Calls_to_Action_English2.pdf. Accessed 2 Sept 2018.
44. Wright A, Wahoush O, Ballantyne M, Gabel C, Jack SM. Selection and use of health services for infants' needs by Indigenous mothers in Canada: Integrative literature review. Can J Nurs Res. 2018;50(2):89–102.
45. Marjerrison S, Antillon F, Bonilla M, Fu L, Martinez R, Valverde P, et al. Outcome of children treated for relapsed acute myeloid leukemia in Central America. Pediatr Blood Cancer. 2014;61(7):1222–6.
46. Vang ZM, Gagnon R, Lee T, Jimenez V, Navickas A, Pelletier J, Shenker H. Interactions between Indigenous women awaiting childbirth away from home and their Southern, non-Indigenous health care providers. Qual Health Res. 2018;28(12):1858–70.
47. Moss A, Racher FE, Jeffery B, Hamilton C, Burles M, Annis RC. Transcending boundaries: Collaborating to improve Northern access to health services in Manitoba and Saskatchewan. In: Kulig J, Williams A, editors. Health in rural Canada. Vancouver, BC: UBC Press; 2012. p. 159–77.
48. Kewayosh A, Marrett L, Aslam U, Steiner R, Lum-Kwong MM, Imre J, Amartey A. Improving health equity for First Nations, Inuit and Métis people: Ontario's Aboriginal cancer strategy II. Law Govern. 2015;17:33–40.
49. Canadian Association of Schools of Nursing. Palliative and end of life care: entry to practice indicators for registered nurses. Ottawa, ON: Canadian Association of Schools of Nursing; 2011. https://casn.ca/wp-content/uploads/2014/12/PEOLCCompetenciesandIndicatorsEn.pdf

Looking Ahead

Lorraine Holtslander, Shelley Peacock, and Jill M. G. Bally

Bringing together the chapters in this book, written by respected authors from around the world, has been exciting and rewarding. It has also given us opportunity to reflect on the most important next steps for nursing students, registered nurses in practice, and nurse educators and researchers to consider. Despite the fact that terms such as hospice and palliative care mean different things around the world, the common concerns are much the same—finding ways and advocating for the provision of quality care to help people live well until they die.

Nursing practice in all sorts of community and home settings would benefit from adopting a *palliative approach to care*, in which any registered nurse feels comfortable having difficult conversations with patients and families about the best next steps, given the situation where a patient is not expected to live more than about 6 months. Optimally, a patient and his/her family who wish to give palliative and end-of-life care at home are provided with the supports, equipment, medications, and guidance they need for the best experience of a "good death" that is recognized as a natural phase of life. Families, who are included in these decisions, receive timely and reliable information and support, and will have more positive outcomes as they journey through bereavement. Unique settings where hospice palliative care and end-of-life care are common practices such as residential long-term care or prisons have unique needs for private spaces that accommodate patients and families toward a dignified and comfortable death. All registered nurses in all settings of care will face situations that involve end of life, either directly or indirectly; how we as nurses approach this can always be improved.

Nursing education can be improved with either mandatory courses in palliative care or a curriculum that embeds aspects of hospice palliative and end-of-life care in every course, be it communication, pediatrics, obstetrics, geriatrics, assessment, education, medical-surgical, or family nursing. Another need concerns continuing nursing education to both expand nursing skills in hospice palliative care and to stay up to date on best practices in symptom management. People spend most of their lives outside of the acute care setting; yet, most nursing education practicums are within the hospital setting, limiting opportunities to provide care within a family and community context. The development and evaluation of additional educational resources such as courses and clinical practice guidelines would assist registered nurses to put research and theory into practice. Many chapters in this book have provided excellent models of care and essential resources for clinical practice. Additionally, there are five chapters which specifically focus on evidence-informed interventions that can be used by registered nurses and nursing students in many settings including the Finding Balance Intervention, Keeping Hope Possible Toolkit, Reclaiming Yourself Tool, the Living with Hope Program, and the COPE Intervention. Case studies are presented for each intervention to support understanding and implementation in practice.

As nursing researchers, we can identify many gaps in what is known about how best to support hospice palliative care in the community. Clinical pathways for all age groups in all settings need to be developed from the best research evidence, as well as evaluating their impact. More research is needed focused on the benefits of excellent hospice palliative care as well as addressing the barriers to meeting the goals of a good death while supporting the family. Research with patients and families at the end of life is not easy; it must be done respectful of the vulnerability of our patients and their families. Many of the contributors to this book have provided excellent ideas for research, and similarly, we encourage you, the readers, to engage in research to inform nursing education and practice which will indeed improve the care and support received by people living with life-threatening or life-limiting illnesses and those at the end of their life and their families. Much more remains to be done and as we look ahead, it is our hope that you will be inspired and equipped to implement the principles, philosophy, concepts, and interventions related to excellent hospice palliative home care across the lifespan and in a variety of settings (Fig. A.1).

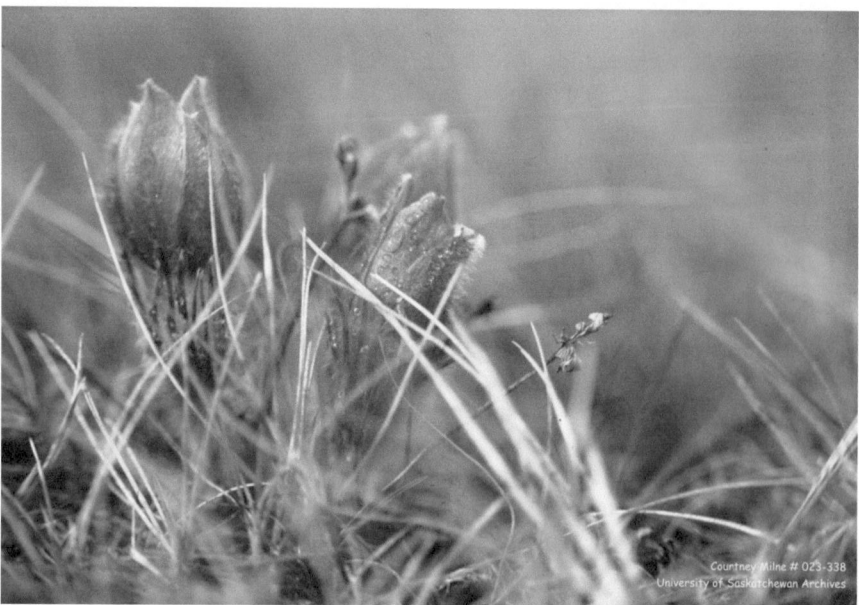

Fig. A.1 #023-338 Spring Crocuses. Image source: Courtney Milne Fonds, University of Saskatchewan Library, University Archives and Special Collections

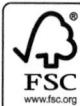

MIX
Papier aus verantwortungsvollen Quellen
Paper from responsible sources
FSC® C105338

If you have any concerns about our products,
you can contact us on
ProductSafety@springernature.com

In case Publisher is established outside the EU,
the EU authorized representative is:
**Springer Nature Customer Service Center GmbH
Europaplatz 3, 69115 Heidelberg, Germany**

Printed by Libri Plureos GmbH
in Hamburg, Germany